T0177313

Manual of Equine Lameness

Manual of Equine Lameness

Gary M. Baxter, VMD, MS, DACVS
Professor Emeritus
University of Georgia College of Veterinary Medicine
Athens, Georgia, USA

Professor Emeritus
Colorado State University College of Veterinary Medicine
Fort Collins, Colorado, USA

Second Edition

WILEY Blackwell

Registered Office
John Wiley & Sons, Inc., 111 River Street, Hoboken, NJ 07030, USA

Editorial Office
111 River Street, Hoboken, NJ 07030, USA

For details of our global editorial offices, customer services, and more information about Wiley products visit us at www.wiley.com.

Wiley also publishes its books in a variety of electronic formats and by print-on-demand. Some content that appears in standard print versions of this book may not be available in other formats.

Library of Congress Cataloging-in-Publication Data

Names: Baxter, Gary M., author.
Title: Manual of equine lameness / Gary M. Baxter.
Other titles: Manual of equine lameness.
Description: Second edition. | Hoboken, NJ : Wiley-Blackwell, 2022. |
  Preceded by Manual of equine lameness / edited by Gary M. Baxter. 2011.
  | Includes bibliographical references and index.
Identifiers: LCCN 2021053064 (print) | LCCN 2021053065 (ebook) | ISBN
  9781119747079 (paperback) | ISBN 9781119747086 (adobe pdf) | ISBN
  9781119747093 (epub)
Subjects: MESH: Horse Diseases | Lameness, Animal | Horses–injuries
Classification: LCC SF959.L25 (print) | LCC SF959.L25 (ebook) | NLM SF
  959.L25 | DDC 636.1/089758–dc23/eng/20211207
LC record available at https://lccn.loc.gov/2021053064
LC ebook record available at https://lccn.loc.gov/2021053065

Cover Design: Wiley
Cover Images: Courtesy of Gary M. Baxter, Abramova_Kseniya/Getty Images, thanaphiphat/Getty Images

Set in 9.5/12.5pt STIXTwoText by Straive, Pondicherry, India

Printed in Singapore
M112521_201221

Contents

Contributors

Some chapters in this book have been revised from material contributed to *Adams and Stashak's Lameness in Horses, 7th Edition,* **by the following authors:**

Gary M. Baxter, VMD, MS, DIPLOMATE ACVS
Colorado State University and University of Georgia
Fraser, CO, USA

James K. Belknap, DVM, PhD, DIPLOMATE ACVS
Department of Veterinary Clinical Sciences
College of Veterinary Medicine
The Ohio State University
Columbus, OH, USA

Alicia L. Bertone, DVM, PhD, DIPLOMATE ACVS
Veterinary Clinical Sciences
Graduate School Columbus, OH, USA

Matthew T. Brokken, DVM, DIPLOMATE ACVS AND ACVSMR
Department of Veterinary Clinical Sciences
College of Veterinary Medicine
The Ohio State University
Columbus, OH, USA

Kathryn V. Dern, DVM, MS DIPLOMATE ACVS
Rood & Riddle Equine Hospital in Saratoga
Saratoga Springs, NY, USA

Randy B. Eggleston, DVM, DIPLOMATE ACVS
Department of Large Animal Medicine
College of Veterinary Medicine
University of Georgia
Athens, GA, USA

Katherine Ellis, DVM, DIPLOMATE ACVSMR
Equine Orthopaedic Research Center
Colorado State University
Ft. Collins, CO, USA

Nicolas S. Ernst, DVM, MS, DIPLOMATE ACVS
University of Minnesota, Leatherdale Equine
Center St. Paul, MN, USA

Anna Dee Fails, DVM, PhD
Department of Biomedical Sciences
Colorado State University
Ft. Collins, CO, USA

Laurie R. Goodrich, DVM, PhD, DIPLOMATE ACVS
College of Veterinary Medicine and
Biomedical Sciences Colorado State University
Ft. Collins, CO, USA

Kevin K. Haussler, DVM, DC, PhD, DIPLOMATE ACVSMR
Orthopaedic Research Center
College of Veterinary Medicine and
Biomedical Sciences Colorado State University
Ft. Collins, CO, USA

Jeremy Hubert, BVSC, MRCVS, MS, DIPLOMATE ACVS
Roberts and Stevenhage Veterinary Surgeons
Bulawayo, Zimbabwe

Chris Kawcak, DVM, PhD, DIPLOMATE ACVS AND ACVSMR
Equine Orthopaedic Research Center
Colorado State University
Ft. Collins, CO, USA

Kevin G. Keegan, DVM, MS, DIPLOMATE ACVS
Program in Equine Lameness, Department of Veterinary Medicine and Surgery
College of Veterinary Medicine
University of Missouri
Columbia, MO, USA

Melissa King, DVM, PhD, DIPLOMATE ACVSMR
Equine Orthopaedic Research Center
College of Veterinary Medicine and Biomedical Sciences
Colorado State University
Ft. Collins, CO, USA

Drew W. Koch, DVM
Department of Clinical Sciences
Colorado State University
Ft. Collins, CO, USA

Stephen E. O'Grady, DVM, MRCVS
Virginia Therapeutic Farriery
Keswick, VA, USA

Kyla F. Ortved, DVM, PhD, DIPLOMATE ACVS AND ACVSMR
Department of Clinical Studies, New Bolton Center
School of Veterinary Medicine University of Pennsylvania
Kennett Square, PA, USA

Andrew H. Parks, MA, VET MB, MRCVS, DIPLOMATE ACVS
Department of Large Animal Medicine
College of Veterinary Medicine
University of Georgia
Athens, GA, USA

W. Rich Redding, DVM, MS, DIPLOMATE ACVS AND ACVSMR
North Carolina State University
College of Veterinary Medicine
Raleigh, NC, USA

Kathryn A. Seabaugh, DVM, MS, DIPLOMATE ACVS AND ACVSMR
Orthopaedic Research Center in the Translational Medicine Institute
College of Veterinary Medicine and Biomedical Sciences Colorado State University
Ft. Collins, CO, USA

Lauren E. Smanik, DVM
Department of Clinical Sciences
College of Veterinary Medicine and Biomedical Sciences Veterinary Teaching Hospital
Colorado State University
Ft. Collins, CO, USA

Ted S. Stashak, DVM, MS DIPLOMATE ACVS
Colorado State University
Santa Rosa, CA, USA

Sara K.T. Steward, DVM
Colorado State University
Veterinary Teaching Hospital
Ft. Collins, CO, USA

Narelle C. Stubbs, b.appsc(pt), m.anim st(animal physiotherapy)
Equine Sports Medicine and Rehabilitation
West Palm Beach, FL, USA

Dane M. Tatarniuk, DVM, MS, DIPLOMATE ACVS
Department of Veterinary Clinical Sciences
Iowa State University – College of Veterinary Medicine
Ames, IA, USA

Troy N. Trumble, DVM, PhD, DIPLOMATE ACVS
College of Veterinary Medicine
Veterinary Medical Center
University of Minnesota
St. Paul, MN, USA

Rob Van Wessum, DVM, MS, DIPLOMATE ACVSMR, cert pract knmvd (eq)
Equine All-Sports Medicine Center PLLC
Mason, MI, USA

Ashlee E. Watts, DVM, PhD, DIPLOMATE ACVS
Director Comparative Orthopedics and Regenerative Medicine Laboratory
Texas A&M University
College Station, TX, USA

Preface

Welcome to the second edition of the *Equine Lameness Manual*. The second edition is a full-color, electronic version that has been updated with new information from the seventh edition of Adams and Stashak's Lameness in Horses. To further condense the second edition, the anatomy and imaging chapters from the first edition were eliminated and relevant information was included within each of the common lameness conditions. Further reorganization and consolidation of material was performed throughout the second edition focusing on physical examination of the horse, common clinical lameness conditions, and potential therapies. The goal of the second edition is to provide the reader with the nuts and bolts of lameness problems in horses. The information is not specifically referenced to individual references but instead a bibliography is included at the end of each chapter.

Also available to the reader are short "how to" video clips that demonstrate a variety of different physical examination (palpation, hoof testing, flexion tests) and perineural and intrasynovial injection techniques. The clips will be available on a companion website intended to complement the text within the book. The select perineural and intrasynovial injection video clips contain extensive anatomic details inserted directly into live demonstrations to better illustrate the techniques. Important anatomic landmarks are clearly labeled on the videos for further clarity.

I wish to thank all of the authors that contributed new information to the second edition as well as to the medical illustrators that helped create the videos for the companion website. I would also like to thank all of the horses, clients, and veterinarians that have provided the case material, knowledge, and experiences that have been included within this text. I hope that the second edition of the Equine Lameness Manual is a succinct lameness text that becomes a must have for both students and more experienced veterinarians alike.

Common Terminologies and Abbreviations

Terminology	Abbreviations
Distal or third phalanx	P3; coffin bone
Middle or second phalanx	P2
Proximal or first phalanx	P1
Metacarpus/metatarsus	MC/MT or MC3/MT3; cannon bone
Second and fourth metacarpal/metatarsal bones	MC2, MC4, MT2, MT4; splint bones
Proximal sesamoid bones	PSB
Distal sesamoidean ligaments	DSL
Distal sesamoidean impar ligament	DSIL
Collateral suspensory ligaments of navicular bone	CSLs
Collateral ligament(s)	CL or CLs
Deep digital flexor tendon	DDFT or DDF
Superficial digital flexor tendon	SDFT or DDF
Accessory ligament of deep digital flexor tendon	ALDDFT, ICL, or inferior check
Accessory ligament of superficial digital flexor tendon	ALSDFT, SCL, or superior check
Digital flexor tendon sheath	DFTS
Common digital extensor tendon	CDET
Long digital extensor tendon	LoDET
Lateral digital flexor tendon	LDFT
Distal interphalangeal joint	DIP joint or coffin joint
Proximal interphalangeal joint	PIP joint or pastern joint
Tarsometatarsal joint	TMT joint
Distal intertarsal joint	DIT joint
Proximal intertarsal joint	PIT joint
Tarsocrural joint	TC joint
Distal tarsal joints	DT joints
Metacarpo/metatarsophalangeal joint	MCP/MTP or fetlock joint
Medial femorotibial joint	MFT joint

Lateral femorotibial joint	LFT joint
Femoropatellar joint	FP joint
Scapulohumeral joint	SH joint or shoulder joint
Sacroiliac joint	SI joint
Computed tomography	CT
Magnetic resonance imaging	MRI
Increased radiopharmaceutical uptake	IRU
Ultrasound/Ultrasonography	US
Cross-sectional area	CSA
Osteochondrosis/osteochondritis dissecans	OC/OCD
Osteoarthritis	OA
Developmental orthopedic disease	DOD
Subchondral cystic lesion	SCL
Angular limb deformity	ALD
Suspensory ligament/suspensory ligament branches	SL/SLBs
Proximal suspensory desmitis	PSD
Medial patellar ligament	MPL
Upward fixation of patella	UFP
Medial patellar ligament desmotomy	MPD
Tarsal sheath	TS
Sustentaculum tali	ST
Peroneus tertius	PT
Palmar digital	PD
Deep branch lateral plantar nerve	DBLPN
Mediolateral	ML
Dorsopalmar/plantar	DP
Nonsteroidal anti-inflammatory drug	NSAID
Hyaluronan or hyaluronic acid	HA
Polysulfated glycosaminoglycans	PSGAG; Adequan
Platelet-rich plasma	PRP
Interleukin receptor antagonist protein/autologous conditioned serum	IRAP/ACS
Mesenchymal stem cell	MSC
Triamcinolone	TA
Methyl prednisolone acetate	MPA or Depo-medrol
Dimethyl sulfoxide	DMSO
Diclofenac cream	Surpass
Extracorporeal shockwave treatment	ESWT or shockwave
Intra-articular	IA
Intravenous	IV
Intramuscular	IM
Regional limb perfusion	RLP

About the Companion Website

The videos in this book have been replicated from *Adams and Stashak's Lameness in Horses, 7th Edition*

This book is accompanied by a companion website:

  www.wiley.com/go/baxter/manual

The website includes: Short "how to" video clips that demonstrate a variety of different physical examination (palpation, hoof testing, flexion tests) and perineural and intrasynovial injection techniques. The goal is for the reader to clearly see these procedures being performed on live horses. The select perineural and intrasynovial injection video clips contain extensive anatomic details inserted directly into the live demonstrations to better illustrate the techniques. Important anatomic landmarks are emphasized and clearly labeled within the videos.

1

Assessment of the Lame Horse

Introduction

- Lameness is an indication of a structural or functional disorder in one or more limbs or the axial skeleton that is evident while the horse is standing or at movement.
- Lameness is a clinical sign, not a disease.
- Lameness can be caused by trauma (single event or repetitive work), congenital or acquired anomalies, developmental defects, infection, metabolic disturbances, circulatory and nervous disorders, or any combination of these.
- It is important to differentiate between lameness resulting from pain and nonpainful alterations in gait, often referred to as "mechanical lameness," and lameness resulting from neurologic (nervous system) dysfunction.
- Most lameness in horses is due to pain during weight-bearing, with shifting of load away from the source limb onto the other non- or less affected limbs.
- The detection of clinical signs of lameness is primarily the recognition of an asymmetric gait in the horse.
- The primary objectives of a lameness examination are to determine:
  1) Whether the horse is lame.
  2) Which limb or limbs are involved?
  3) The site or sites of the problem.
  4) The specific cause of the problem.
  5) The appropriate treatment and/or rehabilitation.
  6) The prognosis for recovery.
- The steps to perform a routine or traditional lameness examination include
  1) Complete history including signalment and use.
  2) Visual exam of the horse at rest.
  3) Palpation of the musculoskeletal system including hoof tester examination of the feet.
  4) Observation of the horse in motion (usually at a straight walk and trot/lope followed by circling) with or without objective lameness evaluation tools.
  5) Observation of the horse under saddle or in work if necessary.
  6) Manipulative tests such as flexion tests.
  7) Diagnostic anesthesia, if necessary.
  8) Diagnostic imaging.

Adaptive Strategies of Lame Horses

- With most lameness conditions, the horse attempts to "unload" the lame limb during weight-bearing or the stance phase of the stride. As an example, in horses with chronic lameness, the limb with the flatter hoof is

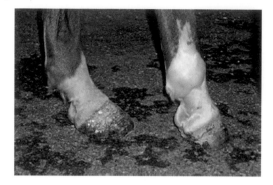

Figure 1.1 Chronic hindlimb lameness that has resulted in a wide flat foot on the sound limb (LH) and a narrow, upright hoof on the lame limb (RH).

thought to exhibit higher vertical loads because it is the non-lame limb (Figure 1.1).

- Horses accomplish this by abnormal movement of a body part (head nod or pelvic hike), weight shifting (to the contralateral or diagonal limb or torso), change in joint angles (lack of fetlock extension), and alterations in foot flight. Detecting these compensatory movements is an integral part of lameness diagnosis.
- The most consistent compensatory movements that are observed in lame horses are the vertical displacement and acceleration of the head in forelimb lameness and of the sacrum and tuber coxae in hindlimb lameness.
- More subtle lameness causes fewer compensatory changes, making lameness diagnosis more difficult. Although these gait changes may be difficult to appreciate during visual examination of a lame horse, it should be remembered that the primary adaptive strategy of the horse is to redistribute load to compensate for pain in a limb without causing an overload situation in other limbs.

Classification of Lameness

- In most cases, there is a primary or baseline lameness that contributes to the most obvious gait abnormalities. Compensatory, secondary, or complementary lameness results from overloading of the other limbs as a result of the primary lameness.
- Lameness may also be classified according to when it occurs (or is best observed) within the stride – i.e. stance, swing, pushoff, etc.
- Visual observation of the gait can usually determine whether the lameness is supporting limb, swinging limb, or mixed. However, because of the many adaptive strategies that occur in lame horses, some clinicians feel that mixed lameness occurs most commonly in horses.
- The different classifications of lameness are:
  1) Supporting limb lameness: Apparent when the foot first contacts the ground or when the limb is supporting weight (stance phase). This is by far the most common type of lameness identified in the horse.
  2) Swinging limb lameness: Evident when the limb is in motion. The majority of these problems are thought to involve the upper limbs or axial skeleton.
  3) Mixed lameness: Evident both when the limb is moving (swing phase) and when it is supporting weight (stance phase).
  4) Primary or baseline lameness: Most obvious lameness or gait abnormality that is observed before flexion or manipulative tests. This can be complicated by lameness in multiple limbs, but the most severe lameness is usually considered the primary lameness.
  5) Compensatory or complementary lameness: Pain in a limb can cause uneven distribution of weight on another limb or limbs, which can produce lameness in a previously sound limb. It is common to have complementary lameness produced in an opposite forelimb or hindlimb.

Anatomic Problem Areas

- The majority of lameness problems in horses occur in the forelimb due to the increased weight-bearing on the forelimbs (60%–65%) and the shock of landing that the forelimbs absorb during movement.

- Breed and occupation can alter these generalizations as horses that pull carts or perform events such as dressage, cutting, and reining, which place greater stress on the hindquarters, often have a higher percentage of hindlimb lameness.
- It is also estimated that approximately 95% of lameness in the forelimb occurs distal to the carpus and approximately 80% of lameness problems in the hindlimbs involve the hock or stifle.
- Although there is considerable overlap, specific lameness conditions are often associated with a specific type of work or occupation. Knowing common problem areas will facilitate a more thorough and complete physical examination that may help detect subtle abnormalities (Table 1.1).

Table 1.1 Occupation-related lameness problems.

Occupation	Lameness conditions
TB and QH racehorse (Fatigue-associated repetitive overuse)	Foot bruising, quarter cracks, heel pain
	Forelimb fetlock synovitis and fractures
	Carpal synovitis and fractures
	Bucked shins in young horses
	Fatigue/stress fractures—MC/MT, P1, humerus, tibia, pelvis
	SDFT tendonitis
	Suspensory injuries
	Coffin joint synovitis/OA—QH
	Proximal suspensory desmitis—QH
	Catastrophic fractures—sesamoids, P1, MC/MT, and humerus
	Palmar/plantar osteochondral disease (POD)
STD racehorse (hindlimb > forelimb)	Front feet bruising and corns
	Hindlimb fetlock synovitis and fractures
	Carpal synovitis and fractures (C3)
	Fatigue/stress fractures—similar to TB and QH but tibia most common
	Suspensory injuries, especially PSD, SDFT tendonitis
	Hock, stifle, and sacroiliac problems
Endurance horse	Muscle disorders including tying-up and muscle spasm, cramps, and strains
	Forelimb and hindlimb suspensory desmitis
	Foot bruising, P3 osteitis, and laminitis
	Fetlock synovitis/OA
	SDFT tendonitis
Show/pleasure horse	Navicular syndrome/disease
	Coffin joint synovitis/OA
	Forelimb and hindlimb PSD
	Distal tarsitis or bone spavin
	Lumbar and sacroiliac problems

(Continued)

Table 1.1 (Continued)

Occupation	Lameness conditions
Western performance horses (Cutting, reining, roping, barrel racing, rodeo, gymkhana, and ranch horses)	Navicular syndrome/disease including DDFT injuries Phalangeal fractures (primarily P2) Pastern ringbone Fetlock and carpal synovitis/OA Distal tarsitis or bone spavin Stifle synovitis/OA Forelimb and hindlimb PSD Thoracolumbar myositis Hindlimb muscle strains
Jumping/dressage/eventing	Navicular syndrome/disease including DDFT injuries Suspensory branch injuries Forelimb and hindlimb PSD Fetlock synovitis/OA SDFT tendonitis Distal tarsitis or bone spavin Stifle injuries Thoracolumbar myositis—back problems Sacroiliac problems
Draft horses	Hoof cracks and laminitis Subsolar abscesses, canker, and thrush Ringbone Sweeny Bone and bog spavin Stifle synovitis/OA Shivers and PSSM
Gaited horses (Hindlimb > Forelimb)	Distal tarsitis or bone spavin Stifle synovitis/OA Thoracolumbar myositis/back problems DSLD

TB, Thoroughbred; QH, Quarter horse; STD, Standardbred.
P1, first phalanx; P2, second phalanx; P3, third phalanx; MC/MT, metacarpus/metatarsus; C3, third carpal bone; PSD, proximal suspensory desmitis; SDFT, superficial digital flexor tendon; OA, osteoarthritis; PSSM, polysaccharide storage myopathy; DSLD, degenerative suspensory ligament desmitis.

Signalment and Use

- Patient age and occupation are important considerations when determining potential lameness conditions (see Table 1.1).
- In general, younger horses are more likely to develop lameness from developmental orthopedic-related conditions (osteochondrosis) and older horses from repetitive-use trauma such as osteoarthritis.

- Certain breeds of horses also appear more prone to foot-related conditions presumably related to their conformation.
- Horses that train and work at speed are more likely to develop lameness conditions related to fatigue-associated repetitive overuse (stress fractures) and high-motion joints.
- Horses that are required to more fully engage their hindlimbs when working (cutting and

reining horses) will not surprisingly have more hindlimb lameness issues.

- Young horses in any type of work may develop lameness problems more easily than older horses due to the immaturity of their musculoskeletal system.
- In general, foals less than four months of age are much more likely to have lameness associated with infection, and older foals are particularly prone to traumatic injuries.

History

- A detailed medical history should be obtained on every horse.
- Specific information that should be obtained regarding the duration and intensity of the lameness, the specific signs observed by the owner or trainer, the activity immediately preceding the lameness, and any previous treatments or therapies employed.
- The minimum questions that should be asked in most cases include
  1) How long has the horse been lame?
  2) Has the horse been rested since the initial lameness?
  3) Has the lameness worsened, improved, or stayed the same?
  4) Was the cause of the lameness observed?
  5) Does the lameness worsen with exercise or does the horse warm out of the lameness?
  6) What treatments have been initiated and have they helped?

Visual Examination at Rest

- Often, the initial part of a lameness evaluation is a visual examination of the horse standing squarely on a flat surface at rest.
- Observations should include the body type and conformation as well as alterations in posture, weight shifting, pointing of limbs, contour of the limbs, and asymmetry between limbs.
- Visual observation of the feet cannot be overemphasized. All four feet should

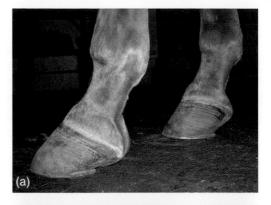
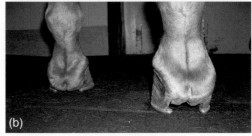

Figure 1.2 Lateral view (a) and dorsopalmar (b) views of both front feet in a horse with forelimb lameness. The front feet have markedly different hoof angles. The right foot has contracted heels resulting in a very upright conformation compared with a low under-run heel with a long toe on the left foot resulting in a low hoof conformation. The medial wall of the right foot is concave with the coronary pushed proximally, suggesting excessive concussion.

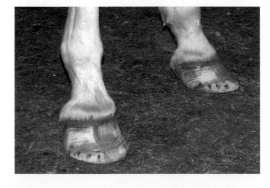

Figure 1.3 Partial thickness dorsal hoof crack associated with a long toe and a concavity of the dorsal hoof wall. Both factors most likely contributed to the development of the crack in this horse.

be observed for abnormal wear, hoof cracks, imbalance, size, shape, and heel bulb contraction (Figures 1.2 and 1.3). Swelling above the coronary band and any alterations in coronary band contour should also be noted.

- All joints and tendons and their sheaths should be visually inspected for swelling and the muscles of the limbs, back, and rump are observed for swelling and atrophy. Comparing one side to the other is most important.
- Significant muscle atrophy and/or asymmetry, especially in the hindlimb is often suggestive of the lame limb (Figures 1.4 and 1.5).

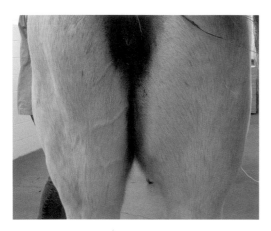

Figure 1.4 Example of atrophy of the inner and outer thigh muscles of the left hindlimb that occurred secondary to an upper hindlimb lameness.

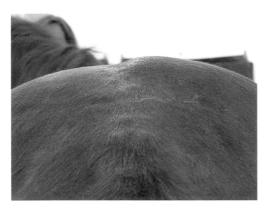

Figure 1.5 Rear view of the pelvis of a horse with a history of an acute onset of right hindlimb lameness. Asymmetry to the sacroiliac region was visible and there was pain on firm palpation of the right tuber sacrale.

Palpation and Manipulation

Overview

- Palpation of the musculoskeletal system is a very important aspect of the lameness evaluation and with experience, subtle abnormalities can be detected that are often indicative of the site of the problem.
- A systematic approach of palpation is recommended to avoid missing abnormalities. One method is to palpate the forelimb proximally to distally with the limb bearing weight, and then distally to proximally with the limb picked up or unweighted (Video 1.1).
- Palpation of the hindlimbs is performed in the same manner, paying close attention to the medial aspects of the stifle and tarsus (Video 1.2).
- The back and axial skeleton are palpated last because some horses become agitated with palpation/manipulation of the back (Video 1.3).
- Hoof tester examination of the feet is usually performed after the entire musculoskeletal system has been palpated or after watching the horse go (Video 1.4).

Foot

- As much information about the foot can be obtained by a thorough visual exam as can be determined with hoof testers. Observations should be compared with what is considered to be normal foot conformation (Figures 1.6 and 1.7).
- The examiner should look for asymmetry in foot size, abnormal hoof wear, hoof ring formation, heel bulb contraction, shearing of the heels and quarters, hoof wall cracks, coronet swellings, and foot imbalances (Figures 1.2, 1.3 and 1.8).
- Visual examination of heel bulb contraction is best performed with the examiner standing or squatting near the flank and looking at both right and left heel bulbs at once (Figure 1.2b).
- Foot imbalances can be dorsopalmar/plantar (DP), lateral medial (LM), or a combination of the two (Figures 1.1 and 1.7).

Figure 1.6 Normal forefoot with structures labeled.

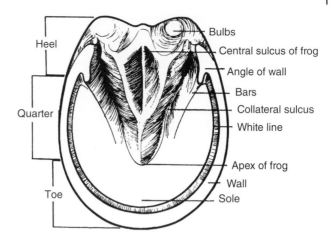

Heel

Quarter

Toe

Bulbs
Central sulcus of frog
Angle of wall
Bars
Collateral sulcus
White line
Apex of frog
Wall
Sole

- The weight-bearing surface of each foot should be examined for abnormal wear of the shoe and/or sole, collapsed heels, heel bulb contraction, heel length and angles, sole contour (concave vs. convex), and the shape and size of the frog.
- Heel contraction and frog atrophy are often common sequelae to chronic foot lameness (Figures 1.2 and 1.9).
- Cleaning the bottom of the hoof and removing debris from the clefts of the frog are necessary to not miss abnormalities and to completely evaluate the hoof.
- A hoof tester is an instrument that permits deep palpation of the sole, frog, and wall of

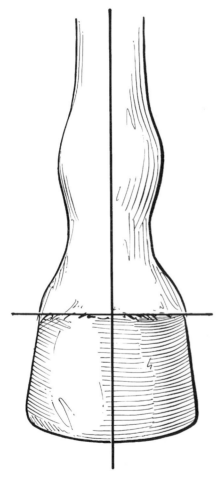

Figure 1.7 A hoof is considered to be in Medial-Lateral (ML) balance when an imaginary line through the coronet is parallel to the ground surface and perpendicular to a line that bisects the limb axis when viewed from the front. Also, each side of the hoof wall has approximately the same angle toward the ground and are of equal length.

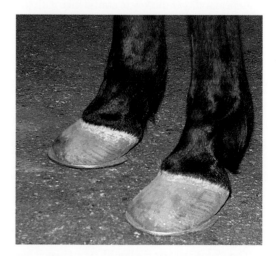

Figure 1.8 Concavity of the left front foot in a horse with chronic laminitis. Abnormal hoof growth rings are also present. This horse was most lame in the left forelimb.

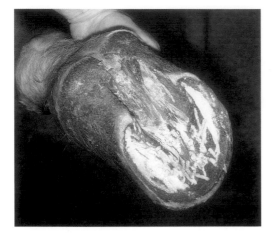

Figure 1.9 A front foot with severely overgrown heels that have resulted in atrophy of the frog. The frog should be prominent and approximately level with the widest part of the heels.

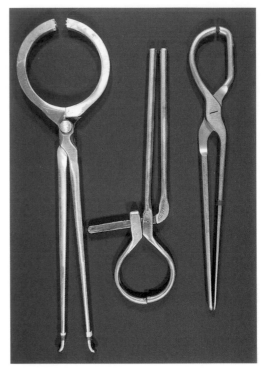

Figure 1.10 Examples of several types of hoof testers. Left, GE Forge and Tool Works, 959 Highland Way, Grover Beach, CA, 93433. Middle, Ryding Hoof Tester, Jorgenson Labs, 2198 W 15th St., Loveland, CO, 80537. Right, Kane Enterprises, AG-TEK Division, P.O. Box 1043, Sioux Falls, SD 57101.

the hoof trying to identify and localize hoof sensitivity (Figure 1.10).

- A systematic approach beginning at the lateral or medial angle of the sole and continuing hoof tester pressure at 2- to 3-cm intervals until the entire surface of the sole is checked is one method. This is followed by applying pressure to the frog (caudal, central, and cranial) from both the medial and lateral heel (Figure 1.11), and then across the heel bulbs (Video 1.4).

- Repeatability is the key to confidence with the findings of a hoof testing exam. True sensitivity is identified by repeated intermittent hoof tester pressure that results in persistent reflexive withdrawal (flexing the shoulder or pulling the foot away) with hoof tester pressure.

- Localized hoof tester sensitivity of the sole can be suggestive of focal sole bruising, puncture wounds, close or hot nail, and localized subsolar abscesses. More diffuse sole sensitivity can be identified in a variety of foot abnormalities.

Coronet and heel bulbs

- The coronary band should be palpated for heat, swelling, and pain on pressure that may indicate a problem within the hoof wall.

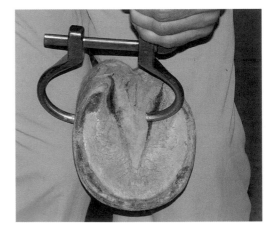

Figure 1.11 Hoof testers are applied over the central third of the frog of the fore foot to produce direct pressure over the navicular region. The author prefers the Ryding Hoof Tester.

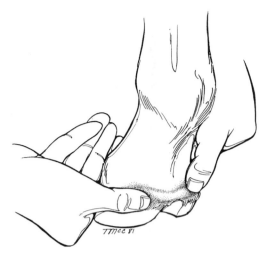

Figure 1.12 Palpation of the heel bulbs to identify heat, pain, and swelling that may be associated with subsolar abscesses.

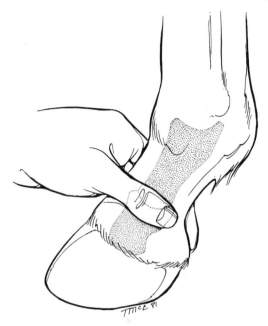

Figure 1.13 Palpation of the pastern. Thickening in this region may suggest the presence of ringbone.

- Point swelling and pain with or without drainage at the coronet in the mid-quarter region may indicate an abscess along the white line or infection of the collateral cartilage of the distal phalanx.
- Palpation of the heel bulbs should be performed as heat, pain, and swelling with or without drainage of one of the heel bulbs can be found in horses with subsolar abscesses (Figure 1.12).
- Symmetrical swelling just proximal to coronary band is suggestive of effusion of the distal interphalangeal (DIP) joint.

Pastern
- The dorsal, medial, and lateral surfaces of the proximal interphalangeal (PIP) joint should be palpated for enlargement, heat, and pain with digital pressure (Figure 1.13).
- Palpable findings should always be compared with the opposite pastern although it is not uncommon for the lateral to medial dimensions of one pastern to be slightly larger than the opposite pastern in normal horses.
- With the limb off the ground, the palmar/plantar aspect of the pastern should be palpated deeply for pain, heat, and swelling (Figure 1.14). Important structures in this

area include the distal sesamoidean ligaments, lateral and medial branches of the superficial digital flexor tendon (SDFT) as

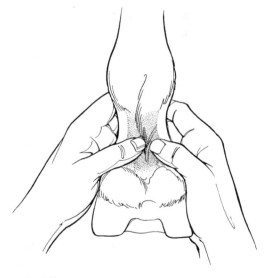

Figure 1.14 Palpation of the distal sesamoidean ligaments, branches of the SDFT, and the DDFT in the palmar/plantar aspect of the pastern. The DDFT should be palpated with digital pressure using your thumb as far distally as possible between the heel bulbs.

they attach to the middle phalanx, the deep digital flexor tendon (DDFT), and digital flexor tendon sheath (DFTS).

- The phalangeal joints should also be rotated medially and laterally to assess the stability of the joints and for evidence of pain (Figure 1.15).

Fetlock

- The dorsal and palmar/plantar joint pouches of the metacarpophalangeal/metatarsophalangeal

(MCP/MTP) joint should be palpated for swelling, effusion, or thickening of the joint capsule (Figure 1.16).

- The dorsal, medial, and lateral surfaces of the PIP joint should be palpated for enlargement, heat, and pain with digital pressure (Figure 1.13).
- The lateral and medial branches of the suspensory ligament just above their attachments to the proximal sesamoid bones, the SDFT, the DDFT, and the DFTS should be palpated for heat, pain, swelling, or effusion (Figure 1.17).
- With the limb off the ground, the basilar, body, and apical portions of the proximal sesamoid bones should be digitally palpated for pain and swelling (Figure 1.18).
- The fetlock should be rotated and stress applied to the collateral ligaments in a manner similar to that of the pastern joint (Figure 1.15).
- The fetlock joint should be passively flexed to identify pain and assess the range of

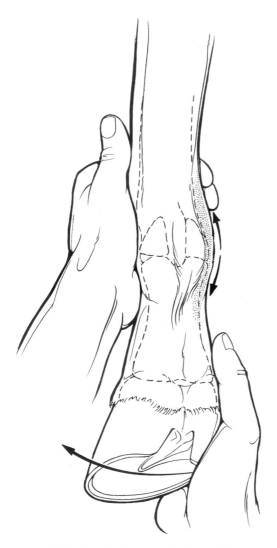

Figure 1.15 Tension is applied to the collateral ligaments supporting the fetlock and interphalangeal joints (pastern and coffin) to identify pain.

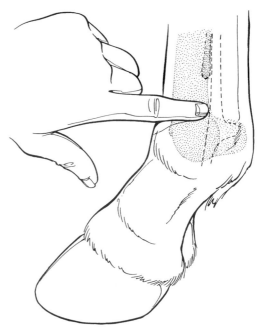

Figure 1.16 The finger marks the palmar recesses of the fetlock joint capsule just distal to the splint bone. Distention at the site indicates synovial effusion of the joint.

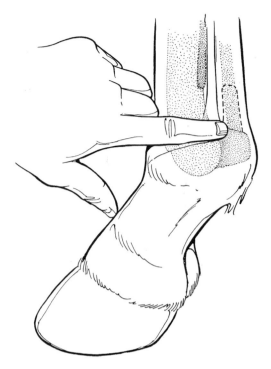

Figure 1.17 Palpation of the digital flexor synovial sheath around the superficial and deep digital flexor tendons is performed behind the branch of the suspensory ligament.

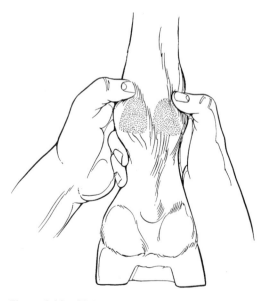

Figure 1.18 Digital pressure applied to the apical sesamoid region to detect pain, heat, and asymmetry. Palpation of the midbody and basilar aspects of the bones also should be performed.

motion by extending the carpus as much as possible with one hand, and then flexing the fetlock with the opposite hand. Either placing your hand on the dorsal aspect of the pastern or on the hoof are acceptable methods to flex the fetlock (Figure 1.19).

Metacarpus/Metatarsus (MC/MT)

- The third MC/MT and each splint bone should be palpated for evidence of swelling, thickness, and pain.
- Palpation of the dorsal aspect of the metacarpus should be performed, especially in racehorses, to detect evidence of dorsal metacarpal disease (buck shins). Firm pressure applied with the fingertips often elicits a painful response in these horses and heat and swelling over the dorsal middle third of the metacarpus also may be present (Figure 1.20).
- The entire length of each small MC/MT bone (splint bone) should be palpated with the limb weighted and unweighted.
- With the limb elevated, the palmar/plantar and axial surfaces of the splint bones can be palpated with the thumb applying pressure as needed by pushing the flexor tendons and suspensory ligament toward the opposite side (Figure 1.21).
- Nonpainful enlargements of the splint bones are often incidental findings but evidence of heat, pain, and swelling together with lameness may indicate a variety of clinical problems.
- Heat, pain, and swelling located in the proximal aspect of MCII in young horses are often referred to as condition called "splints."

Suspensory Ligament

- The suspensory ligament (interosseus medius muscle) lies just palmar/plantar to the splint bones in the MC/MT groove and should be palpated with the limb bearing weight and with the limb flexed.
- Damage to the suspensory ligament tends to occur distally within the branches of the

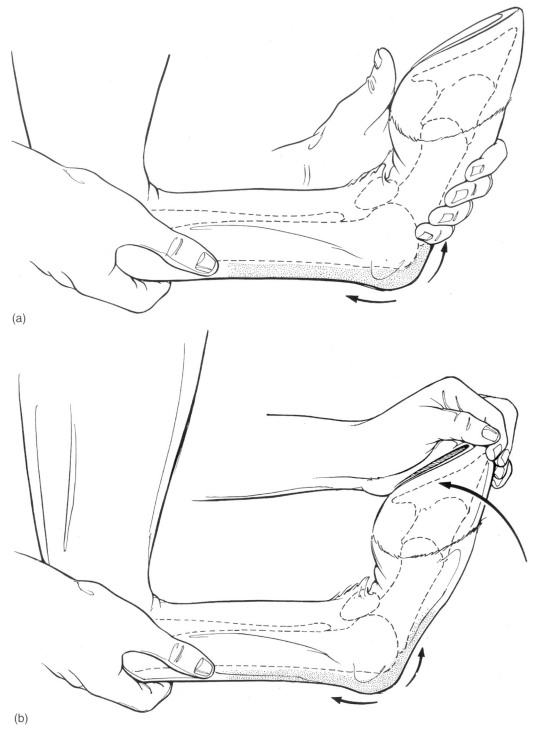

(a)

(b)

Figure 1.19 The fetlock flexion test is performed by extending the carpus and flexing the fetlock joint. Pressure can be applied either on the dorsal aspect of the pastern to try and flex the fetlock without flexing the interphalangeal joints (a) or by using the hoof as is done with a distal limb flexion test (b).

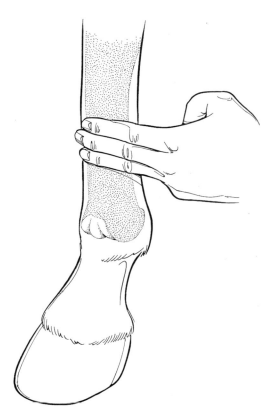

Figure 1.20 Palpation over the dorsal middle third of the metacarpus to identify heat, pain, and swelling associated with dorsal metacarpal disease.

suspensory ligament or at its proximal attachment to the MC/MT, and deep palpation often is needed to identify swelling and pain.

- With the limb held in a flexed position, the proximal attachment of the suspensory ligament can be palpated by pushing the flexor tendons to the side and applying pressure with the thumb (Figure 1.22).
- Alternatively, pressure can be applied to this region by wrapping your fingers around the proximal MC, and using the fingertips to "squeeze" the limb and apply pressure to the proximal palmar MC region (Figure 1.23).
- Palpation of the proximal suspensory is more difficult in the hindlimbs than the forelimbs because the small metatarsal bones closely surround the ligament and the

SDFT is less easily pushed to the side (Figure 1.24).
- A painful withdrawal response that persists and is easily repeatable is suggestive of a problem in the area.

Flexor Tendons
- The flexor tendons (SDFT and DDFT) course along the entire palmar/plantar aspect of the metacarpal/metatarsal regions just palmar/plantar to the suspensory ligament.
- In the metacarpus, the proximal one-third of the flexor tendons (associated with the carpus) and distal one-third (associated with the fetlock) are encased in tendon sheaths, whereas the central one-third is covered by a paratenon only.
- The SDFT and DDFT are intimately associated with each should be palpated carefully for heat, pain, and swelling with the tendons both weighted and relaxed.
- With the limb unweighted, the normal SDFT can be easily separated and differentiated from the DDFT with the thumb and forefinger (Figure 1.25).
- Most horses will respond slightly to "pinching" a normal SDFT between the thumb and index finger, but pain will be elicited easily with palpation in most horses with tendinitis.
- Increased size of the tendons together with palpable pain and an inability to separate the tendons are all common findings in horse with tendinitis.
- The inferior check ligament (accessory ligament of the DDFT) lies directly palmar to the suspensory ligament and can be palpated by holding the ligament between the index finger and the thumb or by applying pressure from the palmar aspect with the thumb.

Carpus
- Important synovial structures around the carpus that should be identified and palpated include the radiocarpal and middle carpal joints, the common digital extensor

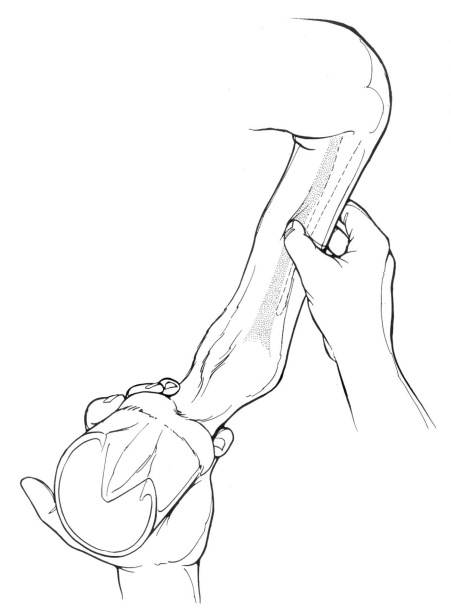

Figure 1.21 Palpation of the medial (axial) surfaces of the small metacarpal bones. The fetlock can be flexed to relax the suspensory ligament to permit easier palpation.

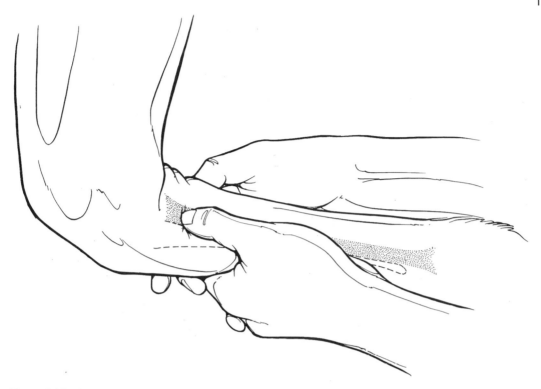

Figure 1.22 Palpation of the origin of the suspensory ligament in the proximal aspect of the metacarpal region. A repeatable painful response may suggest proximal suspensory desmitis.

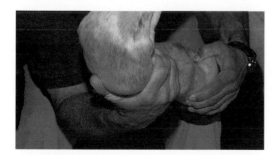

Figure 1.23 Method that can be used to apply digital pressure to the suspensory ligament in the proximal palmar metacarpal region.

tendon sheath, and carpal sheath. Swelling/ effusion of the tendon sheaths course longitudinally on the limb whereas effusion within the joints is more circumferential around the carpus (Figures 1.26 and 1.27).

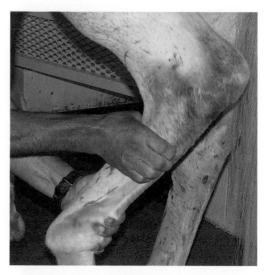

Figure 1.24 Method that can be used to apply digital pressure to the suspensory ligament in the proximal plantar metatarsal region.

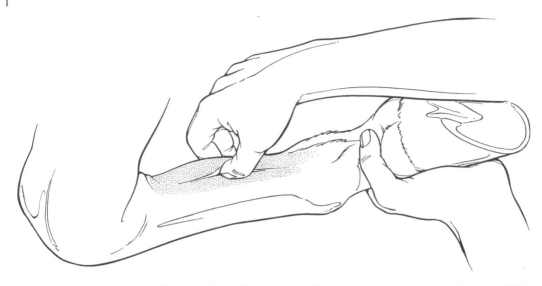

Figure 1.25 Palpation of the flexor tendons with the fetlock flexed to permit separation of the superficial and deep digital flexor tendons. Inability to separate the tendons usually suggests tendinitis.

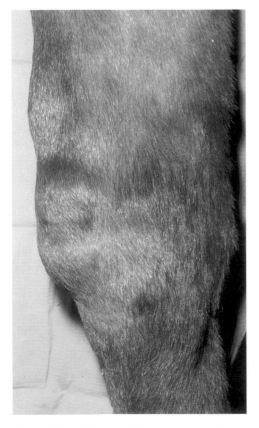

Figure 1.26 Effusion of the extensor carpi radialis tendon sheath is usually characterized by swelling that courses up and down the cranial aspect of the carpus.

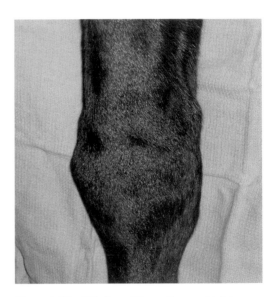

Figure 1.27 Effusion of the radiocarpal joint was visible and easily palpable in both the dorsomedial and palmarolateral joint pouches in this horse.

- If swollen, the external carpus should be closely examined and palpated for swelling/effusion, heat, and pain to determine the origin of the effusion/swelling.
- The degree of carpal flexion or range of motion should be evaluated by lifting the metacarpus upward to the elbow. In the normal horse, the flexor surface of the metacarpal region can

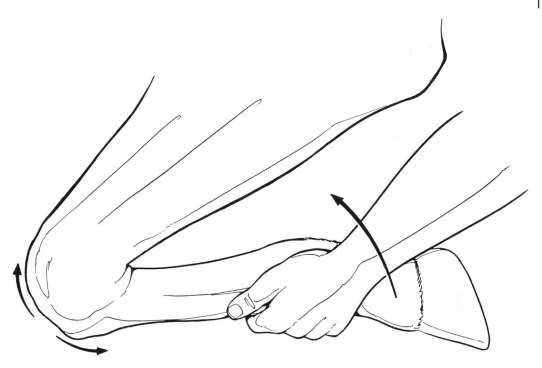

Figure 1.28 Flexion of the carpus to identify a painful response. In the normal horse, the flexor surface of the metacarpus approximates that of the forearm.

approximate that of the forearm when the carpus is flexed (Figure 1.28).

- Palpation of the carpal joints and individual carpal bones, including the accessory carpal bone, is best done with the carpus flexed. With the carpus held in flexion, the individual carpal bones are evaluated by deep digital pressure along the dorsal articular surfaces (Figure 1.29).

- The accessory carpal bone on the palmar aspect of the carpus is most easily palpated with the carpus flexed to relieve the tension of the ulnaris lateralis and flexor carpi ulnaris that attach to the bone (Figure 1.30).

Forearm (Antebrachium) and Elbow

- The soft tissues of the forearm and elbow joint (cubital joint) should be palpated for signs of inflammation, particularly swelling and pain.

- The distal aspect of the radius should also be palpated for swelling, heat, and pain that may be suggestive of a nondisplaced radial fracture.

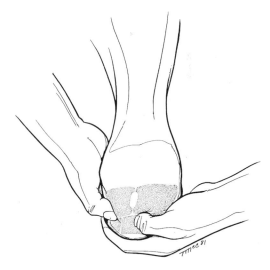

Figure 1.29 The dorsal articular margins of the carpal bones can be palpated after the carpus is flexed to identify pain within the individual carpal bones.

- Palpation of the caudal aspect of the olecranon should not be overlooked and variable degrees of swelling and pain with digital pressure may suggest an olecranon fracture.

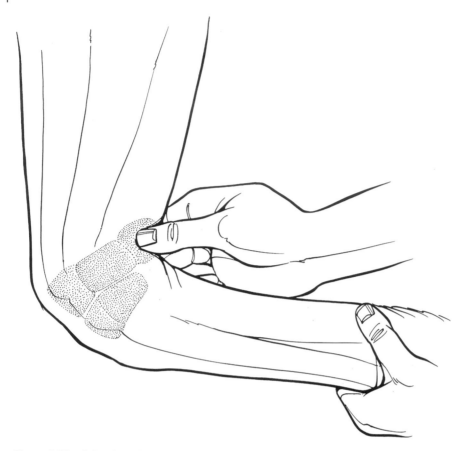

Figure 1.30 Palpation of the accessory carpal bone is best done with the carpus flexed to decrease the tensional influence of the tendinous insertions of the ulnaris lateralis and flexor carpi ulnaris muscles.

- A firm, usually nonpainful but fluctuant swelling at the point of the elbow is consistent with an elbow hygroma, also known as olecranon bursitis. These may or may not be clinically significant.
- Elevation of the limb into extension will often exacerbate any pain within the elbow region although it is not specific for the elbow (Figure 1.31).
- The collateral ligaments of the elbow joint should be evaluated by abducting and adducting the elbow and observing for evidence of pain.

Shoulder and Scapula

- It is very important to observe the shoulder and scapula region for evidence of muscle atrophy or swelling as these often accompany problems in this area (Figure 1.32).
- The two synovial structures in the shoulder region are the scapulohumeral joint and the bicipital bursa. Effusion within these structures can be rarely identified because of the overlying musculature.
- Deep pressure applied directly over the scapulohumeral joint may sometimes elicit a painful response suggesting a problem within the point (Figure 1.33).
- The bicipital bursa region (cranial aspect of shoulder) should also be deeply palpated for evidence of pain in the region. This can be performed by grasping the muscle and tendon with the fingers and thumb and pulling laterad or by squeezing the muscle.

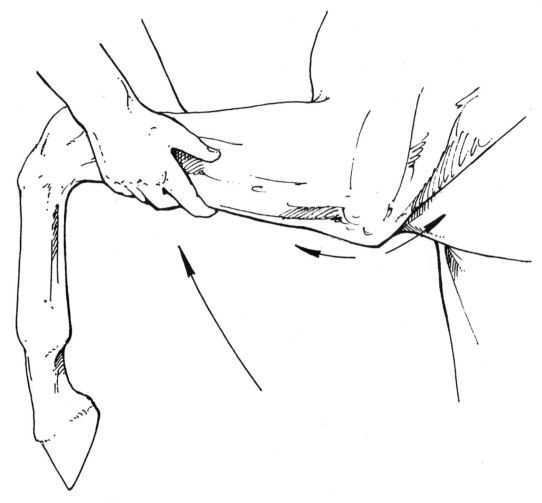

Figure 1.31 Elevating the limb into extension to flex the elbow joint extends the shoulder and increases the tension on the triceps brachii tendon at its insertion on the olecranon process.

- Placing one hand on the olecranon process and pulling the limb caudally or elevating the limb as described for the elbow may also elicit a painful response in the cranial aspect of the shoulder.

Tarsus (Hock)

- The tarsus is a common site contributing to hindlimb lameness and should be closely evaluated by visually and with palpation.
- Synovial structures located in the tarsus include the tarsocrural (TC) joint, tarsal sheath, and calcaneal bursa. It is important to know the anatomic location of each of these and to be able to differentiate them from each other if effusive.
- The TC joint has multiple pouches that can result in tarsal swelling, and this soft, fluctuant swelling is often referred to as "bog spavin" (Figure 1.34).
- Effusion/swelling of the tarsal sheath is often referred to as "thoroughpin," can be located either on the medial or lateral aspect of the tarsus, and courses longitudinally along the tarsus (Figure 1.35).
- Effusion of the calcaneal bursa (calcaneal bursitis) is often characterized by small pockets of fluid on each side of the SDFT

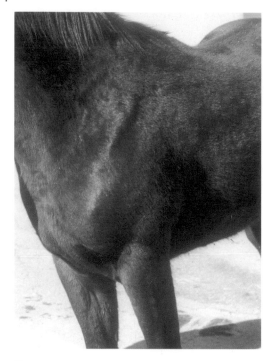

Figure 1.32 Atrophy of the shoulder muscles in young horses is often seen with osteochondrosis of the shoulder joint.

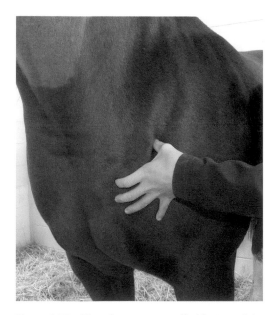

Figure 1.33 Thumb pressure applied just cranial to the infraspinatus tendon may elicit a painful response in horses with shoulder pain.

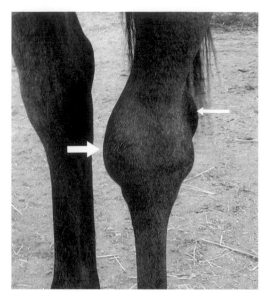

Figure 1.34 Young horse with effusion of the TC joint that is easily compressible and nonpainful (white arrows).

above and below the point of the calcaneus (Figure 1.36).

- The medial aspect of the distal tarsal joints (DIT and TMT) should be closely examined visually and with palpation to detect medial enlargements (tarsal shelves" that are often associated with distal tarsal OA (Figure 1.37).

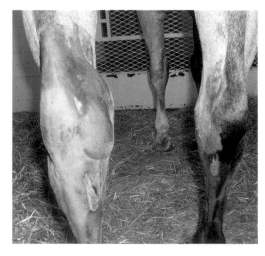

Figure 1.35 Effusion of the tarsal sheath on the medial aspect of the tarsus that was associated with fragmentation of the sustentaculum tali.

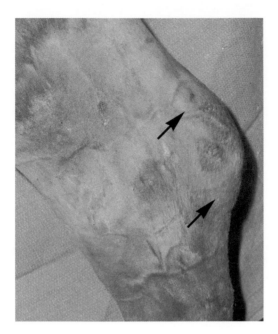

Figure 1.36 Effusion within the calcaneal bursa often can be palpated as fluid outpouchings above and below the retinaculum of the SDFT (black arrows).

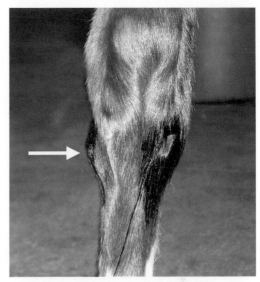

Figure 1.37 Enlargement of the medial aspect of the distal tarsus (arrow).

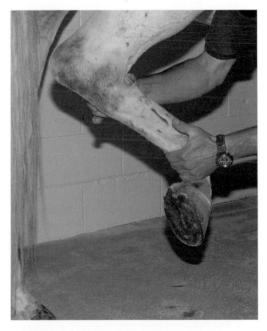

Figure 1.38 Limb and hand positioning to perform the "Churchill" test to detect pain on the medial aspect of the distal tarsal joints.

- The Churchill test can be performed by applying firm pressure using your fingers over the medial aspect of the distal tarsus and plantar aspect of the head of the second metatarsal (splint) bone (Figure 1.38). The test is considered positive if the horse flexes and abducts the limb away from the pressure and if there is a marked difference in the response between the two tarsi.
- The plantar aspect of the tuber calcis can be associated with several abnormalities and should be palpated for enlargement of the plantar ligament, swelling and pain associated with the SDFT (Figure 1.39), displacement of the SDFT (Figure 1.40), effusion within the calcaneal bursa, and for subcutaneous fluid swelling at the point of the hock referred to as "capped" hock.

Tibia

- It can be difficult to detect abnormalities in the tibial region, both visually and with palpation.

- Swelling in the caudal tibial region may indicate myositis of the semimembranosus and semitendinosus muscles or gastrocnemius tendinitis. The gastrocnemius tendon should be palpated for swelling and pain.

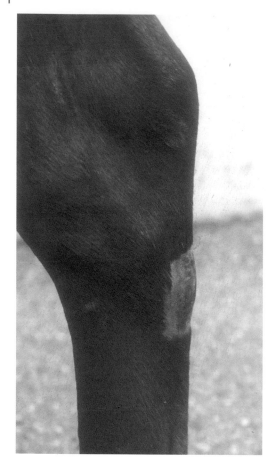

Figure 1.39 Tendinitis of the SDFT in the proximal metatarsal region, which can be misdiagnosed as a curb in some horses.

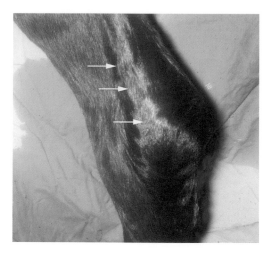

Figure 1.40 Lateral displacement of the superficial digital flexor tendon from the point of the calcaneus (arrows). Effusion of the calcaneal bursa is also usually present in these horses.

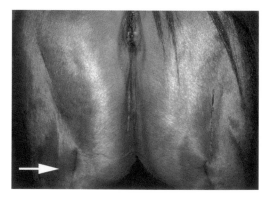

Figure 1.41 Horse with fibrotic myopathy of the left hindlimb. There is atrophy of the semitendinosus muscle and firm scar tissue palpable in the caudal tibial region (arrow).

- Severe pain with deep digital palpation of the distal third of the tibia, together with a severe lamencss and a positive spavin test, may suggest the possibility of an incomplete tibial fracture, especially in racehorses.
- The semimembranosus and semitendinosus muscles should be palpated for any evidence of pain and swelling indicative of myositis (hamstring pull) and for firm scarring/fibrosis that is often present with fibrotic myopathy (Figure 1.41).
- Assessment of the stay apparatus of the hindlimb should be performed if clinical signs consistent with rupture of the peroneus tertius muscle are present during exercise (Figure 1.42). With the stifle flexed, the hock can be extended, and a characteristic dimpling of the gastrocnemius tendon occurs.

Stifle

- The stifle is a common site for lameness problems in horses and should be thoroughly examined and palpated for muscle swelling/ atrophy, synovial effusion, and pain.
- The stifle is comprised of three synovial cavities – femoropatellar (FP) joint, medial

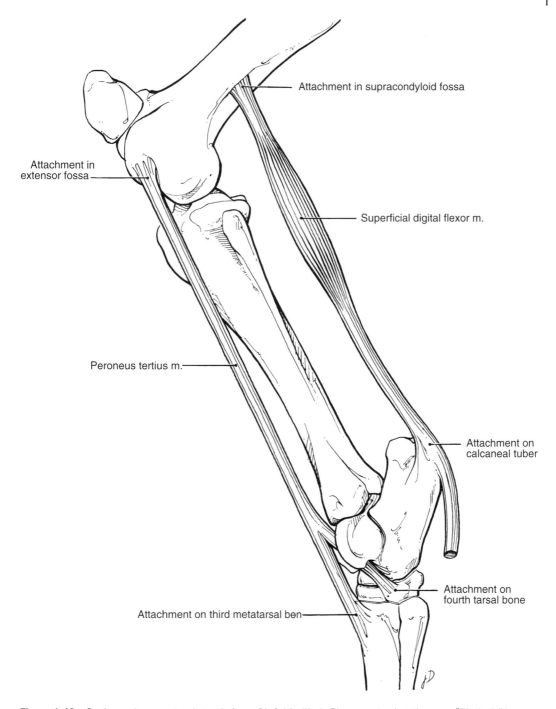

Figure 1.42 Reciprocal apparatus, lateral view of left hindlimb. Please note that the term "fibularis" has superseded "peroneus" (fibular rather than peroneal), although both are widely used.

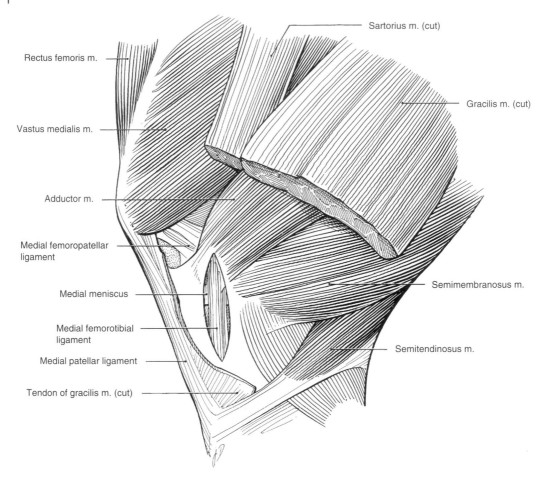

Rectus femoris m.

Vastus medialis m.

Adductor m.

Medial femoropatellar
ligament

Medial meniscus

Medial femorotibial
ligament

Medial patellar ligament

Tendon of gracilis m. (cut)

Sartorius m. (cut)

Gracilis m. (cut)

Semimembranosus m.

Semitendinosus m.

Figure 1.43 Deep dissection of medial aspect of left stifle. The tendon of adductor muscle is incised to reveal medial collateral ligament of the stifle.

femorotibial (MFT) joint, and the lateral femorotibial (LFT) joint, surrounded by an extensive network of ligaments and musculature (Figure 1.43).

- Distention of the FP joint is best seen and palpated on the cranial aspect of the stifle (Figure 1.44) while distention of the MFT joint can be seen and palpated on the medial aspect just behind the medial patella ligament (Figure 1.45). Effusion of the LFT joint can be identified lateral to the lateral patella ligament but is not commonly detected clinically.

- Abnormalities within the stifle joints are usually accompanied with synovial effusion and can be associated with a variety of intra-articular problems.

- The patella and its three patella ligaments (medial, middle, and lateral) are located on the cranial aspect of the stifle and should be palpated for thickening, pain, crepitus, and displacement. The ligaments are easily palpable across the cranial aspect of the stifle, but significant effusion of the FP joint can make palpation of the patella ligaments more difficult.

- The patella displacement test can be performed in horses suspected of upward fixation of the patella by grasping the base of the patella between the thumb and forefinger and

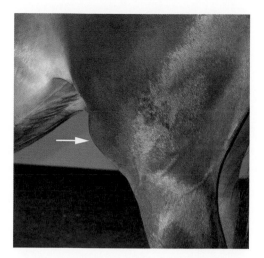

Figure 1.44 Effusion can be seen and palpated within the FP joint cranial to the patella ligaments (arrow).

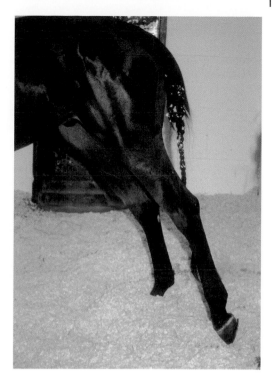

Figure 1.46 The horse is experiencing upward fixation of the patella. The limb is locked in extension and extended caudally and a bit laterally. The digit also is fixed in the flexed position. *Source:* Courtesy of Ken Sullins.

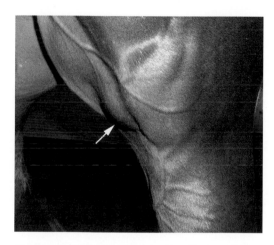

Figure 1.45 Visible and palpable effusion within the MFT joint is present just behind the medial patella ligament (arrow).

pushing proximally (upward) and laterally (outward) in an attempt to engage the medial patellar ligament over the medial trochlea. With complete upward fixation, the horse will be unable to flex its stifle or hock and may drag its limb behind in extension (Figure 1.46).

- A manipulative test to assess the stability of the stifle in horses suspected of damage to the cruciate ligaments can be performed by pushing the tibial tuberosity of the tibia caudally as quickly and forcibly as possible with the limb weight-bearing (Figure 1.47). This is a very subjective assessment of cranial-caudal movement of the stifle and a generalized looseness within the stifle is often the only finding because it is difficult to identify the phase (caudal or cranial) in which the movement occurs.

- A manipulative test to assess the integrity of the medial collateral ligament can be performed by placing the shoulder or outside hand over the lateral aspect of the stifle and abducting the distal limb with the other hand (Figure 1.48). Increased lateral movement of the distal limb usually indicates complete rupture of the ligament.

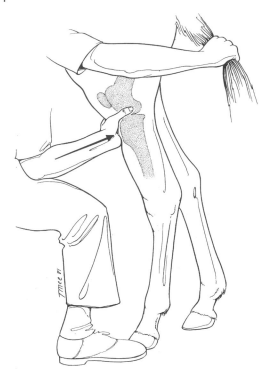

Figure 1.47 Positioning to check for problems with the cranial cruciate ligament. The examiner places one hand on the proximal tibia and forces it caudally (arrow) to check for increased movement (cranial drawer) of the tibia in relation to the femur.

Femur

- The femur is not a common site of lameness problems in horses. However, the muscles surrounding the femur should examined visually and palpated for swelling, atrophy, or evidence of pain.
- Complete femoral fractures are often associated with significant soft tissue swelling and lameness whereas distal physeal fractures and femoral neck fractures are more difficult to diagnose because they typically cause less swelling and lameness.
- Although uncommon, the greater trochanter should be palpated deeply for evidence of pain and swelling that may suggest middle gluteal muscle strain or trochanteric bursitis (whirlbone disease).

- A weak or nonexistent palpable pulse in the femoral artery (medial thigh in the groove between the sartorius muscle cranially and the pectineus muscle) may suggest thrombosis of the iliac artery that could be contributing to the lameness.

Hip and Pelvis

- Visual identification of asymmetry, swelling, and atrophy of the musculature and bones of the hip and pelvis is an important aspect of examination. This includes the coxofemoral joint, tuber coxae, the tuber ischium, the tuber sacrale, and the gluteal muscles on each side.
- With hip problems, swelling over the coxofemoral joint may be visually apparent and pain can often be elicited with deep palpation directly over the joint using the palm of the hand.
- Horses with upper limb lameness problems often have a characteristic stifle-out, hock-in, toe-out stance with an apparent shortening of the limb length (Figure 1.49).
- Asymmetry of the bony pelvis often suggests a pelvic fracture, subluxation of the sacroiliac region, or fracture of the specific bony prominence. Gluteal muscle atrophy often accompanies chronic pelvic fractures but can be seen with any chronic hindlimb lameness (Figure 1.50).
- Manipulation of the limb into extension, flexion, and abduction should be performed to detect for pain and crepitation. Crepitus may also be elicited by swaying the horse from side to side in horses with displaced pelvic fractures.

Back

- Visual assessment of the horse's back should include observing the muscle contour from the side and axial alignment of the spine from the rear specifically looking for swelling, atrophy, or asymmetry in the epaxial musculature.

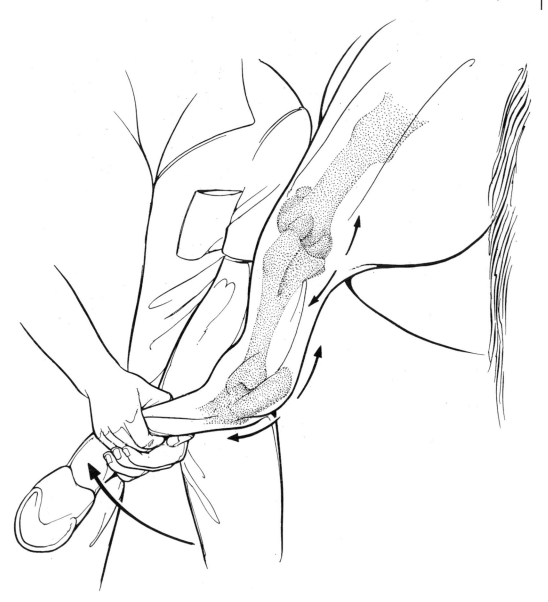

Figure 1.48 Test to stress the medial collateral ligaments of the hock and stifle. Alternatively, one hand can be placed on the medial aspect of the distal tibia to selectively stress the medial collateral ligament of the femorotibial joint. The examiner's shoulder can be placed over the middle of the tibia and both hands on the distal metatarsus to selectively stress the medial aspect of the hock.

- The dorsal spinous processes should be palpated for axial alignment, protrusion or depression, and interspinous distance (Figure 1.51).

- Palpation of the epaxial muscles is usually best performed with firm fingertip pressure using both hands simultaneously or using

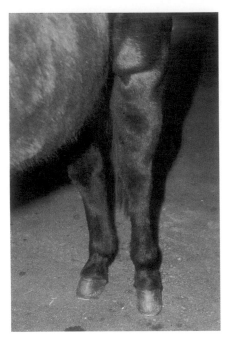

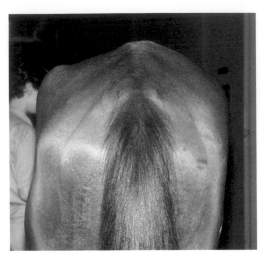

Figure 1.50 Severe atrophy of the left gluteal muscles secondary to a pelvic fracture. Disuse gluteal atrophy tends to occur more quickly and more profoundly with pelvic fractures than other lameness problems more distal in the limb.

Figure 1.49 Typical toe-out, hock-in stance that often accompanies problems within the hip and pelvic region.

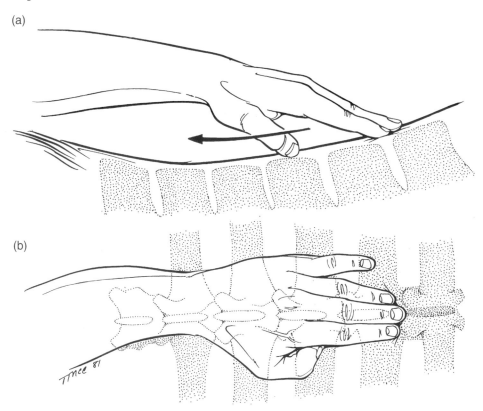

(a)

(b)

Figure 1.51 (a) Palpation of the summits of the dorsal spinous processes to identify depressions or protrusions that may indicate subluxation or fracture. (b) Palpation of the axial alignment of the dorsal spinous processes.

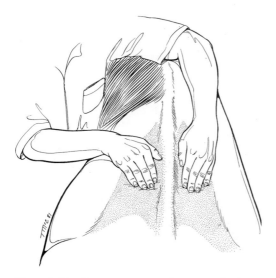

Figure 1.52 Firm pressure applied to the back musculature from the withers to the tuber sacrale to identify a painful response. The fingers should be held flat to prevent "digging in" with the fingertips.

the palms of your hand to apply downward pressure (Figure 1.52). Regardless of the technique, palpation of the equine back is a very subjective exercise.

- In most horses with clinically significant back pain, ventroflexion of the back often is severe and any increase in finger- or palm-applied pressure greatly increases this response. The horse attempts to "drop down" to get away from hand pressure. Palpation may also cause the horse to vocalize, swish its tail, or actually kick out behind.
- In some horses, tightening of the longissimus dorsi muscle may be felt with palpation rather than a painful withdrawal response and may suggest that the horse is attempting to fix the vertebral column because ventroflexion is painful.
- The horse's willingness to ventroflex, dorsiflex, and lateroflex its thoracic and lumbar vertebrae should also be evaluated. Reluctance to flex the back in any of these directions may suggest muscle tightening and back rigidity within the thoracolumbar region.

Neck

- The neck should be visually examined for contour from the side and axial alignment from the front and rear. Abnormalities that should be looked for include ventral arching of the neck, a straight (extended) poll, and axial deviations of the neck.
- The neck musculature and vertebral column should be palpated for signs of swelling, pain, muscle atrophy, and vertebral malalignment. Splinting and spastic contraction of the neck muscles is often suggestive of a painful condition.
- The transverse processes should be assessed for alignment and symmetry, and evidence of pain on firm, deep palpation.
- The neck should be flexed laterally and ventrally and extended to assess flexibility, range of motion, and pain.
- Lateral neck flexion can be encouraged by holding a treat at the horse's shoulder. Most horses should be able to flex their neck laterally enough that the muzzle almost contacts the craniolateral shoulder region.
- Ventroflexion is assessed by feeding the horse from the ground level, and extension is evaluated by elevating the head and neck.
- Resistance to neck movement in any direction usually is due to pain and can be from many potential causes.

Flexion Tests/Manipulation

Overview

- Flexion tests and limb manipulations are subjective methods to further isolate the suspected site of pain and lameness but must be interpreted in light of clinical findings because many otherwise normal horses may demonstrate positive responses.
- The response to flexion tests is based on how the flexion/manipulation changes the severity of the baseline lameness in the horse.

- In general, there are more false-positive results to flexion at any location than false-negative results and false-positive responses are most common in the front fetlock especially in horses in active work.
- Both the amount of force and the duration that it is applied can affect the response to flexion and therefore the procedure should be standardized as much as possible to minimize variability.
- Most flexion tests, regardless of the location, are usually performed for 30–60 seconds although one study found that flexion duration for 5 seconds was comparable to 60 seconds (Videos 1.5 and 1.6).
- Passive flexion usually refers to manipulation of a joint during routine palpation of the horse, and pain detected with passive flexion is often predictive of the response to flexion tests.
- Flexion tests can also be used to subjectively assess the severity of damage within the fetlock, carpus, and stifle as the severity of damage/pathology often is proportional to the severity of the response to the flexion test.
- Flexion tests are not always specific for the joint that is being flexed since it is nearly impossible to flex a single joint without affecting other nearby joints and soft tissue structures.
- Positive responses to hindlimb flexion tests have been shown to significantly change to the objective measurements of pelvic movement even though the individual responses to flexion may be highly variable.
- Changes in lameness in the limb not being flexed (weight-bearing limb) should be assessed as the increased weight-bearing may worsen the contralateral limb lameness.

Distal Limb/Phalangeal/Fetlock Flexion

- It is nearly impossible to only flex the fetlock or only flex the pastern or coffin joints. Flexion of the fetlock joint alone can be

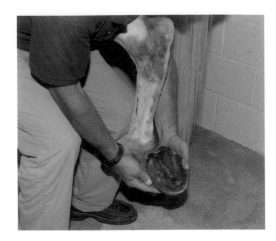

Figure 1.53 Hand and limb positioning to perform distal limb flexion (phalangeal and fetlock joints) of the hindlimb.

performed by placing one hand on the dorsal MC and pulling up on the pastern with the opposite hand (Figure 1.19).
- All three joints are usually flexed together (distal limb flexion) by pulling up on the toe and phalanges with both hands while facing toward the back of the horse (Figure 1.53).
- Fetlock and distal limb flexion tests are usually performed for 30 seconds, after which the horse is trotted off and changes from the baseline lameness are observed (Video 1.5).
- A marked asymmetry in responses to distal limb flexion tests is an important clinical finding, and further indicates a potential problem in the positive distal limb.
- False-positive responses to fetlock flexion are not uncommon especially in horses in work and if excessive force is applied.

Carpal Flexion
- The carpal flexion test is very useful to help isolate a problem to the carpus.
- A negative response does not rule out a problem in the carpus, but a positive response is highly suggestive of a carpal problem (there are few false-positive responses).

- Carpal flexion is performed by grasping the metacarpus with the outside hand while facing the horse and pulling up on the distal limb (Figure 1.28). The carpus is usually held in this position for 30–60 seconds.

Elbow Flexion

- It is nearly impossible to completely separate the elbow from the shoulder when performing upper limb flexion tests in the forelimb.
- Flexion of the elbow (usually 30–60 seconds) can be performed by lifting the antebrachium (forearm) so that it is parallel to the ground and not pulled forward (Figure 1.31). This flexes the elbow and causes the carpus and distal limb to "hang" freely.
- Elbow flexion is not always part of a routine lameness evaluation; it should be performed when an abnormality in the elbow region is found on physical examination.

Shoulder/Upper Forelimb Flexion

- Manipulation of the upper forelimb can be performed either by pulling the limb cranially and upward or by pulling the limb caudally (Video 1.5).
- The cranial approach is performed by standing in front of the limb, grasping the distal limb, and lifting the limb up and forward (Figure 1.54). This will exacerbate lameness problems in the caudal aspect of the elbow and cranial aspect of the shoulder. The more the limb is elevated, the more pressure that is applied to the cranial aspect of the shoulder.
- The caudal approach to flex the shoulder joint is performed by placing one hand on the olecranon process and pulling the limb caudally. Alternatively, the cranial antebrachium may be grasped and pulled caudally together with the distal limb instead of applying pressure to the olecranon (Figure 1.55).

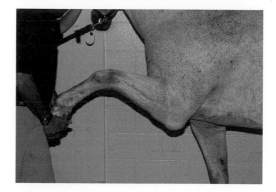

Figure 1.54 Upper limb flexion test in which the limb is pulled cranially and upward to "stress" the shoulder region.

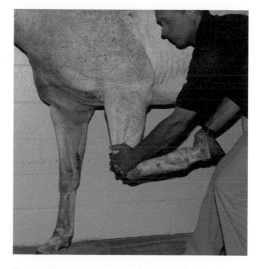

Figure 1.55 Flexion of the upper forelimb can be performed by grasping the antebrachium and foot and pulling the limb caudally.

Tarsal/Hock Flexion

- The tarsal flexion test or spavin test is somewhat of a misnomer because it flexes the fetlock, stifle, and hip in addition to the tarsus (Video 1.6).
- Tarsal flexion is performed by placing the outside hand (when facing the rear of the horse) on the plantar surface of the distal third of the metatarsus and elevating the limb to flex the hock (Figure 1.56). The opposite hand is then

placed around the metatarsus and the limb is held with both hands while facing the back of the horse.

- Alternatively, the tip of the toe can be held so the pastern and fetlock joints are extended, and the hock is flexed (Figure 1.57).
- It may be beneficial in some horses to gradually flex the tarsus to its fullest extent over a 15-second period to avoid resentment.
- Once the tarsus is in full flexion, it is held in this position for 30–60 seconds, the limb is then released gradually, and the horse is trotted off.
- An increase in lameness in the flexed limb should nearly always be compared with the opposite limb since an asymmetrical response often is an important clinical finding.

Stifle Flexion

- The stifle flexion test is used in an attempt to separate stifle pain from tarsal pain in horses that respond to a tarsal flexion test.
- Stifle flexion test is performed by grasping the distal tibia and pulling the limb backward and upward until maximum stifle flexion is achieved (Figure 1.58). It is best to face the back of the horse with the limb in front of the examiner when performing this test (Video 1.6).

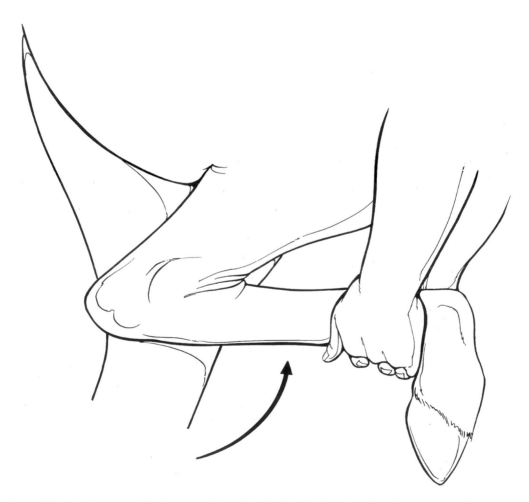

Figure 1.56 Hock or tarsal flexion (spavin) test. The hindlimb is flexed so that the metatarsus is approximately parallel to the ground. This test is not specific for the tarsus because it flexes both the stifle and the fetlock to some degree.

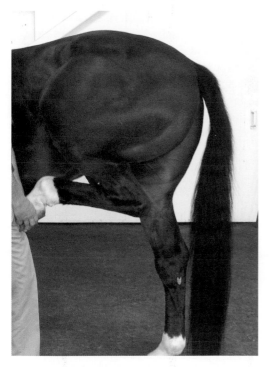

Figure 1.57 Positioning to perform hock or tarsal flexion of the hindlimb, with the limb held by the hoof.

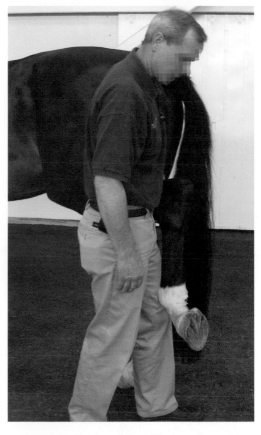

Figure 1.58 Flexion of the stifle is performed by pulling the hindlimb caudally and lifting up on the distal tibia.

- It is thought to flex the hock less and the flex the stifle more than the tarsal flexion, making it more specific for stifle problems, although this is debatable.
- A positive tarsal flexion together with a more positive stifle flexion may suggest that the lameness is due to a stifle problem and vice versa.

Full Limb Forelimb and Hindlimb Flexion

- Full limb forelimb and hindlimb flexion tests can be used as a quick screening test to determine if more isolated flexion tests may be necessary (Videos 1.5 and 1.6).
- Full limb forelimb flexion is performed by grasping the foot and lifting the leg to flex the fetlock, carpus, and elbow. The opposite hand is placed on the metacarpus and the limb elevated and pulled forward to extend the shoulder.

- Full limb hindlimb flexion is performed by grasping the foot and flexing the fetlock, hock, and stifle simultaneously. The hindlimb is pulled out behind the horse to help flex the stifle (Figure 1.59).
- A negative response is thought to suggest that individual flexion responses will also be negative, but this has not been determined definitively for either limb.

Navicular Wedge Test/Distal limb Manipulation

- A navicular wedge test is performed to increase the forces within the palmar aspect of the foot in horses with suspected heel pain. This is usually performed by elevating the toe in relation to the heel by placing a

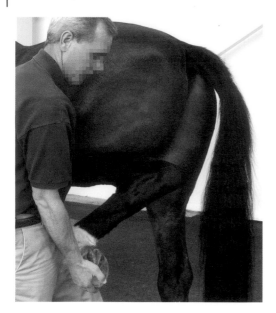

Figure 1.59 Positioning to perform a full limb flexion of the hindlimb.

wooden wedge under the toe (Figure 1.60a). Elevation of the heel may also be performed to assess the structures in the dorsal aspect of the foot (Figure 1.60b).

- The opposite limb is usually held for 30–60 seconds and the change in lameness is detected on the weight-bearing limb.
- The wedge also may be applied to the medial or lateral aspect of the foot to manipulate the soft tissues of the digit (Figure 1.60c and 1.60d).
- Although these tests are often used in horses with suspected navicular syndrome, they are likely not capable of differentiating navicular region pain from other causes of palmar heel pain.

Direct or Local Pressure Plus Movement

- The premise for applying direct pressure to a specific site and watching the horse trot is to confirm the significance of palpation findings. Increasing the baseline lameness by deep palpation of a suspicious area or anatomic structure will often confirm the potential of a problem in the area.

- The limb is usually elevated, direct digital pressure is applied to the site for 15–30 seconds, and the horse is trotted off. The direct pressure test is most commonly performed over swellings of the splint bones, dorsal metacarpus, flexor tendons, suspensory body and branches, and medial aspect of the tarsus.
- A significant exacerbation of the lameness is considered to be a positive response although this can be very subjective.

Subjective Assessment of Lameness

Overview

- Most lameness in horses is caused by pain during weight-bearing, with shifting of load away from the source limb onto the other three, non- or less afflicted, limbs. The result is a decrease in peak vertical ground reaction force on the affected limb.
- Observation of an asymmetrical gait during movement due to the decrease in vertical load on the limb(s) is the main method to detect clinical signs of lameness.
- Observation of how the midline (head and torso) moves is more sensitive and specific for weight-bearing lameness detection than evaluation of limb movements. Exceptions to this generalization include dorsiflexion of the fetlock during weight-bearing and amplitude of hindlimb protraction.
- Horses without pain, neurologic abnormality, or weakness in the limbs or torso usually move symmetrically and are not lame.
- In general, horses with bilateral lameness and those with axial skeletal disease will display less asymmetry of movement than horses with unilateral lameness.
- Some abnormalities may cause pain primarily in the swing (non-weight-bearing) phase of the stride, but there is objective evidence that these conditions also alter the ground reaction forces in the stance phase of the

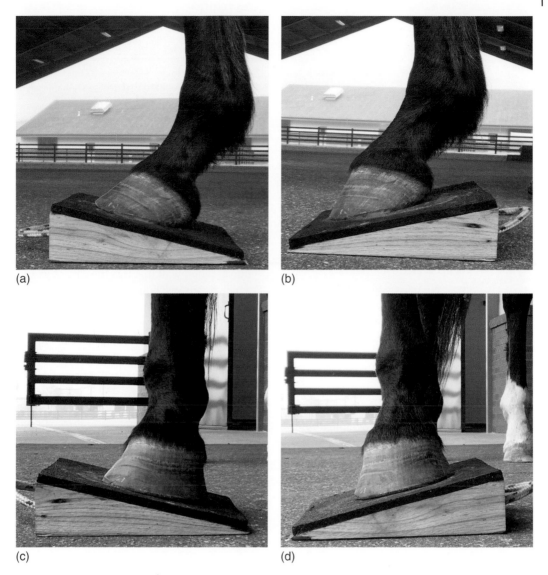

Figure 1.60 A (10″ × 10″) 15° wooden wedge block with a nonslip surface can be used for distal limb manipulation during lameness evaluation. The foot is typically placed in four different orientations: toe wedge (a), heel wedge (b), lateral wedge (c), and medial wedge (d). Depending on the orientation of the block, different tissues within the hoof are placed under compression or tension. *Source:* Courtesy of Randy Eggleston.

stride. Therefore, true swinging limb lameness conditions are uncommon and may be related to conformational differences.

Subjective Scoring Methods

- There are primarily two scoring methods that can be used to subjectively describe

lameness in horses – the AAEP lameness scale (Table 1.2) and the United Kingdom lameness scale (Table 1.3). The scoring systems are very similar except the United Kingdom scale splits each grade of the AAEP scale into two separate categories.

- These lameness scales are viewed as relatively accurate yet imprecise methods to

Table 1.2 American Association of Equine Practitioners Lameness Scale.

Grade	Description
0	Lameness not perceptible under any circumstances.
1	Lameness is difficult to observe and is not consistently apparent, regardless of circumstances (e.g. under saddle, circling, inclines, hard surface).
2	Lameness is difficult to observe at a walk or when trotting in a straight line but consistently apparent under certain circumstances (e.g. weight-carrying, circling, inclines, hard surface).
3	Lameness is consistently observable at a trot under all circumstances.
4	Lameness is obvious at a walk.
5	Lameness produces minimal weight-bearing in motion and/or at rest or a complete inability to move.

Table 1.3 United Kingdom Lameness Scale.

Grade	Description
0	Not lame
1–2	Lameness hard to detect at walk or trot
3–4	Lameness barely detectable at walk, easy to see at the trot
5–6	Lameness easily detectable at the walk
7–8	Hobbling at the walk, unwilling to trot
9–10	Non-weight-bearing

assess the severity of lameness since the lameness amplitude can change significantly within a single grade.

- The consistency and severity of lameness are also assessed under different conditions (walk, trot, circling, etc.).
- The lameness scales are primarily used as communication tools that estimate the overall lameness severity and consistency.

Evaluation of Lameness at the Walk

- Because limb and torso movements are slower when walking, it is the easiest gait in which to observe lameness provided that the lameness is severe enough to reach the minimum threshold for pain.
- Many/most lameness conditions will require movement at speed (increased ground reaction forces) to cause an asymmetrical gait to become visible.
- Vertical head movement is the best method to detect a forelimb lameness if it exists at the walk, although other forelimb lameness characteristics may also be evident (Box 1.1).
- Using vertical pelvic movement (VPM) to detect a hindlimb lameness at the walk is

---

Box 1.1 Observations that may be used to detect lameness in the forelimb.

1) Vertical head movement – highest vertical head position occurs at the beginning of stance of lame limb and the lowest head position occurs at stance of sound or less lame limb.
2) Reduced dorsiflexion of fetlock during weight-bearing – lack of fetlock "drop."
3) Reduced stride length or limb protraction (primarily with bilateral forelimb lameness).
4) Vertical movement of the withers – less sensitive than vertical head movement.

5) Front to back rocking of torso in an attempt to unweight the forelimbs (primarily with bilateral forelimb lameness).
6) Tensing of the shoulder musculature: shoulder of lame limb fixes or "props" just before it hits the ground.
7) Asymmetrical joint flexion angles and/or limb movement (i.e. reduced carpal flexion, paddling, winging, etc.).
8) Abnormal limb posture (i.e. "pointing" of limb).

problematic and alterations in hindlimb movement like decreased hindlimb protraction, lack of fetlock dorsiflexion, or abnormal limb posture are usually more obvious than asymmetry of VPM (Box 1.2).

- Lameness conditions that can usually be recognized and diagnosed almost solely by evaluation of the gait at the walk include:
  1) Fibrotic myopathy
  2) Stringhalt
  3) Upward fixation of the patella
  4) Gastrocnemius muscle injury
  5) Peroneus tertius rupture
  6) Shivers

Evaluation of Lameness at the Trot

- Detection of lameness in quadrupeds is easiest during the symmetrical gaits, like the trot. A normal expected symmetry provides a standard against which amplitudes of asymmetry between right and left halves of a stride can be compared within the individual horse.
- Decreased loading and weight shifting off a painful limb is more easily accomplished in the symmetrically moving horse and helps explain why lameness is not only easiest but also more accurately and more precisely evaluated using symmetric gaits such as the trot compared with the canter or gallop.

- Speed of movement at the trot has been shown to affect the amplitude of lameness but when using subjective evaluation, it appears that lameness is greater at slower trotting speeds because it is easier to see.
- There is an optimum speed of movement when lameness amplitude is greatest and stride-by-stride variation is least and finding this optimal speed is usually achieved by allowing the horse to move naturally.
- To prevent changes in the amplitude of lameness due to speed of movement, one should attempt to keep speed of movement the same throughout the lameness evaluation, especially after manipulations and blocking.
- The most sensitive body-movement indicators of lameness in quadrupeds are the vertical movement of the head for forelimb lameness and vertical movement of the entire pelvis for hindlimb lameness.
- Limb movement parameters are useful in some cases but are generally too variable and inconsistent to be considered more sensitive and specific indicators of lameness than vertical movement of the head and pelvis (Boxes 1.1 and 1.2).

Box 1.2   Observations that may be used to detect lameness in the hindlimb.

1) Vertical pelvic movement (VPM) – upward movement of entire pelvis during stance phase of lame limb; can be impact or pushoff-type hindlimb lameness.
2) Pelvic rotation method (PRM) – detecting asymmetric pelvic movement by observing vertical movement of the tuber coxae (often referred to as "hip hike" of "hip dip").
3) Reduced dorsiflexion of fetlock during weight-bearing – lack of fetlock "drop."
4) Reduced hindlimb protraction (stride length) as viewed from the side.
5) Drifting or leaning away from lame limb during movement.
6) Asymmetrical joint flexion angles and/or limb movement (i.e. reduced tarsal flexion, toe dragging, plaiting, etc.).
7) Abnormal limb posture (i.e. toe-out, tarsus-in posture for upper hindlimb lameness problems).
8) Exaggerated downward movement of the head and neck on stance phase of lame hindlimb; often accompanied by obvious VPM and usually only seen with severe lameness.

Use of Vertical Movement of the Head for Forelimb Lameness

- Symmetrical up and down movement of the head occurs with every stride and there should be no difference in the lowest positions of the head during stance or in the highest positions of the head before and after stance.
- The horse will always try to move the head upward during pain with maximum effect at the moment of peak pain causing an asymmetrical vertical head movement.
- The overall head trajectory or movement is the summation of the normal head movement associated with the stride combined with the exaggerated head movement intended to reduce the ground reaction forces and pain (Figure 1.61).
- With both impact and pushoff types of lameness, the amplitude of forelimb lameness is reflected in a combination of the difference in low and high heights of the head. The classic description of "head nod" as only "down on sound" or only as "up on bad" neglects consideration of differences in both the minimum and maximum head positions and will therefore underestimate the true amplitude of forelimb lameness.
- Random causes of vertical head movement (shaking or jerking head by misbehaving horses) must somehow be extracted and ignored by the examiner when detecting forelimb lameness.

Use of Withers Movement for Forelimb Lameness

- Vertical movement of the withers may also be used to detect and measure the amplitude of forelimb lameness, and there is evidence that the character of withers vertical movement may help to differentiate compensatory from primary lameness in the multiple limb lameness situation.
- When asymmetry of withers movement is in the same sign (same limb) with asymmetry of head movement, a primary forelimb lameness should be suspected.
- In general, asymmetric withers movement is less sensitive than asymmetric head movement at detecting amplitude of forelimb lameness.

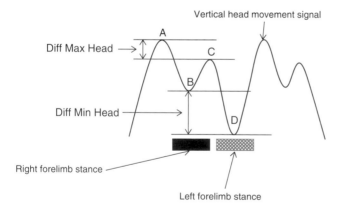

Figure 1.61 Overall vertical head trajectory pattern for horse with impact-type right forelimb lameness or lameness with pain greatest in the first half of, in this case, right forelimb stance. Peak (highest maximum) head vertical position occurs near beginning of stance of the lame or more lame forelimb. Diff Max Head or first maximum head height (A: near beginning of stance of the right forelimb) minus second maximum head height (C: near beginning of stance of the left forelimb) is a positive value. Lowest head position occurs during stance of the not or less lame forelimb. Diff Min Head or first minimum head height (B: during stance of the right forelimb) minus second minimum head height (D: during stance of the left forelimb) is a positive value. Diff Max Head and Diff Min Head are the same sign. For right forelimb lameness, both Diff Max Head and Diff Min Head are positive.

Use of Vertical Pelvic Movement (VPM) for Hindlimb Lameness

- Movement of the posterior half of the horse's torso can be modeled as a simple single free body (pelvis) moving down and up in response to resultant and applied ground reaction forces. However, the amplitude of vertical movement of the pelvis is smaller and more difficult to see than movement of the head in the forelimb.
- The most direct observational sign of hindlimb lameness is asymmetric vertical movement of the entire posterior end (pelvis) of the horse.
- To decrease force on the hindlimbs, the pelvis either falls less (like dropping a ball from a lower height), if the pain is greatest in the first half of stance (impact-type lameness), or rises less, from decreased hindlimb vertical propulsion, if pain is greatest during the second half of stance (pushoff-type lameness).
- Hindlimb lameness can be both impact and pushoff, which becomes more common as hindlimb lameness increases in severity.
- Decreased pelvic fall during hindlimb lameness is accomplished by complex muscular activity in the proximal hindlimb, by shifting weight to the contralateral forelimb, and by "hip hiking" as the horse attempts to use the lame-side hemipelvis in a similar (but not so successful) manner as it uses the head in forelimb lameness, elevating the lame-side hemipelvis immediately before weight-bearing.
- Decreased pelvic rise during pushoff-type hindlimb lameness is primarily caused by reduced extensor muscle activity, resulting in decreased propulsion of the body mass upward and forward. This increase limb flexion during swing creates the "hip dip" that occurs after stance of the lame-side hindlimb.
- The VPM method is very versatile because it can be observed equally well from the side as well as behind the horse. An easily visible marker fixed to the most dorsal aspect of the pelvis between the tuber sacrale may aid detection of the asymmetric movement.

Use of Pelvic Rotation Method (PRM) for Hindlimb Lameness

- An alternative to the VPM method to detect hindlimb lameness, some clinicians assess the amount of "hip hike" and "hip dip," which are manifestations of asymmetric pelvic rotation and are actually due to movements of the tuber coxae and not the hip itself.
- With most hindlimb lameness, total vertical movement of the tuber coxae is greatest on the lame or more lame side. This is thought to be due to both a "hip dip" (a low position of the tuber coxae) right after pushoff of the lame hindlimb and a "hip hike" (a high position of the tuber coxae) right before impact of the lame limb.
- A "hip hike" occurs in an attempt to prevent or dampen pelvic fall before lame hindlimb impact. As such, the "hip hike" signifies an impact-type hindlimb lameness and "hip dip" signifies a pushoff hindlimb lameness.
- "Hip hike" has also been defined as the total movement upward of the tuber coxae on the lame side instead of the relative differences in tuber coxae height from the ground between right and left stances. This definition does not account for the type of hindlimb lameness (impact or pushoff).
- Most practitioners today use the PRM in some form for detection and evaluation of hindlimb lameness. The best position for the evaluator to use the PRM is behind the horse with the horse moving away from the evaluator.
- Many clinicians likely use a combination of the VPM and the PRM to help detect hindlimb lameness without actually realizing the differences. Figure 1.62 compares and contrasts the observations for hindlimb lameness using the VPM and PRM.

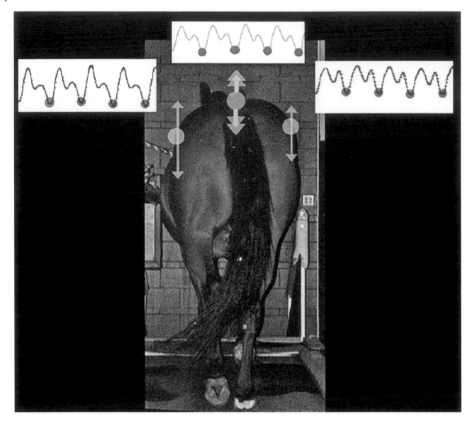

Figure 1.62 Two methods of hindlimb lameness detection and evaluation. Vertical pelvic movement method evaluates imaginary "ball" on midline of pelvis between the tuber sacrale. Pelvic rotation method evaluates imaginary "balls" located at left and right tuber coxae. Vertical pelvic movement method relies on temporal asymmetry of movement of entire pelvis, with less downward movement of the pelvis (pelvis stops downward movement at higher height) during stance phase of lame limb and/or less upward movement of the pelvis (pelvis stops upward movement at lower height) after pushoff of the lame limb, depending on whether the lameness is impact or pushoff or both. Top curve (green) indicates dorsal pelvic movement through four strides of horse with left hindlimb lameness with black circle at time of sound (right) hindlimb stance (synchronous with picture). Pelvic rotation method relies on greater total vertical movement of the tuber coxae on the lame hindlimb side. Curve on left (black) indicates left tuber coxae vertical movement through four strides in horse with left hindlimb lameness with black circles at time of sound (right) hindlimb stance (synchronous with picture). Curve on right (red) indicates right tuber coxae vertical movement through four strides in horse with left hindlimb lameness with black circles at time of sound (right) hindlimb stance (synchronous with picture).

Observing Movement of the Limbs

- Many motion parameters have been measured and studied as lameness indicators in horses, and there are many limb movement parameters that have been associated with lameness.
- Kinematic studies have measured different limb motion parameters, but few have been found to be significantly associated with lameness, and there is contradiction between studies as to which motion parameters are sensitive indicators of lameness in horses.
- Despite these qualifications, there are some limb movement parameters that can be used as indicators of lameness in horses.
- Due to high variability and low consistency, observing limb movement changes is less critical for detecting and evaluating lameness in most cases.

- Other subjective observations that are thought to indicate lameness in the horse include the amount of head flexion when ridden, overall straightness of movement, sequence and timing of foot fall cadence, being "on the bit," amount of "engagement" of the hindlimbs, "ease" of transition from one gait to another, overall willingness to move, and many others. These observations are often utilized in horses with subtle lameness where vertical movement of the head and pelvis and other abnormalities cannot be detected.

Joint Angle Measurements Associated with Lameness

- Decreased weight-bearing due to lameness in the forelimbs or hindlimbs will decrease maximum fetlock extension and maximum coffin joint flexion during the stance phase of the lame limb compared with the stance phase of the contralateral sound limb (Figure 1.63).
- Maximum fetlock extension and coffin joint flexion during stance are sensitive indicators of both forelimb and hindlimb lameness in the horse.
- If fetlock joint angle could be detected sensitively and accurately, it would be an excellent visual clue for the detection and evaluation of both forelimb and hindlimb lameness. Fetlock extension during lame limb stance was 8° less than sound limb stance in a sole pressure-induced lameness model of a grade 2 (out of 5) lameness.
- Other joint angles appear to be less sensitive to reduced weight-bearing, and for the most part not helpful in detecting lameness.

Stride Timing and Length Variables Associated with Lameness

- Stride timing variables (stance duration, swing duration, etc.) are relatively insensitive and inconsistent indicators of lameness.
- Stride timing variables are strongly dependent on the speed of forward movement and training, which makes them less useful for detecting lameness before and after blocking or treatment.
- Stride length is usually shortened significantly only in moderate-to-severe lameness.
- Height of foot flight arc may be increased or decreased in the lame forelimb compared with the sound forelimb, and the shape may be different, depending on the cause of lameness.
- Dragging the hindlimb toe is commonly thought to be a sign of subtle hindlimb lameness, but this may not always be true. In the hindlimb, the height of hoof flight arc is determined by the competing factors of decreased torso rise from reduced propulsion during pushoff and the resultant increased limb flexion that occurs.
- Although the amount of limb abduction or adduction during the swing phase of the limb has been thought to be indicative of certain lameness conditions, this has not been objectively studied.

Hoof Trajectory Associated with Lameness

- The length and shape of forelimb and hindlimb hoof trajectory during the swing phase of the stride are commonly perceived to be associated with lameness even though

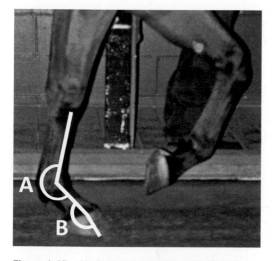

Figure 1.63 (A) Fetlock extension and (B) coffin flexion angles during full weight-bearing. With lameness (A) decreases and (B) decreases.

objective measurements of these perceptions have yet to be confirmed.

- Forelimb protraction, the cranial phase of the hoof flight arc, may either decrease or increase with lameness, depending upon the type of lameness.
- One consistent finding as that hindlimb protraction is usually decreased in most cases of hindlimb lameness.
- Unilateral decreased hindlimb protraction is easy to recognize in the lame limb at the walk or trot by visualizing the increased distance between the affected hindlimb at full protraction and the ipsilateral forelimb at full retraction (Figure 1.64).

Evaluation of Lameness at the Lunge

- Evaluation for lameness during the lunge, on either soft or hard ground, is thought to exacerbate lameness that may not be seen when the horse is moving in a straight line.
- Because the torso and limbs are tilted relative to ground surface, the distribution of ground reaction forces both within a single limb and between right and left limbs is altered.

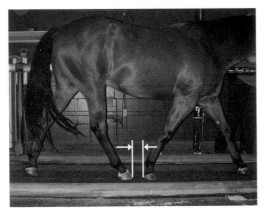

Figure 1.64 Hindlimb protraction is easily seen when viewing from the side of the horse. The hoof of the retracted ipsilateral forelimb acts as a point of reference. Hindlimb protraction is reduced in most hindlimb lameness; thus, the space between the retracted forelimb and protracted hindlimb is greater (arrows) on the lame hindlimb side.

- However, because the torso is tilted relative to the ground, there are normal asymmetrical peak vertical forces between the inside and outside limbs and normal vertical movement of both the head and pelvis. These asymmetries must be appreciated and understood as normal.
- Large horses, small diameter circles, and high speed of movement will exacerbate these asymmetries.
- It has also been determined that the amplitude and characteristics of vertical head and pelvic asymmetries are dependent on the type of ground surface on which the horse is lunged, and because of high normal horse-to-horse variability, an asymmetry observed in one direction should not be identified as abnormal until lunging in the other direction is also observed.
- The increased variability of observing horses at the lunge makes detecting lameness more complicated compared with straight-line evaluation. Disagreement between veterinarians of the existence, side, and amplitude of lameness observed during the lunge is higher than that for evaluation of lameness in the straight line.
- Horses that show consistent lameness during a straight-line trot, will most commonly show lameness in the same limb during the lunge on the same surface and rarely only in the opposite side limb.

Evaluation of Lameness Under Saddle

- Lameness evaluation under saddle should be performed in certain circumstances if practical but it should not be expected that lameness under saddle would always be worse or more visible than lameness without a rider.
- In some environments, for example, in a large arena with an appropriate surface, evaluation for lameness under saddle is easier and often preferred.
- Although the extra weight and back extension may induce more pain, the influence of

the rider and excitement of the horse may serve to mask lameness.

- Rider position and activity can also create artifactual (i.e. "false") lameness that will interfere or confuse veterinary examination for clinical abnormalities.
- Effects of posting and moving in a circle are frequently additive and, depending on the surface characteristics, may either exacerbate or mask existing lameness when the rider posts while riding in small circles.
- As with lunging, if a horse displays lameness consistently without a rider, it will usually display lameness in the same limb with the rider, and it is uncommon for lameness to be displayed in only a different limb.
- Hindlimb and concurrent hindlimb and forelimb lameness has also been shown to be associated with saddle slip, slightly more frequently toward the lame than the non-lame or less lame side. Saddle slip increased when lame horses were ridden in circles and when the rider was posting.

Objective Assessment of Lameness

Overview

- The standard of practice to detect and assess severity of lameness in horses is observing the horse in motion with the naked eye and then scoring using a discrete scale, for example, the AAEP or UK lameness scales/grades.
- Clinical studies suggest that detection and evaluation of mild lameness in horses using the naked eye is insufficient in many cases. Multiple limb involvement and compensatory movement in the opposite half of the body, and observation of different movement parameters, contribute to variability in assessment.
- Limited temporal resolution of the human eye to detect fast events and small amounts of asymmetry in the movement of the horse predisposes to lack of agreement in

lameness detection. In addition, unblinded subjective assessment is predisposed to bias.

- Objective assessments of lameness by precise and accurate measurement of ground reaction forces (kinetics) or asymmetry of movement at high sampling rates (kinematics) can help mitigate the limitations of visual lameness assessment.

Kinetics – Measurement of Ground Reaction forces

- In most lameness situations, the horse will bear less weight on an affected limb to decrease pain, resulting in decreased ground reaction forces, which can be objectively measured.
- The stationary force plate, force-measuring treadmill, and force-measuring devices are attached to the bottom of the hoof, and pressure-sensitive mats have been used to measure ground reaction forces in moving horses.
- The stationary force plate is the most commonly used method for kinetic studies (Figure 1.65). Ground reaction forces can be measured in all three directions—vertical, horizontal, and transverse (Figure 1.66).
- Decreased vertical ground reaction force and, to some extent, altered horizontal

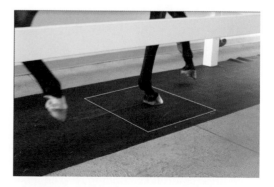

Figure 1.65 Stationary force plate set for evaluation of lameness in horses. White line outlines approximate area of top of force plate, which is embedded into the ground and covered with a rubber mat to prevent shying. *Source:* Courtesy of Dr. Michael Schoonover.

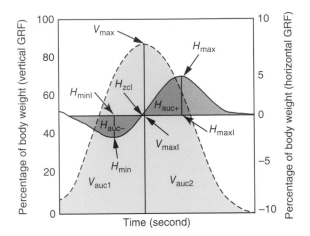

Figure 1.66 Stationary force plate data (from a single hoof strike) of relevance for determination of lameness. V_{max} = peak vertical ground reaction force. V_{auc1} = vertical impulse (force × time) in first half of stance. V_{auc2} = vertical impulse (force × time) in second half of stance. H_{min} = peak negative (deceleratory) horizontal ground reaction force in first half of stance H_{max} = peak positive (acceleratory) horizontal ground reaction force in second half of stance. H_{auc-} = deceleratory horizontal impulse. H_{auc+} = acceleratory horizontal impulse. V_{maxl} = time index of V_{max}. H_{minl} = time index of H_{min}. H_{maxl} = time index of H_{max}. H_{zcl} = time index of horizontal ground reaction force cross over from deceleratory to acceleratory force. No transverse forces are shown.

ground reaction forces are most often associated with lameness in the horse. Lower peak forces and impulse (area under the force vs. time curve) are associated with increasing severity of lameness.

- The shape of the vertical and horizontal ground reaction force curves contains information relevant to determining timing of lameness and differentiating whether pain is maximum during limb impact, in the first half of stance or during pushoff, in the second half of stance.

- The stationary force plate is a precise and accurate instrument with low variability between trials and sensitivity high enough to detect subclinical lameness.

- The stationary force plate is considered to be the gold standard for objective lameness evaluation in horses, but acquiring data requires controlled conditions. The hoof must strike completely within a relatively small area and speed of movement must be controlled, both to increase the chance of successful hoof strike and to decrease variability between hoof strikes (Figure 1.65).

- The force plate is not used clinically that often because of the controlled conditions that are required to obtain consistent data, logistics of its use, and the associated cost.

Kinematics – Measurement of Movement

- If pain predominates in one side of the body, the normal symmetric movement between right and left parts of the stride will become asymmetric. Kinematics is used to quantify absolute movement measures that may correlate well with lameness.

- Many different motion parameters have been studied and used to detect and evaluate forelimb and hindlimb lameness in horses, including vertical movement of the torso (head bob, pelvic fall, and rise), stride and step length and timing, pelvic rotation (hip hike and dip), limb and hoof flight pattern, and joint angle extremes and range of motion.

- Asymmetric vertical movement of the torso (head and pelvis), because it is more directly associated with vertical ground reaction force, is the most sensitive kinematic indicator of lameness.

- Body motion changes of lameness are more variable stride by stride than changes in ground reaction forces, increasing the variability of kinematic assessment. This variability can be decreased by strictly controlling conditions of evaluation and by collecting data from a high number of contiguous strides.

- Despite the higher variability compared with the force plate, results of kinematic evaluation of lameness are generally more intuitive and easier to understand for most veterinary practitioners.

- The original kinematic technique was camera based with the horse filmed while moving on a treadmill and body motion quantified by analyzing trajectories of markers attached to the body of the horse.

- Newer kinematic systems with automatic calibration and tracking of markers and user-friendly software to collect and display results greatly simplify use of this technique, but the requirement for dedicated space and multiple cameras to collect multiple strides with adequate spatial resolution limits this practice to research centers and technologically advanced clinics.

- Asymmetry of motion can be more readily measured using inertial sensors attached to the horse's body with sensor data wirelessly transmitted to the evaluator.

- Wireless transmission of body-mounted inertial sensor data allows clinicians to objectively evaluate lameness in horses in a natural clinical environment and is more intuitive and practical than other methods.

- The Q® (hardware) and Lameness Locator® (software) is one such body-mounted inertial sensor data system that was specifically designed to aid veterinarians in the detection and evaluation of lameness in horses.

The Q® and Lameness Locator®

- The Q consists of three inertial sensors: a tablet PC for data collection, analysis, and archiving; a sensor battery charger; and accessories for attaching the sensors to the horse's body (Figure 1.67).

- The inertial sensors are attached to the head, right forelimb pastern, and dorsum of the pelvis between the tuber sacrale. Each sensor is 1.5 inches by 1.25 inches by 0.75 inches and weighs 28 g.

- Vertical accelerations of the head and pelvis and angular velocity of the right distal forelimb are measured and wirelessly transmitted (Bluetooth Class 1) in real time to a handheld tablet computer.

- Sensor data (acceleration) is algorithmically converted to vertical position relative to the ground, which is the data of interest to the evaluator. Additional custom-designed algorithms are used to detect and quantify forelimb and hindlimb lameness when the horse is moving in a symmetrical gait, which is usually the trot.

- An additional sensor can be attached to the lower waist of the rider to evaluate rider activity, to determine if the rider is sitting or posting correctly, and to assess how rider activity affects the measurement of lameness.

- Automatic Interpretation and Degree of Evidence (AIDE) algorithms, developed from studies of induced lameness and from contemporary clinical cases, for straight-line evaluation, lunging, flexions, effect of blocking and treatment, under-saddle evaluation, and compensatory lameness, simplify interpretation of kinematic values related to lameness for the practitioner.

- Lameness is detected and quantified by reporting means and standard deviations of maximum and minimum height differences of the head (for forelimb lameness evaluation) and pelvis (for hindlimb lameness evaluation) positions. Location of lameness to limb (or limbs) and timing of peak lameness within the stride phase of a limb are determined by the association of head and pelvic movement to movement (angular velocity) of the right forelimb.

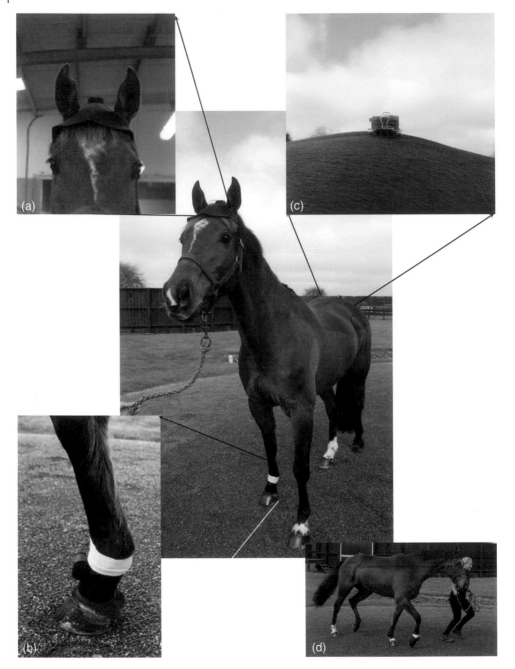

Figure 1.67 The Q™ (hardware) with Lameness Locator® (software) on standing horse. (a) Head accelerometer attached to head bumper. (b) Right forelimb gyroscope attached to dorsal pastern in pouch. (c) Pelvic accelerometer attached with foam pad and rubberized grip device. (d) Instrumented horse in motion.

- Lameness evaluation results are reported in a graphical display that depicts amplitude of impact and propulsion asymmetry in each stride. Compensatory or multiple limb lameness patterns can be determined by studying the distribution of impact and pushoff asymmetry in all four limbs.
- Lameness can be evaluated with the horse trotting in a straight line, while lunging (at the trot), trotting under saddle, and in response to flexion tests and blocking.

Measuring Forelimb Lameness Using the Lameness Locator®

- The forelimb lameness display provides a qualitative description of the forelimb lameness by representing each analyzed stride as a single ray directed outward from the plot origin.
- The length of the ray is representative of the amplitude of asymmetric head motion for that stride. The direction of the ray on the plot represents the side and timing of lameness for that stride.
- Using polar coordinate terminology, rays in quadrant 1 (upper right) represent lameness in the right forelimb during the first half of stance, from impact to midstance; rays in quadrant 2 (upper left) represent lameness in the right forelimb during second half of stance, midstance to pushoff; rays in quadrant 3 (lower left) represent lameness in the left forelimb during the first half of stance; and rays in quadrant 4 (lower right) represent lameness in the left forelimb during the second half of stance.
- Diff Max Head and Diff Min Head are calculated for every stride selected for analysis, and the mean and standard deviation over all strides are reported.
- As an example, the display in Figure 1.68 indicates a right forelimb lameness as the predominance of rays (strides) are pointing toward quadrant 1.

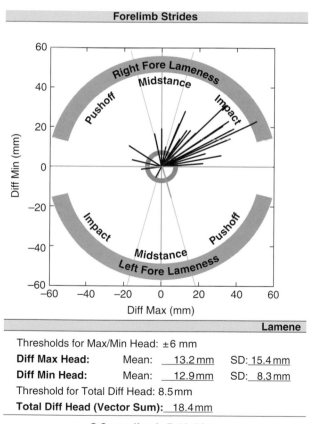

Forelimb Strides

Thresholds for Max/Min Head: ±6 mm
Diff Max Head: Mean: ___13.2 mm___   SD: _15.4 mm_
Diff Min Head: Mean: ___12.9 mm___   SD: _8.3 mm_
Threshold for Total Diff Head: 8.5 mm
Total Diff Head (Vector Sum): _18.4 mm_

Q Score (fore): R 18.4 Imp

Figure 1.68 Output of Lameness Locator® indicating right forelimb impact lameness. Predominance of rays pointing in quadrant 1 (upper right) have Diff Max Head and Diff Min Head > reference range of ±6 mm and Vector Sum or Total Diff Head > 8.5 mm. Standard deviations of Diff Min Head less than mean Diff Min Head indicating consistent right-sided lameness.

Measuring Hindlimb Lameness Using the Lameness Locator®

- Hindlimb lameness is reported in a graphical display that depicts deficiency of right and left hindlimb impact (first half of stance) or pushoff (second half of stance; Figure 1.69). The left side of the display represents qualities of the left hindlimb function. The right side of the display represents qualities of the right hindlimb function.
- Each vertical line on the display moving from left to right is a measure of either the deficiency of impact (pelvic fall) or the deficiency of pushoff (pelvic rise) for that stride.

The length of the line is representative of the amplitude of lameness (Figure 1.69).

- Hindlimb lameness is quantified by calculation of the difference in maximum pelvic position between left and right hindlimb strides (Diff Max Pelvis) and the difference in minimum pelvic position between left and right hindlimb strides (Diff Min Pelvis).
- Diff Max Pelvis and Diff Min Pelvis are calculated for every stride collected, and the mean and standard deviation over all strides are reported. The signs of Diff Max Pelvis and Diff Min Pelvis determine side and timing of lameness.

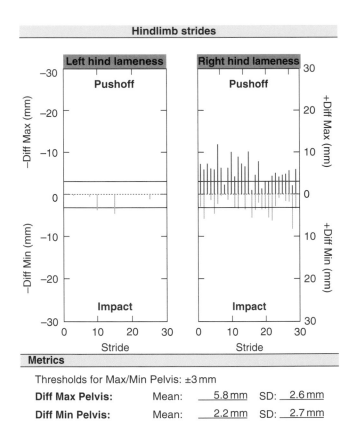

Metrics

Thresholds for Max/Min Pelvis: ±3 mm

Diff Max Pelvis:	Mean: 5.8 mm	SD: 2.6 mm
Diff Min Pelvis:	Mean: 2.2 mm	SD: 2.7 mm

Q Score (hind): R 5.8 Push / R 2.2 Imp

Figure 1.69 Output of Lameness Locator® indicating right hindlimb pushoff lameness. Most red rays (Diff Max Pelvis) are on the right side. This indicates most Diff Max Pelvis are + in sign, i.e. the pelvis is thrust up less after pushoff of right hindlimb compared with left hindlimb. Diff Max Pelvis > reference range of ± 3 mm. Standard deviation of Diff Max Pelvis is less than mean of Diff Max Pelvis, indicating consistent lameness.

- Positive values indicate right hindlimb lameness, and negative values indicate left hindlimb lameness. High Diff Max Pelvis absolute values indicate pushoff-type hindlimb lameness. High Diff Min Pelvis absolute values indicate impact-type hindlimb lameness (Figure 1.69).

Detecting Compensatory Lameness
- In trotting quadrupeds, a primary lameness in the front half of the body will sometimes cause compensatory movements in the back half of the body and vice versa, such that an apparent multiple limb lameness is present.
- Interpretation of these compensatory movements is sometimes referred to as the "law of sides" (Figure 1.70).
- The first principle of the "law of sides" states that an apparent ipsilateral lameness, i.e. forelimb and hindlimb lameness on the same side of the body, is likely a primary hindlimb lameness and a compensatory but false forelimb lameness (Figure 1.70).
- Pain during stance in the hindlimb will cause the horse to shift weight forward onto the simultaneously weight-bearing contralateral forelimb, and the head will fall more than normal. Normal falling of the head during weight-bearing of the opposite forelimb will be less, giving the appearance of an ipsilateral forelimb lameness ("low on sound").
- The second principle of the "law of sides" states that an apparent contralateral lameness, i.e. forelimb and hindlimb lameness on opposite sides of the body, is likely primary forelimb lameness and a compensatory but false hindlimb lameness.
- Primary forelimb lameness causes the horse to shift its center of gravity slightly toward the back half of the body during the stance phase of the affected forelimb potentially mimicking an ipsilateral hindlimb impact-type lameness but contralateral pushoff-type hindlimb lameness (Figure 1.70).
- Compensatory pelvic movement patterns with primary forelimb lameness are not commonly observed subjectively but are regularly measured with the increased sensitivity of the inertial sensors, and these patterns

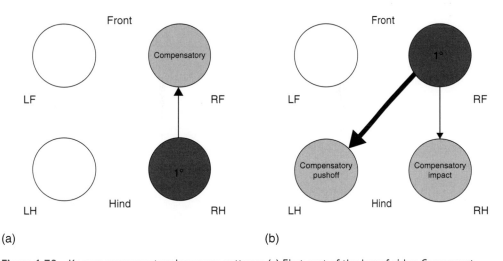

(a)   (b)

Figure 1.70 Known compensatory lameness patterns. (a) First part of the law of sides. Concurrent apparent ipsilateral forelimb and hindlimb lameness is usually a primary hindlimb lameness and an ipsilateral compensatory (false) forelimb lameness. (b) Second part of the law of sides. Concurrent forelimb and either compensatory contralateral hindlimb pushoff or ipsilateral hindlimb impact (or both) lameness. Compensatory contralateral compensatory hindlimb pushoff lameness is more common and usually more prominent.

are useful in evaluating forelimb and multiple limb lameness.

- Experimental studies have determined that the first principle of the law of sides is, for the most part, true but the second principle is less true and less straightforwardly explained.

Perineural Anesthesia

Overview

- Local anesthesia is important to document the region of the lameness and pain so that diagnostic imaging can be used to determine the specific cause of the problem.
- Local anesthesia may be accomplished by perineural infiltration (local nerve block), ring block, direct infiltration of a painful region, or intrasynovial injection (joints, tendon sheaths, and bursae).
- Perineural infiltration and ring blocks are used to localize the source of pain to a specific region and, therefore, should be performed in a systematic manner starting with the distal extremity and progressing proximally (Table 1.4).
- Direct infiltration and intrasynovial anesthesia are used to identify the involvement of a specific structure or synovial cavity and do not necessarily have to be performed in a systematic manner.
- In general, the accuracy of desensitizing a nerve is greater in the distal limb (distal to the carpus and tarsus) than more proximally where the nerves are deeper and covered with soft tissue. Also, the more distal the nerve, the more specific or smaller the region is that is anesthetized.
- Perineural anesthesia should not interpreted as particularly accurate for a number of reasons – local diffusion of the anesthetic, difficulty in interpreting the success of the block, and the presence of aberrant nerves. This should be remembered when interpreting the response to a perineural nerve block.

Types of Anesthetics

- The local anesthetics most frequently used are 2% lidocaine hydrochloride (Xylocaine hydrochloride) and 2% mepivacaine hydrochloride (Carbocaine).
- Mepivacaine is used most frequently because it is thought to last longer and be less irritating than lidocaine. Lidocaine is thought to last only 60 minutes with the maximum effect at 15 minutes and may not resolve lameness despite the loss of skin sensation.
- Mepivacaine's duration of action is variable, being reported to last anywhere from one to six hours with most studies suggesting that the effects of the block begin to subside after two hours.
- Bupivacaine hydrochloride (Marcaine) may be used if the goal is to provide a longer duration of analgesia (four–six hours), such as following surgery but is rarely used for lameness evaluation.

Skin Preparation and Restraint

- The only skin preparation necessary for most sites of perineural anesthesia is scrubbing/wiping the area with gauze soaked in alcohol until clean.
- A more thorough skin preparation is recommended for a few nerve blocks that are adjacent to synovial structures where the needle may inadvertently enter the synovial cavity, or the solution may diffuse into these structures. These exceptions include the low four-point and 6-point blocks, the medial and lateral approaches to the lateral palmar nerve, the high two-point block, the subtarsal block, and the deep branch of the lateral plantar nerve (DBLPN) block (Table 1.4).
- Most perineural blocks of the distal limb can be performed with minimal restraint without the use of stocks.
- The horse should be haltered and restrained by an attendant who is standing on the same side of the horse. Twitch restraint should be used only if necessary.

Table 1.4 Guidelines for perineural local anesthesia.

Specific block	Needle size	Volume of anesthetic	Sterile skin prep recommended (Yes or No)	Location
Palmar/plantar digital (PD)	25 g, 5/8″	1–1.5 mL	No	Just above collateral cartilages
Basisesamoid (high PD)	25 g, 5/8″	1.5–2 mL	No	At the base of the proximal sesamoid bone
Abaxial sesamoid	25 g, 5/8″	1.5–2 mL	No	Abaxial surface of proximal sesamoid bone
Low palmar or 4-point	22–25 g, 5/8–1″	2–3 mL/site	Yes	Distal metacarpus (above buttons of splint bones)
Lateral palmar (lateral approach)	20–22 g 1″	4–6 mL	Yes	Distal to accessory carpal bone
Lateral palmar (medial approach)	25 g, 5/8″ or 22 g 1″	3–4 mL	Yes	Medial aspect of accessory carpal bone
High 2-point	25 g, 5/8″ + 22 g 1″	3–4 mL/site	Yes	Medial aspect of accessory carpal bone and proximal medial metacarpus
Ulnar	20 g 1.5″	10 mL	No	4″ above accessory carpal bone
Median	20–22 g 1.5–2.5″	10 mL	No	Caudal to radius below pectoralis muscle
Medial cutaneous antebrachial	22–25 g 1–1.5″	5–10 mL	No	Mid-radius near cephalic and accessory cephalic veins
Low plantar or 6-point	25 g, 5/8″ or 22 g 1″	2–3 mL/site	Yes	Distal metatarsus and each side of long digital extensor tendon
Deep branch of lateral plantar nerve (DBLPN)	20–22 g 1.0″	3–5 mL	Yes	Lateral aspect of proximal metatarsus
Tibial/peroneal	20–22 g 1.5″	10–20 mL/site	No	4″ above point of hock on lateral and medial aspects of limb

- When using local anesthesia in the hindlimb, the practitioner should always be in a position so that minimal bodily harm will result if rapid movement occurs.
- In general, the least amount of anesthetic possible should be used to reduce tissue irritation and to prevent local diffusion of anesthetic that may complicate the interpretation of the block.

Assessment of Response to Perineural Blocks

- Accurately determining whether the nerve has been completely desensitized by the block is often the first step in interpreting the result.
- Complete desensitization of the nerve is often evaluated by checking the skin sensation distal to the point of injection. This can be performed with a blunt object such as a pen, hemostat, or needle cap.
- These objects should not be jabbed into the skin but applied gently at first with a gradual increase in pressure. Most horses are receptive to this technique and will quietly respond if the nerves are not totally desensitized.
- Some horses are very difficult to read, and skin sensation may persist even with an

effective block making accurate assessment of a block somewhat subjective.

- In general, the more proximal the perineural block, the less accurate skin sensation is to evaluate the success of the block. Skin sensation is typically not reliable with blocks above the fetlock.

- Other manipulative tests that previously caused pain (such as hoof tester examination, deep palpation, and flexion) can be used to help determine if the block worked.

- The ultimate test is whether lameness is no longer present, but for those horses that have not improved, accurate interpretation of complete nerve desensitization is important and multiple approaches may be necessary to make this decision.

Palmar Digital (PD) Block (Figures 1.71 and 1.72)

- The injection is performed with the foot elevated in most cases. Some prefer to stand with their back toward the animal's hind end while holding the hoof between their knees. Others prefer holding the pastern with one hand while injecting with the other, while assuming either a lateral or frontal position in relation to the limb (Video 1.7).

- The PD nerves should be anesthetized just distal to or at the proximal border of the collateral cartilages. If the PD block is performed 2 to 3 cm above the collateral cartilages, the pastern joint can be desensitized in addition to the foot.

- A 25-gauge, 5/8-inch needle is inserted in a proximal to distal direction over the nerve, and local anesthetic (1–1.5 mL) is injected perineurally (Figure 1.72).

- Loss of skin sensation at the coronary band in the heel region and loss of deep sensation between the heel bulbs after 5 to 10 minutes is a reliable indication that the block was successful.

- Structures that are desensitized with a biaxial PD nerve block include the entire sole, the navicular apparatus and soft tissues of the heel, the entire DIP joint of the forelimb, the distal portion of the DDFT, and some of the distal sesamoidean ligaments.

- **Pitfalls:**
  1) Blocking too high in the pastern – desensitize pastern.
  2) Using too much anesthetic—diffusion decreases specificity.

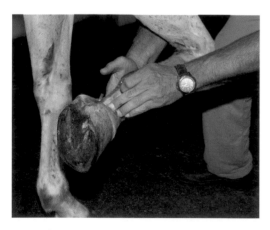

Figure 1.71 This image illustrates the positioning to perform a PD nerve block when facing the back of the horse and holding the limb with one hand. The needle is directed toward the hoof and is inserted at or below the level of the collateral cartilages.

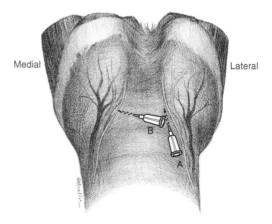

Medial   Lateral

Figure 1.72 Injection sites for a PD nerve block. In (A), the needle is inserted parallel to the lateral PD nerve, while in (B), the needle enters just off midline and is inserted in the subcutaneous tissues to approximate the medial PD nerve.

3) Assuming that the PD block only desensitizes the palmar aspect of the foot.

Basisesamoid or High PD Block (Figures 1.73 and 1.74)

- This block is performed similarly to the PD block, except it is more proximal on the limb at the base of the proximal sesamoid bones (why it is referred to as a high PD block).
- The PD nerves are digitally palpated at this location and 1.5 to 2 mL of anesthetic is deposited directly over the nerves (Video 1.8).
- Because the block is performed at the base of the sesamoid bones, it is unlikely to desensitize any of the fetlock joint but will desensitize the dorsal branch of the PD nerve.
- This block will desensitize the palmar/plantar soft tissue structures of the pastern, the PIP joint, and all structures of the foot.
- **Pitfalls:**
  1) Using too much anesthetic—proximal diffusion decreases specificity.

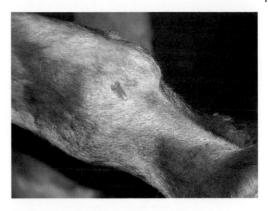

Figure 1.74 Location of needle insertion to perform a high PD nerve block in the forelimb. This block is best performed with the limb held.

2) Difficulty in palpating the PD nerves at base of sesamoids—they are not as superficial in this location compared with more distally.

Abaxial Sesamoid Block (Figure 1.75)

- The neurovascular bundle is easily palpable along the abaxial surface of the proximal sesamoid bone.
- With the limb elevated and holding the fetlock in the palm of the hand, isolate the palmar nerve by rolling it away from the artery and vein with the thumb or forefinger.
- A 5/8-inch (1.5-cm), 25-gauge needle is used to inject 1.5–2 mL of anesthetic perineurally in a proximal to distal direction (Figure 1.75a; Video 1.9).
- Alternatively, the block can be performed with the horse standing (Figure 1.75b; Video 1.10).
- It is best to use a small volume of anesthetic and direct the needle distally to avoid partial desensitization of the fetlock joint.
- The biaxial block desensitizes the foot, middle phalanx, PIP joint, distopalmar aspects of the proximal phalanx, distal portions of the SDFT and DDFT, distal sesamoidean ligaments, and the digital annular ligament.
- Loss of skin sensation at the coronary band in the toe region together with loss of skin sensation on the palmar pastern is used to determine the success of the block.

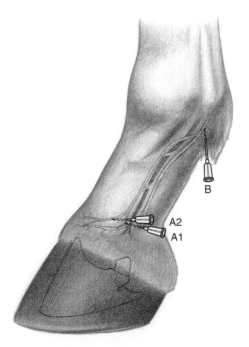

Figure 1.73 Injection sites for local anesthesia. A1 and A2. Sites for the pastern ring block. B. Site for the digital nerve block at the base of the sesamoid bones (basisesamoid block).

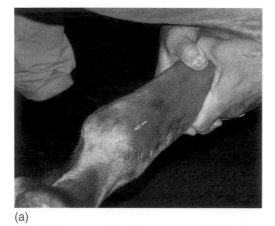

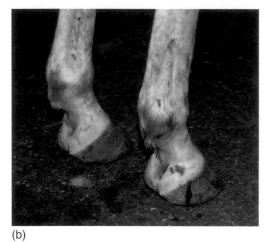

(a)

(b)

Figure 1.75 Needle location to perform an abaxial sesamoid nerve block in the forelimb with (a) the limb held or (b) in the standing horse.

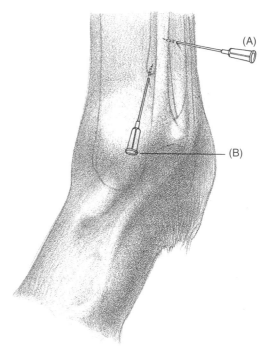

(A)

(B)

Figure 1.76 Low palmar or 4-point block. a. Site for palmar nerve block; it is recommended to go 1 cm proximal to the distal end of the small metacarpal bones. b. Site for palmar metacarpal nerve block at the distal end of the splint bones.

- **Pitfalls:**
  1) Using too much anesthetic—diffusion can desensitize the fetlock joint and/or the sesamoid bones.
  2) May not completely desensitize the skin over the dorsal aspect of the pastern.

Low Palmar or 4-point Block (Figure 1.76)

- The low palmar block is often referred to as the low 4-point block because both palmar and palmar metacarpal nerves are anesthetized at the distal aspect of the MC/MT (Figure 1.76; Video 1.11).
- The lateral and medial palmar nerves lie between the suspensory ligament and the DDFT, and the medial and lateral palmar metacarpal nerves course parallel and axial to the second and fourth metacarpal bones.
- The 4-point block is performed while the horse is bearing full weight or the limb can be held with the opposite hand, although it is usually easier to perform in the standing position.
- The palmar nerves are relatively deep but can be reached in most cases with a 5/8-inch (1.5-cm), 25-gauge needle (a 1-inch, 22-gauge needle may also be used), after which 2 to 3 mL of local anesthetic is deposited.
- It is best to block the palmar nerves 1 cm proximal to the distal ends of the splint bones to avoid injection into the DFTS.
- The palmar metacarpal nerves are blocked in similar manner as they emerge distal to the ends of the second and fourth metacarpal bones. The proximal palmar pouches of the fetlock joint should be avoided.

- Anesthesia of these four nerves effectively desensitizes the deep structures of the fetlock region and all structures distally.
- Anesthesia of the skin over the dorsal aspect of the pastern and fetlock indicates that the block was successful.
- **Pitfalls:**
  1) Inadvertent injection of the fetlock joint or DFTS (Figure 1.77).
  2) Proximal diffusion of anesthetic that may desensitize the body of the suspensory or other more proximal structures.
  3) Difficulty in assessing whether all nerves have been desensitized.

Lateral Palmar Block (Lateral Approach; Figures 1.78 and 1.79)

- At the proximal end of the fourth metacarpus, the lateral palmar nerve gives off its deep branch that detaches branches to the origin of the suspensory ligament and

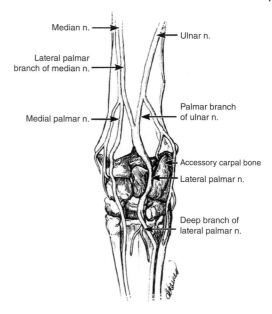

Figure 1.78 Neuroanatomy of the palmar aspect of the carpus illustrating the course of the lateral palmar nerve. The lateral palmar nerve can be anesthetized just below the accessory carpal bone (lateral approach) or axial to the accessory carpal bone in a more proximal location (medial approach). *Source:* Castro FA., Schumacher JS, Pauwels F, et al.: 2005. A New Approach for Perineural Injection of the Lateral Palmar Nerve in the Horse. *Vet Surg* 34(6): 539–542. Reprinted with permission from John Wiley & Sons.

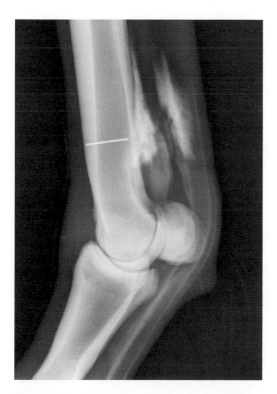

Figure 1.77 Contrast material within the DFTS after a low palmar nerve block.

divides into the lateral and medial palmar metacarpal nerves (Figure 1.78).
- The lateral palmar nerve can be anesthetized just below the accessory carpal bone (lateral approach) or axial to the accessory carpal bone in a more proximal location (medial approach).
- The lateral palmar nerve is anesthetized with 4 to 6 mL of anesthetic administered through a 1-inch (2–3 cm), 20-gauge needle midway between the distal border of the accessory carpal bone and the proximal end of the fourth metacarpal bone on the palmar border of the accessoriometacarpal ligament (Figure 1.79; Video 1.12).
- The needle is directed in a palmarolateral-to-dorsomedial direction and must penetrate the 2- to 3-mm thickness of the flexor retinaculum of the carpus (Video 1.12).

- This block may be performed with the horse standing or with the carpus slightly flexed.
- Skin sensation is not useful to evaluate the effect of the block. Instead, lack of any response to deep palpation of the proximal suspensory ligament often suggests an effective block.
- Performing this block avoids the necessity of direct infiltration of the suspensory ligament or anesthesia of the palmar and palmar metacarpal nerves independently.
- **Pitfalls:**
  1) Injection into the carpal sheath or middle carpal joint.
  2) Difficulty in injecting—needle must penetrate the fascia below accessory carpal bone.
  3) Difficulty in assessing success of the block. Best done by palpating the absence of pain in the suspensory ligament.
  4) More difficult to palpate the anatomy to locate injection site compared with the medial approach.

Lateral Palmar Block (Medial approach; Figures 1.78 and 1.80)

- The lateral palmar nerve may also be blocked medial to the accessory carpal bone, which is thought to reduce the risk of inadvertent injection into the carpal sheath.
- The site of injection is a longitudinal groove in the fascia palpable over the medial aspect of the accessory carpal bone, palmar to the insertion of the flexor retinaculum that forms the palmaromedial aspect of the carpal canal (Figure 1.80).
- With the limb weight-bearing, a 25-gauge, 5/8-inch needle is inserted into the distal third of the groove in a mediolateral direction perpendicular to the limb. The author uses a 22-gauge, 1-inch (2.5 cm) needle and 3–4 mL of anesthetic for this technique (Video 1.13).
- Skin sensation is not useful to evaluate the effect of the block and lack of pain on palpation of the suspensory ligament is often the best indicator of success.

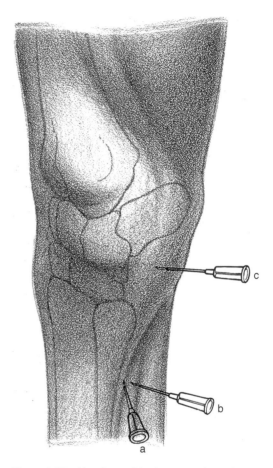

Figure 1.79 Needle positioning to perform the lateral approach to block the lateral palmar nerve below the accessory carpal bone (C). Needles A and B indicate positioning to block the lateral and medial palmar nerves in the proximal metacarpus. The high two-point block is a combination of the lateral palmar block (C) and the high medial palmar block (B).

Pitfalls:
1) Difficulty in injecting—needle in fascia or against the medial aspect of the accessory carpal bone.
2) Difficulty in assessing success of the block. Best done by palpating the absence of pain in the suspensory ligament.
3) Diffusion of anesthetic proximally to the distal third of the antebrachium following the block.

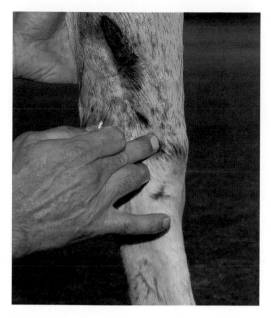

Figure 1.80 The medial approach to desensitize the lateral palmar nerve is located on the axial border of the accessory carpal bone.

High Two-point Block (Figure 1.79)

- The high two-point block is a combination of the lateral palmar block (medial or lateral approach) and the high medial palmar block. The author prefers to use the medial approach to the lateral palmar nerve with this block.
- The lateral palmar blocks have been described previously. The high medial palmar block is performed in the proximal metacarpus just dorsal to the flexor tendons analogous to the low palmar nerve block.
- When performed, all deep and superficial structures on the palmar aspect of the metacarpus distal to the block should be desensitized including the proximal aspects of the second and fourth metacarpal bones and the origin of the suspensory ligament.
- Some clinicians have found it unnecessary to block the medial palmar nerve in conjunction with blocking the lateral palmar nerve.
- **Pitfalls:**
  1) Similar to those for the lateral palmar block.
  2) Difficulty in assessing success of the block. Best done by palpating the absence of pain in the suspensory ligament and metacarpal region.
  3) Blocking the high medial palmar nerve may be an unnecessary step.

Ulnar, Median, and Medial Cutaneous Antebrachial Nerve Blocks (Figure 1.81)

- The entire carpus and distal aspect of the limb can be desensitized by blocking the ulnar and median nerves. The median and ulnar nerve blocks may be used to locate a painful condition in the distal limb and could be used to rule out lameness of the distal limb if lameness in the proximal forelimb was suspected.
- The medial cutaneous antebrachial nerve innervates only the skin and it is primarily used to anesthetize the limb for a surgical procedure.
- The ulnar nerve is anesthetized approximately four inches (10 cm) proximal to the accessory carpal bone on the caudal aspect of the forearm in the groove between the flexor carpi ulnaris and ulnaris lateralis muscles (Figure 1.81C).
- A 20-gauge, 1.5-inch (3.8-cm) needle is inserted through the skin and fascia perpendicular to the limb to a depth of about 0.25 to 0.5 inches (1 to 1.5 cm). The local anesthetic (10 mL) is infused both superficially and deeply in the region.
- The accessory carpal bone and surrounding structures, palmar carpal region, carpal canal, proximal metacarpus, SDFT, and suspensory ligament are partially blocked by this technique. Lame horses with lesions in the very proximal aspect of the SDFT may only improve after an ulnar block.
- The median nerve is anesthetized on the caudomedial aspect of the radius, cranial to the origin of the flexor carpi radialis muscle just below the elbow joint where the ventral edge of the posterior superficial pectoral muscle inserts in the radius (Figure 1.81A).

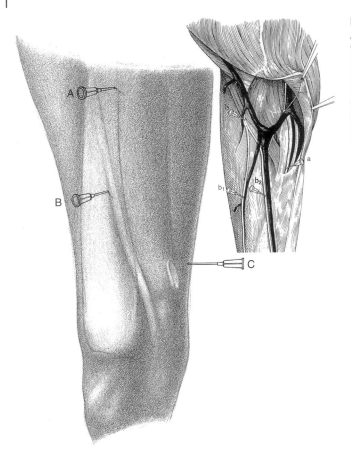

Figure 1.81 Upper forelimb blocks. A. Site for median nerve block. B. Site for medial cutaneous antebrachial nerve block. C. Site for ulnar nerve block. Inset: a. Site for median nerve block. b. Site for medial cutaneous antebrachial nerve block as nerve crosses the lacertus fibrosus, which blocks both the cranial (b1) and the caudal (b2) branches.

- A 2- to 2.5-inch (5- to 6.2-cm), 20-gauge needle is inserted obliquely through the skin and fascia to a depth of 1 to 2 inches (2.5 to 5 cm) staying behind the radius to avoid the median artery and vein which lie caudal to the nerve. Approximately 10 mL of anesthetic is usually injected.
- The two branches of the medial cutaneous antebrachial nerve can be blocked on the medial aspect of the forearm halfway between the elbow and the carpus, just cranial to the accessory cephalic vein (Figure 1.81b). The nerve is usually just below the skin; however, its location can vary. It is best to block the subcutaneous tissues both cranial and caudal to the cephalic vein. A 1-inch, 22-gauge needle is used to deposit 5 mL of anesthetic in both locations.

Pitfalls:

1) Difficulty locating injection sites – inject too proximally or distally on the limb.
2) Injecting the anesthetic too superficially for both ulnar and median nerve blocks.
3) Difficulty in assessing success of the block.
4) Inadvertently hitting the median artery or vein or the cephalic vein.

The Hindlimb

- The neuroanatomy of the distal hindlimb below the tarsus is somewhat similar to that of the forelimb below the carpus. The plantar digital, basisesamoid, abaxial sesamoid, and low plantar nerve blocks are performed in a similar manner to those in the forelimb.
- The plantar digital and basisesamoid blocks are more difficult to perform in the hindlimb because the distal limb flexes

when the limb is held off the ground due to the reciprocal apparatus. These blocks are best performed with the limb extended behind the horse in a position similar to that when performing a fetlock flexion test or applying a horseshoe.

- When dealing with the hindlimb, proper restraint and body positioning are important to prevent bodily harm. In most cases a twitch is used, and the handler should stand on the same side as the veterinarian.
- All blocks should be performed with the veterinarian facing toward the back of the horse and many times it is best to securely hold the limb when performing the block.

Low Plantar Block

- The plantar and plantar metatarsal nerves in the distal metatarsus are blocked in a similar manner to the corresponding nerves in the distal metacarpus.
- The nerves are usually blocked using a 1 inch, 22-gauge needle with the limb weight-bearing and the horse properly restrained. Holding the limb while performing this block in the hindlimb is usually more difficult.
- One difference in the neuroanatomy in the hind fetlock compared with the front fetlock is that the lateral and medial dorsal metatarsal nerves from the deep peroneal (fibular) nerve course over the dorsolateral and dorsomedial surfaces of the third metatarsal bone and digit. Theoretically, these nerves should be anesthetized to completely desensitize the fetlock and distal limb, although there is debate as to whether this is necessary.
- This is accomplished by injecting 2 to 3 mL of anesthetic subcutaneously, lateral and medial to the long digital extensor tendon using a 5/8-inch (1.5-cm), 25-gauge needle. Blocking these nerves when performing a low plantar nerve block is why this block is referred to as the 6-point block.
- Not all clinicians feel that blocking the two dorsal nerves is necessary for the low plantar block to be effective.

- **Pitfalls:**
  1) Inadvertent injection into the fetlock joint or DFTS.
  2) Difficulty in assessing the success of the block.
  3) Resentment by the horse if the periosteum of the dorsal metatarsus is contacted with the needle.

Deep Branch of the Lateral Plantar Nerve (DBLPN) Block

- The DBLPN innervates the proximal suspensory in the hindlimb and can be selectively desensitized to aid more accurate diagnosis of this condition (Figure 1.82).
- Two different techniques have been described although the perpendicular approach is easier to perform and used by most (Figures 1.82 and 1.83). With this approach, a 20–22-gauge,

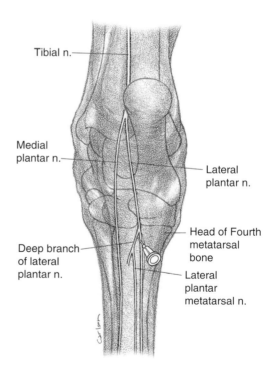

Figure 1.82 Innervation of the proximal suspensory ligament in the hindlimb and the location and positioning of the needle following the perpendicular approach to block the DBLPN just below the tarsus.

1-inch (2–3 cm) needle is inserted 15 mm distal to the head of the fourth metatarsus and directed perpendicular to skin between the axial border of the fourth metatarsus and the SDFT to a depth of approximately 25 mm.

- Alternatively, a 20–22-gauge, 1.5-inch (3.8-cm) needle can be inserted 20 mm distal and plantar to the head of the fourth metatarsus and directed proximodorsally and axial to the bone to a depth of 1 to 2 cm (Figure 1.83).

- It is usually best to hold the limb to perform either of these techniques, and with the perpendicular approach the flexor tendons can be pulled medially to facilitate needle placement (Figure 1.84).

- Diffusion of anesthetic both proximally and distally in the limb can occur following injection, and the amount of diffusion is volume dependent suggesting that a small volume of anesthetic (5 mL or less) should be used to prevent inadvertent desensitization of other structures.

- The single injection technique is thought to provide a reliable method for perineural analgesia of the DBLPN (and therefore the proximal suspensory region) with minimal risk of inadvertently desensitizing other tarsal structures.

- **Pitfalls:**
  1) Difficulty in injecting—needle in origin of suspensory, overlying fascia or against bone.
  2) Difficulty in assessing success of the block— best done by palpating absence of pain in the suspensory ligament.
  3) Inadvertent desensitization of distal tarsal joints or tarsal sheath.
  4) Proximal and distal diffusion of anesthetic.

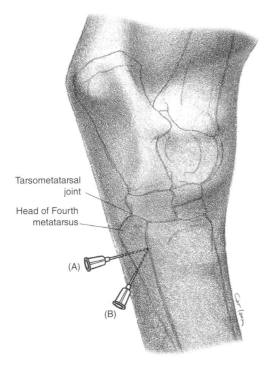

Figures 1.83 The deep branch of the lateral plantar nerve (DBLPN) can be desensitized by inserting a needle 15 mm below the head of the lateral splint bone directed perpendicular to the limb (A) or 20 mm below the head of the lateral splint and directing the needle proximodorsally and axial to the bone (B).

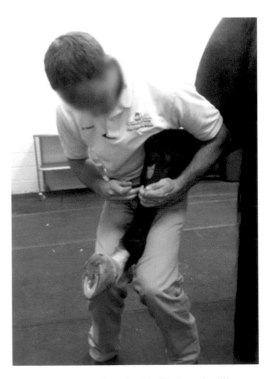

Figure 1.84 Cradling the hindlimb and pulling the flexor tendons medially can help facilitate needle placement when performing the perpendicular approach to block the DBLPN.

Tibial and Peroneal Block (Figure 1.85)

- Anesthetizing the tibial and deep and superficial peroneal nerves above the point of the hock essentially desensitizes the entire distal limb. These blocks can be helpful to diagnose some horses with hock lameness, or they can be used to rule out whether the pain causing the lameness is located within the hock or distal limb.
- The site for injection of the tibial nerve is approximately 4 inches above the point of the hock on the medial aspect of the limb, between the Achilles tendon and the deep

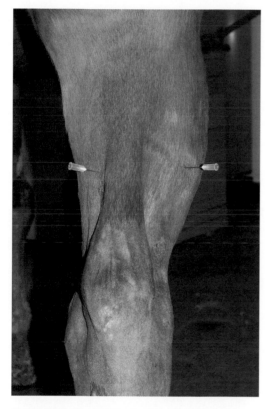

Figure 1.85 Image illustrating the locations to block the tibial and peroneal nerves. The site for injection of the tibial nerve is approximately 4 inches (10 cm) above the point of the hock on the medial aspect of the limb, between the Achilles tendon and the deep digital flexor muscle. The location to block the peroneal nerves is approximately 4 inches (10 cm) above the point of the hock on the lateral aspect of the limb in the groove formed by the muscle bellies of the lateral and long digital extensor muscles.

digital flexor muscle. A 1.5-inch, 20- to 22-gauge needle is used to deposit 15 to 20 mL of anesthetic in several tissue planes in the fascia that overlies the deep digital flexor muscle.

- Blocking the tibial nerve provides anesthesia to the plantar tarsus, metatarsus, distal Achilles tendon, calcaneus, suspensory ligament, and most of the foot.
- The deep and superficial peroneal (fibular) nerves can be anesthetized approximately 4 inches above the point of the hock on the lateral aspect of the limb in the groove formed by the muscle bellies of the lateral and long digital extensor muscle. A 1.5- to 2-inch, 20-gauge needle is inserted in a slightly caudal direction until the needle contacts the caudal edge of the tibia. Ten to 15 mL of anesthetic is injected on the lateral border of the cranial tibial muscle close to the tibia. The needle is then retracted and another 10 to 15 mL of local anesthetic is injected more superficially in several planes to be sure that the superficial peroneal nerve is blocked.
- **Pitfalls:**
  1) Difficulty in palpating the tibial nerve and determining the location of the injections.
  2) Placing the anesthetic too proximal or distal on the leg and missing the nerves.
  3) Placing the anesthetic too superficially to block both branches of the peroneal nerves.
  4) Anesthesia of the peroneal nerve may affect the ability of the horse to extend the limb and may cause dragging of the toe or knuckling of the fetlock.

Direct Infiltration of Anesthetic

- Direct infiltration of anesthesia to document pain in a region is used most often at sites of insertions of ligaments and tendons (e.g. the proximal interosseous muscle), or at bony prominences (i.e. splints or swellings).

- This approach often permits the clinician to be more definitive regarding whether a painful region is contributing to the lameness.
- The amount of local anesthetic administered depends on the location and dimensions of the area involved.
- One of the more common locations to use direct infiltration of anesthetics is the origin of the suspensory ligament. However, perineural anesthesia using the lateral palmar nerve block in the forelimb and the DBLPN block in the hindlimb is preferred.
- Direct infiltration of the proximal suspensory is best performed with the limb held with the opposite hand. A 1-inch (2–3 cm), 20- to 22-gauge needle is inserted between the attachments of the suspensory ligament and the inferior check ligament in the forelimb or between the fourth metatarsus and the SDFT in the hindlimb.
- The needle is directed toward the origin of the suspensory ligament and 3–5 mL of anesthetic is injected. Both the lateral and medial sides can be blocked in the same manner, but this is usually unnecessary.
- Direct infiltration will likely desensitize some of the nerves that are located in the proximal metatarsal/metacarpal region.
- **Pitfalls:**
  1) Inadvertently injecting the carpometacarpal or tarsometatarsal joints or the tarsal sheath.
  2) Diffusion of anesthetic to other tissues.
  3) Difficulty in assessing the success of the block.

Intrasynovial Anesthesia

Overview

- The use of intrasynovial anesthesia plays an important role in the diagnosis of equine lameness.
- In most cases, it is more specific and efficient to anesthetize the specific synovial structure (joint capsule, tendon sheath, or bursa) that is thought to be the cause of the lameness than performing local perineural anesthesia.
- Intrasynovial anesthesia is commonly performed above the carpus and tarsus where perineural anesthesia becomes more difficult and is thought to be more specific than perineural anesthesia because if the lameness improves, the synovial cavity is considered the site of the problem.
- The three major exceptions to the specificity of intrasynovial blocks are the DIP joint, middle carpal joint, and the TMT joint, and in general, the more anesthetic that is used, the greater the likelihood of inadvertent analgesia of surrounding structures.
- Mepivacaine is the anesthetic of choice to use intrasynovially because it is considered to be less irritating and knowing several different approaches to the synovial cavities can be very beneficial depending on the circumstances (Table 1.5).

Skin Preparation and Restraint

- Proper preparation of the site for injection is necessary to prevent subsequent infection within the synovial cavity even though the reported risk of infection is very low (1/1279 injections or 0.08%).
- Clipping the hair is usually unnecessary if the site is prepared with a 5-minute sterile antiseptic scrub. However, if the hair is very long and soiled, it is best to clip the hair overlying the injection site, and clipping is recommended when using spinal needles with stylets.
- Clipping a very small area (1–2 cm square) has the advantage of marking the site of injection so that a helper knows exactly where to prep the skin.
- An experienced helper makes performing intrasynovial injections much easier and safer. Proper restraint of the horse is also required to prevent injury to personnel and damage to the articular cartilage and to reduce the risk of needle breakage.

Table 1.5 Guidelines for intrasynovial anesthesia.

Synovial cavity	Needle size	Volume of anesthetic	Approaches and limb position (standing or held)
Coffin joint	20–22 g, 1–1.5″	4–5 mL	Dorsal approaches: standing Lateral approach: standing or held
Pastern joint	20–22 g, 1.5″	4–5 mL	Dorsal and dorsolateral approaches: standing Palmar/plantar approach: held
Fetlock joint	20–22 g, 1–1.5″	8–12 mL	Proximal palmar/plantar approaches: standing or held Collateral sesamoidean approach: held Distal palmar/plantar approach: standing Dorsal approach: standing
Carpal joints	20–22 g, 1–1.5″	8–10 mL	Doral approaches: held Palmar approaches: standing
Elbow	20 g, 1.5″ or 20 g, 3.5″	20–30 mL	All approaches: standing
Shoulder	18–20 g, 3.5″	20–40 mL	All approaches: standing
Tarsometatarsal joint	20 g, 1–1.5″	4–6 mL	All approaches: standing
Distal intertarsal joint	25 g, 5/8″ or 22 g, 1″	3–5 mL	All approaches: standing
Tarsocrural joint	20–22 g, 1.5″	15–20 mL	All approaches: standing
Femoropatellar joint	20 g, 1.5–3.5″	30–40 mL	All approaches: standing
Medial femorotibial joint	20 g, 1.5″	20–30 mL	All approaches: standing
Lateral femorotibial joint	20 g, 1.5″	20–30 mL	All approaches: standing
Coxofemoral joint	16–18 g, 6–8″ spinal	30–60 mL	All approaches: standing
Digital flexor tendon sheath	20–22 g, 1–1.5″	8–15 mL	Proximal approach: standing All other approaches: held
Carpal sheath	20 g, 1.5–3.5″	15–30 mL	Medial approach: standing Lateral approach: held
Tarsal sheath	20 g, 1.5″	15–20 mL	Medial approach: standing
Extensor carpi radialis sheath	20 g, 1.5″	10–20 mL	All approaches: standing or held
Podotrochlear (navicular) bursa	18–20 g, 3.5"	2–4 mL	All approaches: standing or held
Calcaneal bursa	20 g, 1.5″	10–15 mL	Distal approach: standing Proximal approach: standing or held
Bicipital bursa	18–20 g, 3.5–5″ or 20 g, 1.5″	20–30 mL	All approaches: standing
Trochanteric bursa	18–20 g, 1.5–3.5″	7–10 mL	All approaches: standing

- Twitch restraint is recommended by the author for all intrasynovial injections unless it is not tolerated by the horse or if the horse has been sedated.

- In general, the smallest possible gauge needle (usually 20 gauge or smaller) should be used to minimize objection by the horse.

- Sterile gloves are recommended to permit careful palpation of the anatomic landmarks and to be able to handle the shaft of the needle without contamination.
- The injection should be done carefully but also as rapidly as possible and synovial fluid draining from the needle hub is the only definitive method to confirm that the needle is in the correct location.

Assessment of Response to Intrasynovial Blocks

- Most intrasynovial blocks take effect quickly and their effects wear off quickly. The response to the block should be assessed no later than 10 minutes after performing the block and then again at 20 to 30 minutes if no improvement in the lameness is observed at the initial reevaluation.
- Evaluation of the effectiveness of the block should include repeating the exercise that resulted in the most significant signs of lameness and possibly re-performing the manipulative/flexion test that suggested there was a problem.
- In general, at least a 50% improvement in lameness should be observed to suggest that the synovial structure is the primary location of the lameness.
- False-negative intrasynovial blocks have been reported but tend to be uncommon. If there is minimal improvement within 60 minutes, it is unlikely that the site is contributing to the lameness.
- Diffusion of anesthetic to local structures, inadvertent anesthesia of peripheral nerves closely associated with the synovial cavity outpouchings, and the possibility that the injection was not in the synovial cavity should all be considered when assessing the response to intrasynovial anesthesia.

Distal Interphalangeal (DIP) Joint – Dorsolateral Approach

- The dorsolateral approach to the DIP joint is performed with the horse standing.

- The site of injection is 1/2 inch above the coronary band and 3/4 to 1 inch lateral (or medial) to midline.
- A 1- to 1.5-inch, 20-gauge needle is inserted from a vertical position and directed distally and medially toward the center of the foot at approximately a 45° angle (Figure 1.86; Video 1.14).
- The needle should enter the DIP joint capsule at the edge of the extensor process.

Pitfalls:
1) Inadvertent blocking of the palmar/plantar digital nerves (using > 5 mL).
2) Interpreting a positive DIP joint block as only a coffin joint problem.
3) Contacting bone due to incorrect angle of needle.
4) Inability to obtain synovial fluid.

Distal Interphalangeal (DIP) Joint – Dorsal Perpendicular Approach

- The dorsal perpendicular approach to the DIP joint is performed with the horse standing.
- The injection site is just above the coronary band, 1/2 inch above the edge of the hoof wall on the dorsal midline of the foot. A 1- to 1.5-inch, 20-gauge needle is directed downward perpendicular to the bearing surface of the foot to enter the dorsal outpouching of the DIP joint (Figure 1.87; Video 1.15).

Pitfalls:
1) Inadvertent blocking of the palmar/plantar digital nerves (using > 5 mL).
2) Contacting bone by placing needle too far proximal.
3) Inability to obtain synovial fluid.

Distal Interphalangeal (DIP) Joint – Dorsal Parallel Approach

- The dorsal parallel approach to the DIP joint is performed with the horse standing.
- The injection site is just above the coronary band, 1/4 above the edge of the hoof wall on the dorsal midline of the foot. A 1- to 1.5-inch, 20-gauge needle is inserted just above the coronary band parallel to the bearing surface of

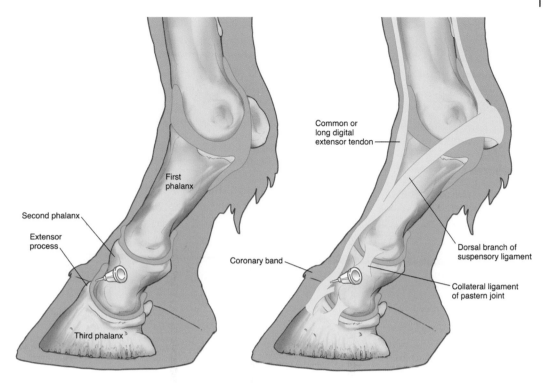

Figure 1.86 Dorsolateral approach to the coffin joint.

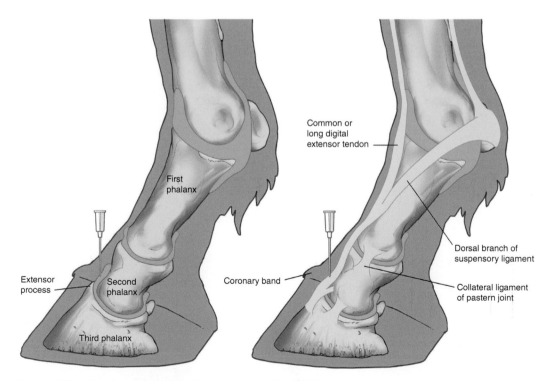

Figure 1.87 The dorsal perpendicular approach to the DIP joint.

the foot to enter the dorsal outpouching of the DIP joint (Figure 1.88; Video 1.16).

- The needle can be inserted in a slight downward angle to ensure hitting the dorsal recess of the DIP joint.
- The dorsal parallel approach usually is considered to be easier to perform than other techniques and is recommended by many clinicians.

Pitfalls:

1) Inadvertent blocking of the palmar/plantar digital nerves (using > 5 mL).
2) Inserting needle too far proximally and missing the dorsal pouch.
3) Excessive bleeding if insert needle through coronary band.

Distal Interphalangeal (DIP) Joint – Lateral Approach

- The lateral approach to the DIP joint is performed with the limb held in slight flexion.
- The site for injection is bounded distally by a depression along the proximal border of the collateral cartilage approximately

midway between the dorsal and palmar/plantar border of P2. A 1-inch, 20-gauge needle is directed downward at a 45° angle toward the medial weight-bearing hoof surface (Figure 1.89; Video 1.17).

- Most horses appear to tolerate the technique, but the specificity of the lateral approach is thought to be less than the other approaches (anesthetic can enter the DFTS or subcutaneous tissue).

Pitfalls:

1) Inadvertent blocking of the palmar/plantar digital nerves (using > 5 mL).
2) Difficulty in palpating anatomic landmarks and directing needle at correct angle.
3) Entering the DFTS.

Proximal Interphalangeal (PIP) Joint – Dorsolateral Approach

- The dorsolateral approach to the PIP joint is performed with the horse standing or with the limb extended and the sole supported on the knee (author prefers standing).

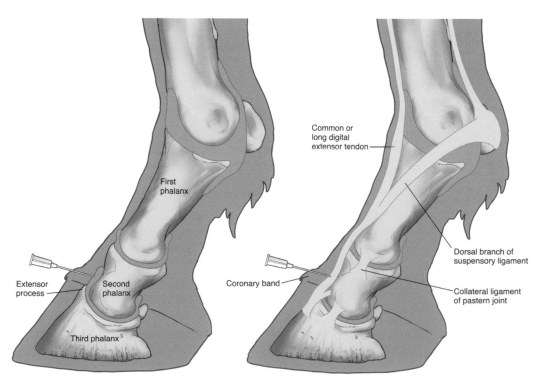

Figure 1.88 Dorsal parallel approach to the DIP joint.

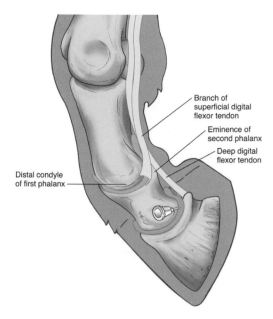

Figure 1.89 Lateral approach to the DIP joint.

- The condylar eminences of the distolateral aspect of the first phalanx (P1) are identified and a 1.5- inch, 20-gauge needle is inserted parallel to the ground surface 1/2 inch distal to the palpable eminence.
- The needle is directed underneath the edge of the extensor tendon dorsal to the collateral ligament to enter the dorsal joint pouch at a depth of 1/2 inch (Figure 1.90; Video 1.18).
- 3–5 mL of anesthetic is all that can usually be injected without excessive pressure.

Pitfalls:
1) No easily palpable joint pouch dorsally because of extensor tendon.
2) Difficult to "feel" the needle penetrate the joint space.
3) Condylar eminences not always that easy to palpate in horses with OA.

Proximal Interphalangeal (PIP) Joint – Palmar/Plantar Approach

- The palmar/plantar approach to the PIP joint is performed with the limb held in flexion – carpus flexed and distal limb relaxed.

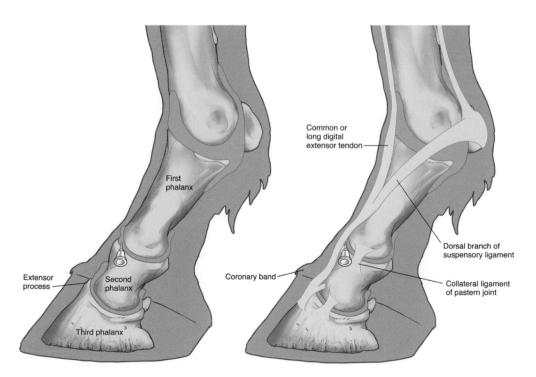

Figure 1.90 Dorsolateral approach to the PIP joint.

- A 1.5-inch, 20-gauge needle is inserted perpendicular to the limb into the palpable V-depression formed by the palmar aspect of P1 dorsally, the distal eminence of P1 distally, and the lateral branch of the SDFT as it inserts on the eminence of P2 palmarodistally (Figure 1.91; Video 1.19). This corresponds to the transverse bony prominence on the proximopalmar/plantar border of P2 that is usually easily palpable.
- The author prefers to angle the needle slightly dorsally to contact P1, and then direct the needle along the palmar/plantar aspect of the bone. This ensures that the needle is just behind P1 where it will enter the PIP joint capsule at a depth of approximately 1 inch (2.5 cm).

Pitfalls:
1) No easily palpable palmar/plantar joint pouches because of the ligaments/tendons on the palmar/plantar aspect of the pastern.
2) Placing the needle too distally – use eminence of P2 as landmark.
3) Inadvertent injection of the DFTS.
4) Inability to obtain synovial fluid.

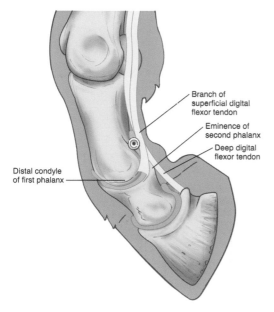

Branch of
superficial digital
flexor tendon

Eminence of
second phalanx

Deep digital
flexor tendon

Distal condyle
of first phalanx

Figure 1.91 Palmar/plantar approach to the PIP joint.

MCP/MTP (Fetlock) Joint – Proximal Palmar/Plantar Approach

- The proximal palmar/plantar approach to the fetlock joint can be performed with the horse standing (Figure 1.92) or with the limb held in flexion (Figure 1.93).
- The boundaries of the palmar/plantar pouches of the fetlock joint are the apical border of the proximal sesamoid bones distally, the distal ends of the splint bones proximally, the third metacarpal/metatarsal bone dorsally, and the branch of the suspensory ligament palmar/plantarly.
- In the normal horse, these palmar/plantar pouches appear as a depression, and attempts to retrieve synovial fluid may be difficult but are often easily identified in horses with fetlock effusion.
- When performing this approach in the standing patient, a 1- to 1.5-inch, 20-gauge needle is inserted from lateral to medial and directed distally at a 45° angle to the long axis of the limb (Figure 1.92; Video 1.20).
- The disadvantages of the standing approach are contamination of the synovial fluid with blood because of the highly vascular synovial membrane and the inability to aspirate synovial fluid because the synovial villi plug the needle.
- Performing the proximal palmar/plantar approach with the fetlock flexed can potentially minimize these complications.
- With the fetlock flexed, there is a very palpable depression at the very distal aspect of the joint pouch just above the branch of the suspensory ligament. A 1-inch (2–3 cm), 20-gauge needle is inserted at this location and directed distally at a 45° angle (Figure 1.93; Video 1.21).

Pitfalls:
1) Difficulty palpating landmarks/joint pouch with the absence of synovial effusion.
2) Blood contamination and/or inability to aspirate synovial fluid.

MCP/MTP (Fetlock) Joint – Collateral Sesamoidean Ligament Approach

- The collateral sesamoidean ligament approach to the fetlock joint is performed with the limb held in flexion – carpus flexed and distal limb relaxed.

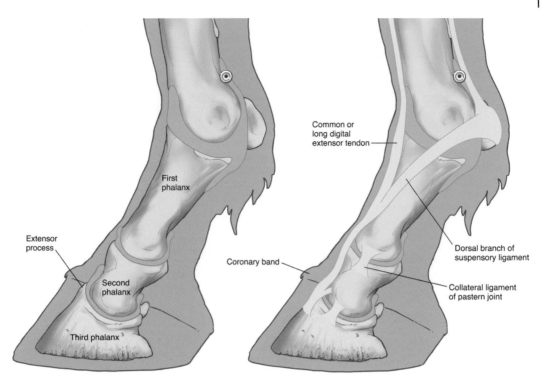

First
phalanx

Extensor
process

Second
phalanx

Third phalanx

Common or
long digital
extensor tendon

Coronary band

Dorsal branch of
suspensory ligament

Collateral ligament
of pastern joint

Figure 1.92 Proximal palmar/plantar approach to the fetlock joint in the standing horse.

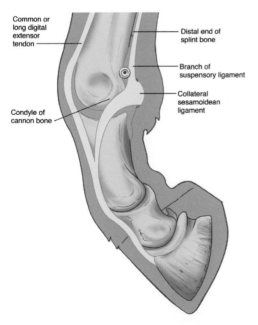

Common or
long digital
extensor
tendon

Condyle of
cannon bone

Distal end of
splint bone

Branch of
suspensory ligament

Collateral
sesamoidean
ligament

Figure 1.93 Injection of the proximal palmar/plantar pouch of the fetlock joint with the limb flexed.

- The space (depression) between the articular surfaces of the proximal sesamoid bones and the MC/MT is palpated and a 1-inch, 20-gauge needle is inserted through the collateral sesamoidean ligament perpendicular to the limb (Figure 1.94; Video 1.22).
- If the needle fails to advance, it is most likely contacting bone and will need to be redirected to enter the joint space.
- Arthrocentesis of the fetlock through the lateral collateral sesamoidean ligament is probably the best approach to obtain a hemorrhage-free synovial fluid sample.
- **Pitfalls:**
  1) Difficulty palpating the depression between the proximal sesamoid bones and the MC/MT.
  2) Contacting bone – need to redirect needle.

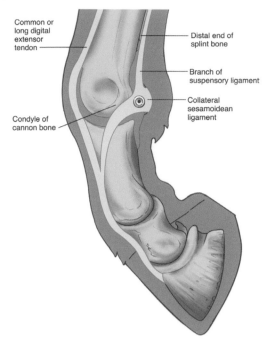

Common or long digital extensor tendon

Distal end of splint bone

Branch of suspensory ligament

Collateral sesamoidean ligament

Condyle of cannon bone

Figure 1.94 Lateral view of the injection site through the collateral sesamoidean ligament into the fetlock joint. Synovial fluid is reliably obtained with this technique.

MCP/MTP (Fetlock) Joint – Distal Palmar/Plantar Approach

- The distal palmar/plantar approach to the fetlock joint is performed with the horse standing.
- The landmarks are the distal aspect of the proximal sesamoid bone and collateral sesamoidean ligament proximally; the proximal palmar/plantar eminence of P1 distally; and the digital vein, artery, and nerve palmar/plantarly.
- The injection site is in the palpable depression formed by the distal aspect of the proximal sesamoid bone, the proximopalmar/plantar eminence of P1, and dorsal to the palmar/plantar digital artery, vein, and nerve.
- A 1.5-inch, 20-gauge needle is inserted in the depression and directed slightly dorsally (10 to 20°) and proximally (10°) until the joint is entered (Figure 1.95; Video 1.23).

Pitfalls:
1) Difficulty palpating anatomic landmarks.
2) Contacting bone – incorrect needle angle.

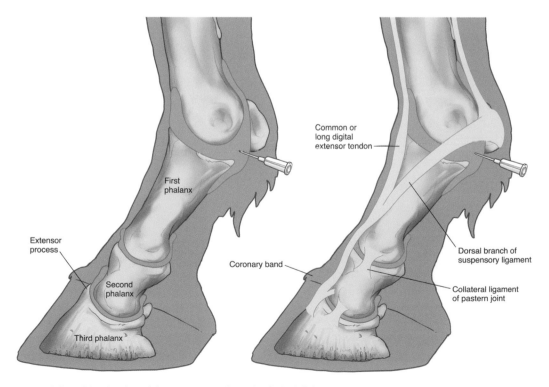

Common or long digital extensor tendon

First phalanx

Extensor process

Second phalanx

Third phalanx

Coronary band

Dorsal branch of suspensory ligament

Collateral ligament of pastern joint

Figure 1.95 Distal palmar/plantar approach to the fetlock joint.

3) Penetration of the DFTS if needle is inserted palmar/plantar to the neurovascular bundle.

MCP/MTP (Fetlock) Joint – Dorsal Approach

- The dorsal approach to the fetlock joint is performed with the horse standing.
- The injection site is proximal to the proximodorsal limits of P1 in the palpable joint space in a slightly oblique manner, either lateral or medial to the extensor tendon.
- A 1.5-inch, 20-gauge needle is inserted perpendicular to the limb along the dorsal aspect of the fetlock joint (Figure 1.96; Video 1.24). 8–10 mL of anesthetic is adequate.
- The fetlock joint capsule is thicker in this location than in the palmar/plantar pouch and appears to cause greater discomfort to the horse than the other techniques.

Pitfalls:

1) Difficulty palpating joint pouch with minimal effusion.
2) Damage to articular surfaces with needle.

Middle Carpal Joint – Dorsal Approach

- The dorsal approach to the middle carpal joint is performed with the carpus fully flexed.
- The site of injection is located in palpable depressions lateral or medial to the extensor carpi radialis tendon on the dorsal aspect of the carpus.
- A 1–1.5 inch, 20- or 22-gauge needle is inserted midway between the proximal and distal rows of carpal bones directed slightly proximally to avoid hitting the articular surface (Figure 1.97b; Video 1.25).
- Approximately 10 mL of anesthetic is recommended.

Pitfalls:

1) Damage to the articular cartilage.
2) Inadvertent anesthesia of the proximal metacarpal region.

Middle Carpal Joint – Palmarolateral Approach

- The palmarolateral approach to the middle carpal joint is performed with the horse standing.
- This approach is best used when the joint is distended because the joint capsule is

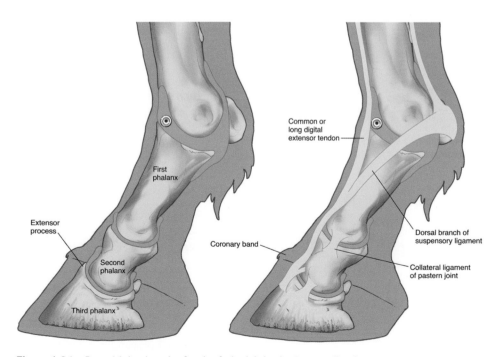

Figure 1.96 Dorsal injection site for the fetlock joint in the standing horse.

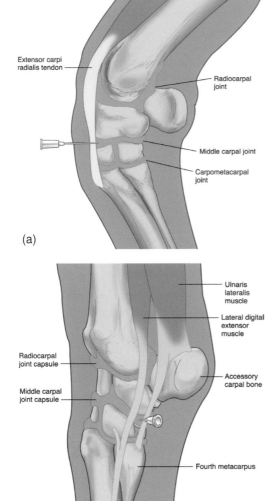

Extensor carpi
radialis tendon

Radiocarpal
joint

Middle carpal joint

Carpometacarpal
joint

(a)

Ulnaris
lateralis
muscle

Lateral digital
extensor
muscle

Radiocarpal
joint capsule

Accessory
carpal bone

Middle carpal
joint capsule

Fourth metacarpus

(b)

Figure 1.97 Dorsal flexed (a) and palmarolateral standing (b) approaches to the middle carpal joint.

usually more easily palpable on the palmarolateral aspect of the carpus.
- The injection site is palmar and lateral to the ulnar and fourth carpal bones distal to the accessory carpal bone approximately 1 inch distal to the site of injection of the palmarolateral radiocarpal joint. A 1-inch 20-gauge needle is inserted perpendicular to the skin to a depth of about 1/2 inch (Figure 1.97b; Video 1.26).

Pitfalls:
1) Placing the needle too distally.
2) Inability to palpate the palmar pouch.

Radiocarpal Joint – Dorsal Approach
- The dorsal approach to the radiocarpal joint is performed with the carpus fully flexed.
- The site of injection is located in palpable depressions lateral or medial to the extensor carpi radialis tendon on the dorsal aspect of the carpus.
- The injection is made with a 1-inch, 20- or 22-gauge needle midway between the distal radius and proximal row of carpal bones directed slightly proximally to avoid hitting the articular surfaces (Figure 1.98a; Video 1.27).
- Approximately 10 mL of anesthetic is recommended.

Pitfalls:
1) Damage to the articular cartilage.

Radiocarpal Joint – Palmarolateral Approach
- The palmarolateral approach to the radiocarpal joint is performed with the horse standing.
- This approach is best used when the joint is distended because the joint capsule is more easily palpable on the palmarolateral aspect of the carpus.
- The landmarks for the palmarolateral approach to the radiocarpal joint are the palmarolateral aspect of the radius, proximolateral aspect of the accessory carpal bone, and palmarolateral aspect of the ulnar carpal bone.
- A 1–1.5 inch (2–3 cm), 20-gauge needle is inserted in this palpable depression at 90° to the long axis of the limb, and the needle is directed dorsomedially (Figure 1.98b; Video 1.28).
- Another palmarolateral approach is at the midaccessory carpal bone level in a palpable "V" between the tendons of the ulnaris lateralis and the lateral digital extensor. The needle is inserted perpendicular to the skin

in a small depression 1/2 to 1 inch distal to the "V" in the space between the distal lateral aspect of the radius (vestigial ulna) and the proximal lateral aspect of the ulnar carpal bone (Figure 1.98b).

Pitfalls:

1) Difficulty in palpating the palmar pouch of the radiocarpal joint.
2) Placing the needle too far distally.

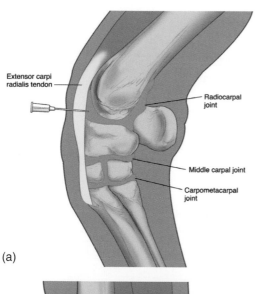

(a)

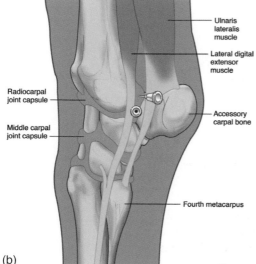

(b)

Figure 1.98 Dorsal flexed (a) and palmarolateral standing (b) approaches to the radiocarpal joint.

Elbow Joint – Lateral Approach

- The lateral approach to the elbow joint is performed with the horse standing.
- The elbow joint is fairly large, and 20–30 mL of anesthetic is recommended.
- The landmark is the lateral collateral ligament that extends across the joint from the lateral epicondyle of the humerus to the lateral tuberosity of the radius. The elbow joint can be entered either cranial or caudal to the collateral ligament.
- The site for injection is 2/3 the distance distally measured from the lateral epicondyle of the humerus to the lateral tuberosity of the radius. A 1.5-inch, 20-gauge needle is inserted at a 90° angle to the skin just cranial or caudal to the lateral collateral ligament (Figure 1.99).
- If injected caudally, the needle may enter the bursa of the ulnaris lateralis muscle, which is thought to communicate with the elbow joint in about 1/3 of horses.

Pitfalls:

1) Difficulty in palpating the radial tuberosity or the lateral humeral epicondyle.
2) Hitting bone when advancing the needle between the radius and humerus.
3) Radial nerve paralysis from injecting anesthetic outside the joint when using the cranial injection site.
4) Inability to obtain synovial fluid.

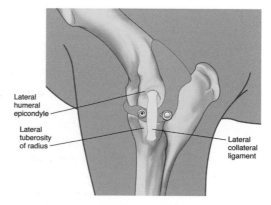

Figure 1.99 Lateral approaches cranial or caudal to the collateral ligament of the elbow joint.

Elbow Joint– Caudolateral Approach

- The caudolateral approach to the elbow joint is performed with the horse standing.
- The caudolateral approach is an alternative to placing the needle directly caudal to the collateral ligament using the lateral approach.
- The injection site is caudal to the palpable humeral epicondyle in the anconeal notch within the humero-ulna joint.
- This palpable V-shaped depression is usually just below the triceps muscles and 6 to 8 cm cranio-distal from the point of the olecranon process. A 1.5- to 3-1/2-inch, 20-gauge needle is inserted at a 45° angle to the skin and directed craniomedially (Figure 1.100).

Pitfalls:

1) Difficulty in palpating the anconeal notch.
2) Hitting bone when advancing the needle between the humerus and ulna.
3) Inability to obtain synovial fluid.

Elbow Joint– Caudal Approach

- The caudal approach to the elbow joint is performed with the horse standing and ultrasound can be used to help facilitate the injection.
- The large caudal joint pouch of the elbow can be entered from a more proximal location. The landmarks are the lateral supracondylar crest of the distal humerus

and the most proximal point of the olecranon process.

- The injection site is 1/2 inch proximal to and 1/3 of the distance measured caudally from the supracondylar eminence to the point of the olecranon. A 3-1/2-inch, 18- to 20-gauge spinal needle is directed distomedially through the triceps musculature at a 45° angle to the long axis of the limb into the olecranon fossa (Figure 1.101).

Pitfalls:

1) Difficulty in palpating landmarks for injection.
2) Inaccurate needle placement – more challenging than other techniques.
3) Inability to obtain synovial fluid.

Scapulohumeral (Shoulder) Joint – Craniolateral Approach

- The craniolateral approach to the shoulder joint is performed with the horse standing and many clinicians utilize ultrasound to help guide the injection.
- The shoulder joint is large, and therefore 30–40 mL of anesthetic is recommended.

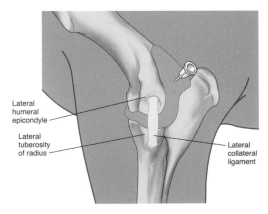

Figure 1.101 The approach to the large caudal outpouching of the elbow joint is 0.5 inch (1 cm) proximal to and one-third of the distance measured caudally from the supracondylar eminence to the point of the olecranon. A 3.5-inch (8.9-cm), 18- to 20-gauge spinal needle is directed distomedially through the triceps musculature at a 45° angle to the long axis of the limb into the olecranon fossa.

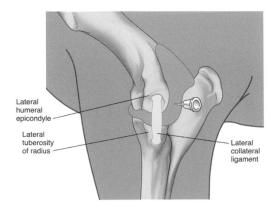

Figure 1.100 Caudolateral approach to the humeral-ulnar joint.

- The injection is located in the notch formed between the cranial and caudal prominences of the lateral tuberosity of the humerus. The caudal prominence (point of the shoulder) is easiest to palpate, and by exerting deep finger pressure, the depression for needle insertion can be palpated 3.5–4 cm cranial to the caudal prominence.
- A 3.5-inch (8.8-cm), 18- to 20-gauge spinal needle is inserted into this notch and directed parallel to the ground in a caudomedial direction toward the opposite elbow. The depth of penetration depends on the size of the horse, but the joint capsule is usually entered at a depth of 2–3 inches (5–7 cm) (Figure 1.102).
- Alternatively, the spinal needle may be inserted slightly more proximal on the limb in a distinct depression located cranial to the infraspinatus tendon and slightly proximal and cranial to the point of the shoulder. The needle is placed parallel to the ground or slightly downward and directed caudomedially at a 45° angle until bone is contacted.
- Synovial fluid usually can be aspirated and is the only definitive method to document correct needle placement.

Pitfalls:
1) Needle directed too proximally contacting the glenoid of scapula.

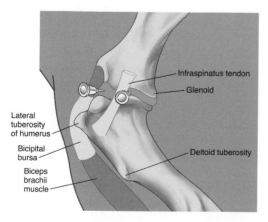

Figure 1.102 Craniolateral (left needle) and lateral (right needle) approaches to the shoulder joint.

2) Needle directed too medial to lateral and diverges across the cranial aspect of the humeral tuberosity.
3) Inadvertent anesthesia of the bicipital bursa; communicates with the shoulder joint in some horses.
4) Temporary anesthesia of the suprascapular nerve with periarticular injection.
5) Inability to aspirate synovial fluid.

Scapulohumeral (Shoulder) Joint – Lateral Approach

- The lateral approach to the shoulder joint is performed with the horse standing and many clinicians utilize ultrasound to help guide the injection.
- The landmarks for the lateral approach to the shoulder are the lateral humeral tuberosity and the infraspinatus tendon.
- A 3-1/2-inch, 18- to 20-gauge spinal needle is inserted 1 to 2 cm caudal and distal to the infraspinatus tendon in line with the lateral humeral tuberosity (Figure 1.102). The needle is directed slightly caudally and upward toward the lateral aspect of the humeral head.
- In general, the lateral approach is more difficult than the craniolateral approach.

Pitfalls:
1) Needle directed too proximally contacting the glenoid of scapula.
2) Inadvertent anesthesia of the bicipital bursa; communicates with the shoulder joint in some horses.
3) Inability to aspirate synovial fluid.

Tarsometatarsal (TMT) Joint – Plantarolateral Approach

- The plantarolateral approach to the TMT joint is performed with the horse standing.
- The landmarks for injection are the proximal head of the fourth metatarsal (MTIV) bone and the lateral edge of the SDFT.
- A 1- to 1.5-inch, 20-gauge needle is inserted in the small palpable depression just proximal to the head of MTIV. The needle is directed toward the dorsomedial aspect of the tarsus

in a slightly downward direction to a depth of 1/2 to 1 inch (Figure 1.103; Video 1.29).

● 3–5 mL of anesthetic is recommended.
   Pitfalls:
   1) Placing the needle too distally and contacting the head of MTIV.
   2) Directing the needle too medial to lateral or caudal to cranial.
   3) Inadvertent anesthesia of the proximal suspensory region.

Distal Intertarsal (DIT; Centrotarsal) Joint – Medial Approach

● The medial approach to the DIT joint is performed with the horse standing.
● The landmarks are midway between the plantar and dorsal aspect of the medial distal tarsus, just below the palpable distal border of the cunean tendon in a notch between the combined first and second tarsal bones and the third and the central tarsal bones (Figure 1.104a).
● Another approach to find the landmarks is to identify the medial eminence of the talus and medial eminence of the central tarsal bone. The site for injection is halfway between these landmarks and 1/2 inch distal to the eminence of the central tarsal bone.
● A 5/8 to 1 inch, 22- to 25-gauge needle is directed parallel to the ground and slightly

caudally, and 3–4 mL of anesthetic is recommended (Figure 1.104a; Video 1.30).

● The needle is determined to be within the DIT joint by low resistance to injection without developing a subcutaneous swelling.
● This is a difficult joint to inject with an accuracy rate of only 42% in a recent report.

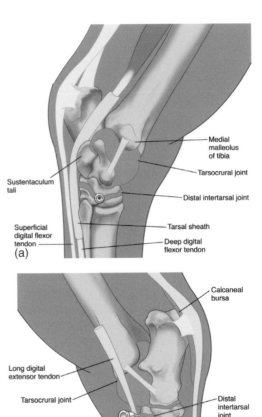

(a)

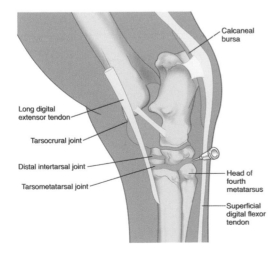

(b)

Figure 1.104 Medial (a) and dorsolateral (b) approaches to the DIT joint. The dorsolateral injection site is 2 to 3 mm lateral to the long digital extensor tendon and approximately 6 to 8 mm proximal to a line drawn perpendicular to the axis of MTIII through the head of MTIV. The needle is directed plantaromedially at an angle of approximately 70° from the sagittal plane until bone is contacted.

Figure 1.103 Lateral approach to the TMT joint.

Pitfalls:

1) Inability to advance the needle—joint space is difficult to hit.
2) Excessive pressure when injecting—usually not within joint space.
3) Injecting the proximal intertarsal joint by placing needle too proximal.
4) Placing needle too far caudally and missing the notch between the tarsal bones.

Distal Intertarsal (DIT; Centrotarsal) Joint – Dorsolateral Approach

- The dorsolateral approach to the DIT joint is performed with the horse standing.
- The injection site is 2 to 3 mm lateral to the long digital extensor tendon and 6 to 8 mm proximal to a line drawn perpendicular to the axis of the third metatarsal bone through the head of the fourth metatarsal bone. This is usually distal to the palpable lateral trochlear ridge of the talus.
- A 2–3.5" 20 g needle is directed plantaromedially at an angle of approximately 70° from the sagittal plane until bone is contacted (Figure 1.104a; Video 1.31).
- This approach is considered to be safer for the clinician because it is performed on the lateral aspect of the tarsus but is more technically difficult than the medial approach.

Pitfalls:

1) Injection site is difficult to accurately identify.
2) Placing needle too proximal and entering the TC joint.
3) Inability to obtain synovial fluid.

Tarsocrural (TC) Joint – Dorsomedial and Dorsolateral Approaches

- The TC joint has two large dorsal outpouchings that are easily accessible for injection. The dorsomedial pouch is largest and is therefore used most frequently.
- The dorsomedial approach to the TC joint is usually performed in the weight-bearing limb from the opposite side of the horse but can be performed from the same side.

- For the dorsomedial approach, a 1- to 1.5-inch (2–3 cm), 20-gauge needle is inserted 1–1.5 inches (2–3 cm) distal to the medial malleolus of the tibia, medial, or lateral to the cranial branch of the medial saphenous vein (Figure 1.105; Video 1.32).
- The needle is advanced in a plantarolateral direction at approximately a 45° until synovial fluid flows from the needle. 15–20 mL of anesthetic is recommended.
- For the dorsolateral approach, a 1- to 1.5-inch (2–3 cm), 20-gauge needle is inserted 1–1.5 inches (2–3 cm) distal to the lateral

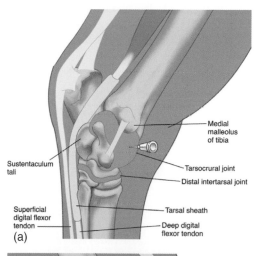

(a)

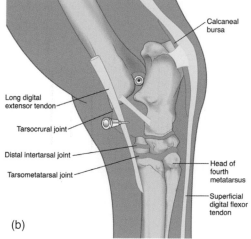

(b)

Figure 1.105 Dorsomedial (a), dorsolateral (b), and plantarolateral (b) approaches to the tarsocrural joint.

malleolus of the tibia, lateral to the extensor tendon branches (Figure 1.105b).

Pitfalls:
1) Inadvertent puncture of the saphenous vein with the dorsomedial approach.
2) More difficult to palpate the joint pouch with the dorsolateral approach.

Tarsocrural (TC) Joint – Plantarolateral and Plantaromedial Approaches

- The TC joint has medial and lateral plantar outpouchings that can be used for arthrocentesis, especially if there is significant effusion. The plantarlateral pouch is more easily accessible and used most frequently.
- The palpable landmarks of the lateral plantar pouch are bordered by the tuber calcis caudally, the caudal aspect of the distal tibia cranially, and the proximal aspect of the lateral trochlear ridge of the talus distally.
- Confirmation that fluid swellings in this location are part of the TC joint can be determined by applying finger pressure to the swellings and feeling the dorsal pouches of the TC joint distend even further.
- A 1-inch, 20-gauge needle is inserted perpendicular to the skin at the site of the effusion with the limb bearing weight (Figure 1.105b; Video 1.33).

Pitfalls:
1) Difficult to palpate the plantar pouches with minimal joint effusion.
2) Landmarks for plantar pouches more challenging than for dorsal approaches.

Medial Femorotibial (MFT) Joint – Medial Approach

- The medial approach to the MFT joint is performed with the limb weight-bearing usually from the opposite side of the horse reaching under the belly but can be performed from the same side.
- The injection is located in the space between the medial patellar and medial collateral ligaments just above the palpable proximomedial edge of the tibia.

- A 1.5 inch, 20-gauge needle is inserted just caudal to the medial patellar ligament, 1 cm proximal to the tibia, and directed perpendicular to the long axis of the limb (Figure 1.106a). The needle may need to be repositioned slightly cranially or caudally to help obtain synovial fluid. 20–30 ml of anesthetic is recommended.
- An alternative injection site for the medial approach is located 1/2 to 1 inch proximal to the medial tibial plateau in the depression between the medial patella ligament and the tendon of insertion of the sartorius muscle.
- A 1.5 inch, 20-gauge needle is directed in a cranial to caudal direction parallel to the

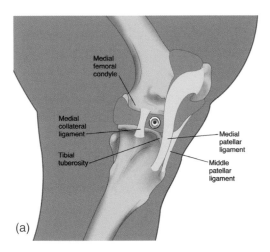

(a)

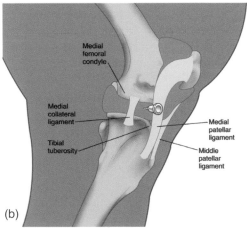

(b)

Figure 1.106 Medial approaches (a and b) to the MFT joint.

ground and parallel to a plane that bisects the limb. The needle enters a medial outpouching of the MFT joint and avoids inadvertent penetration of the medial meniscus and the medial femoral condyle (Figure 1.106b).

Pitfalls:

1) Hitting bone—needle inserted too distally (tibia) or too proximally (medial condyle).
2) Inability to obtain synovial fluid—needle may be entering meniscus.
3) Inserting needle into medial meniscus.
4) Difficulty finding the medial outpouching of the MFT joint.

Femoropatellar (FP) Joint – Cranial Approach

- The cranial approach to the MFT joint can be performed with the limb weight-bearing or with the limb slightly flexed.
- A 3-1/2-inch, 20-gauge needle is inserted approximately 1 to 1.5 inches proximal to the tibial crest between the middle and medial patella ligaments and is directed proximally under the patella. This is best performed with the limb in a partial weight-bearing (slightly flexed) position. The needle can also be directed parallel to the ground with the limb weight-bearing (Figure 1.107a).
- The FP joint can also be entered just distal to the apex of the patella on either side of the middle patellar ligament with the limb bearing weight. The joint capsule is superficial at this location and a 1.5-inch, 20-gauge needle is directed at right angles to the skin (Figure 1.107a). 30–40 mL of anesthetic is recommended.

Pitfalls:

1) Hitting bone—needle inserted too distal (tibial crest) or too proximal (patella).
2) Inability to obtain synovial fluid—needle may be within fat pad.

Femoropatellar (FP) Joint – Lateral Approach

- The lateral approach to the FP joint can be performed with the limb weight-bearing.
- The lateral cul-de-sac of the FP joint is located caudal to the lateral patellar

ligament and approximately 2 inches proximal to the lateral tibial condyle.

- A 1.5-inch, 20-gauge needle is inserted into the recess perpendicular to the long axis of the femur until the nonarticular portion of the lateral trochlea is contacted (Figure 1.107b).
- Synovial fluid can be retrieved in most cases, and this approach is usually well tolerated by the horse.

Pitfalls:

1) Placing needle too proximally or distally and missing joint cul-de-sac.

Lateral Femorotibial (LFT) Joint – Lateral Approach

- The lateral approach to the LFT joint is performed with the limb weight-bearing.

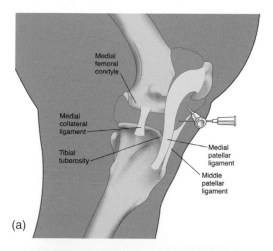

(a)

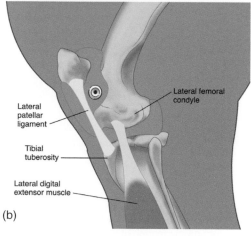

(b)

Figure 1.107 Cranial (a) and lateral (b) approaches to the femoropatellar joint.

- The injection site is slightly caudal to the palpable edge of the lateral patellar ligament just above the proximolateral edge of the tibia. A 1.5-inch, 20-gauge needle is inserted at right angles to the long axis of the femur and directed from lateral to medial to a depth of 1 inch (Figure 1.108). 20–30 mL of anesthetic is recommended.
- An alternative site just proximal to the tibia in the space between the lateral collateral ligament of the LFT joint and the tendon of origin of the long digital extensor tendon. The palpable head of the fibula helps to identify these structures. A 1.5-inch, 20-gauge needle is inserted to a depth of approximately 1 inch until the joint capsule is entered (Figure 1.108).

Pitfalls:
1) Hitting bone—needle inserted too low (tibial crest) or too high (lateral condyle).
2) Inability to obtain synovial fluid.
3) Difficult to find anatomic landmarks for tendon of origin of long digital extensor tendon and lateral collateral ligament.

Coxofemoral Joint – Craniodorsal Approach

- The craniodorsal approach to the coxofemoral joint is performed with the horse standing and usually restrained within stocks.
- Ultrasound guidance of the injection is commonly performed and recommended because the block is very difficult to perform blindly.
- The greater trochanter is an important landmark and is approximately 4 inches (10 cm) wide with a notch between the cranial and caudal protuberances that can be difficult to palpate (Figure 1.109).
- The site for injection is about 0.5 inches (1–2 cm) above the middle of the proximal summit of the greater trochanter. A small bleb of anesthetic is injected subcutaneously over the injection site, and a small stab incision may aid needle insertion.
- A 6- to 8-inch (15- to 20-cm), 16- to 18-gauge spinal needle is directed in a horizontal plane perpendicular to the vertebral column (Figure 1.109). The needle should be directed slightly downward to stay close to the femoral neck so that it is approximately 0.5 inches (1–2 cm) lower than the insertion site after it has been advanced 3–4 inches (8–10 cm).
- Firm fibrous tissue is often felt just before the needle penetrates the joint capsule at approximately 4–6 inches (10–15 cm). Synovial fluid can often be aspirated and 30–60 mL of anesthetic is recommended.

Pitfalls:
1) Inability to palpate the greater trochanter.

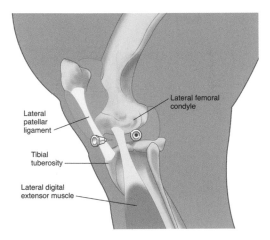

Figure 1.108 Injection sites for the lateral femorotibial joint just proximal to the tibia in the space between the lateral collateral ligament of the joint and the tendon of origin of the long digital extensor (right needle) or just caudal to the lateral patellar ligament (left needle).

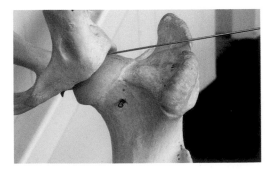

Figure 1.109 Lateral view of the injection site for the coxofemoral joint. The needle is inserted in the trochanteric notch and directed along the femoral neck until the joint is entered.

2) Directing the needle too proximally and hitting the acetabulum.

3) Inadvertent needle bending and not knowing location of the needle tip.

4) Not contacting bone—needle usually directed too far cranially or caudally and not along the femoral neck.

Digital Flexor Tendon Sheath (DFTS) – Proximal Approach

- The proximal approach to the DFTS can be performed with the limb weight-bearing or with the limb slightly flexed.
- The site for injection is 1 cm proximal to the palmar/plantar annular ligament and 1 cm palmar/plantar to the lateral branch of the suspensory ligament (Figure 1.110).
- A 1- to 1.5-inch, 20-gauge needle is directed slightly distally until the sheath is

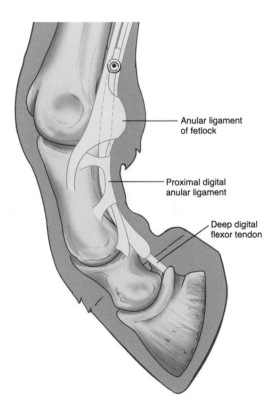

— Anular ligament of fetlock

— Proximal digital anular ligament

— Deep digital flexor tendon

Figure 1.110 The proximal approach to the DFTS can be performed with the limb slightly flexed or with the limb weight-bearing.

penetrated. 10–15 mL of anesthetic is recommended (Video 1.34).

Pitfalls:

1) Difficulty in palpating the proximal pouch of the DFTS.

2) Inability to obtain synovial fluid.

3) Inadvertent anesthesia of lateral palmar/plantar nerve.

Digital Flexor Tendon Sheath (DFTS) – Distal Approach

- The distal approaches to the DFTS are performed with the limb held and the fetlock slightly flexed.
- The distal outpouching of the DFTS is located in the pastern between the proximal and distal digital annular ligaments and between the diverging branches of the SDFT where the DDFT lies close to the skin. It is often visible and easily palpable as a distinct "bubble" when effusion is present.
- A 1-inch, 20-gauge needle is directed in a lateral to medial direction just beneath the skin so as not to penetrate the DDFT (Figure 1.111; Video 1.35).

Pitfalls:

1) Difficulty in locating DFTS outpouchings below sesamoid bones.

2) Inability to obtain synovial fluid – often against tendon.

Digital Flexor Tendon Sheath (DFTS) – Basilar Sesamoidean Approach

- The basilar sesamoidean approach to the DFTS can be performed either with the limb held and the fetlock slightly flexed or with the limb weight-bearing.
- The landmarks for injection are outpouchings of the DFTS that are located abaxial and distal to the sesamoid bones between the annular and proximal digital annular ligaments.
- A 1- to 1.5-inch, 20-gauge needle is inserted into one of the outpouchings (medial or lateral) in a distal to proximal direction at approximately a 45° angle to the sagittal plane (Figure 1.111; proximal needle).

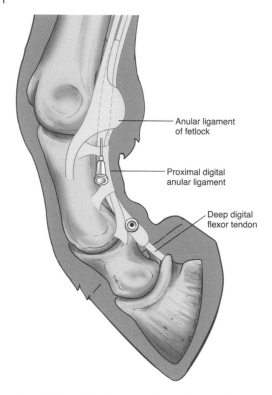

Figure 1.111 Distal approaches to the DFTS.

- This approach has been reported to be more reliable to obtain synovial fluid than the axial sesamoidean approach.

Pitfalls:
1) Difficulty in palpating the landmarks for injection.
2) Inability to aspirate fluid—needle against tendon of bone.

Digital Flexor Tendon Sheath (DFTS) – Axial Sesamoidean Approach

- The axial sesamoidean approach to the DFTS is performed with the limb held and the fetlock slightly flexed and can be used in both the distended and non-distended DFTS.
- The injection is performed 3 mm axial to the palpable border of the midbody of the lateral proximal sesamoid bone directly through the annular ligament on the palmar/plantar aspect of the fetlock. A 1- to 1.5-inch, 20-gauge needle is directed at a 45° angle to the

sagittal plane to a depth of approximately 1.5 to 2 cm (Figure 1.112; Video 1.36).

- This approach is often best used when the DFTS is non-distended since no palpable synovial outpouching is a necessary landmark for injection.

Pitfalls:
1) Difficulty in palpating the abaxial border of sesamoid bone.
2) Inability to aspirate fluid—needle against tendons.
3) Contacting bone—needle inserted too far abaxially and against sesamoid bone.
4) Minor damage to flexor tendons from needle.

Tarsal Sheath – Medial Approach

- The medial approach to the tarsal is usually performed with the limb weight-bearing.

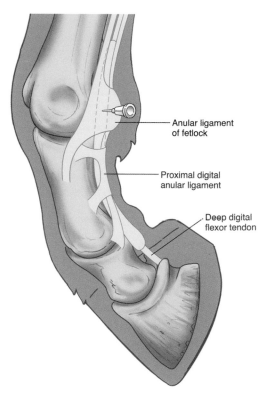

Figure 1.112 Injection site for the DFTS on the axial surface of the proximal sesamoid bone through the annular ligament.

- The tarsal sheath is located on the medial aspect of the tarsus and begins approximately 5 to 8 cm proximal to the medial malleolus and extends distally to the proximal 1/3 of the metatarsus. It encloses the DDFT of the hindlimb as it courses over the sustentaculum tali on the medial aspect of the tarsus.
- The tarsal sheath can be accessed for synoviocentesis anywhere along its course when distended. The easiest location is usually either above or below the palpable sustentaculum tali on the medial aspect of the tarsus (Figure 1.113).
- A 1.5-inch, 20-gauge needle is directed proximolaterally or distolaterally at about a 45° angle with the long axis of the limb. 15 to 20 mL of anesthetic is recommended.
  Pitfalls
  1) Difficult to palpate injection site if no effusion.
  2) Inability to obtain synovial fluid.

Podotrochlear (Navicular) Bursa – Palmar/Plantar Approach
- The palmar/plantar approach to the navicular bursa can be performed with the limb weight-bearing or with the carpus flexed and the distal limb relaxed.

- The injection site is between the heel bulbs just proximal to the coronary band. Local anesthesia at the site of the injection or perineural anesthesia may be used to provide skin analgesia prior to the injection.
- A 3-1/2-inch, 18- or 20-gauge spinal needle is inserted between the heel bulbs and advanced along a sagittal plane aiming for a point 1 cm below the coronary band, midway between the toe and the heel (Figure 1.114).
- The needle is advanced until bone is contacted, and radiographic or fluoroscopic documentation of the needle's location is recommended in most cases.
- Usually only 2 to 3 mL of anesthetic can be injected and flexing the lower limb will decrease the resistance to injection (Figure 1.114; Video 1.37).
- Placing the limb on a wooden block that unweights the heel and flexes the distal limb or placing the forelimb within a padded hoof stand can help facilitate the injection.

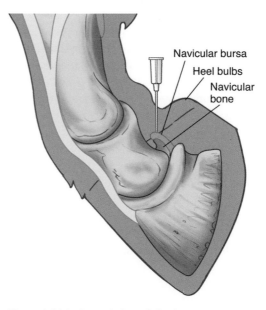

Figure 1.114 Lateral view of the foot demonstrating the correct angulation of the spinal needle to enter the navicular bursa using the palmar approach between the heel bulbs.

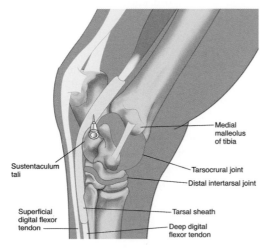

Figure 1.113 Injection site for the tarsal sheath.

Pitfalls:
1) Needle directed too proximally and enters the DIP joint.
2) Excessive pressure when injecting—unweight the limb or needle may be against the navicular bone.
3) Anesthesia of palmar soft tissues of the foot due to extravasation of anesthetic.
4) Damage to DDFT from spinal needle.

Podotrochlear (Navicular) Bursa – Abaxial Approach (Medial or Lateral)
- The abaxial approach to the navicular bursa is typically performed with the limb weight-bearing either from the medial or lateral sides just proximal to the collateral cartilages but can also be done with the carpus flexed and the distal limb relaxed.
- Two lateral techniques that do not penetrate the DDFT have been described – one technique was performed in the standing horse using radiographic guidance, and the other used ultrasound to guide the needle into the bursa with the foot placed in a navicular block.
- The injection site for both approaches is along the proximal and dorsoproximal margin of the collateral cartilage, and an 18- to 20-gauge, 3.5-inch (8.9-cm) needle is angled approximately 45° to the horizontal plane toward the 10 o'clock (right front) or 2 o'clock (left front) position (Figure 1.115). The needle is directed beneath the DDFT and DFTS to enter the bursa.
- The primary advantage of the abaxial approach is that the needle does not penetrate the DDFT, which may decrease the morbidity associated with the injection.
- A similar technique can also be performed with the limb unweighted (Video 1.38) and is the same approach that is used for endoscopic entry.

  Pitfalls:
  1) Difficulty of placing the needle at the correct angle and entering DFTS and DIP joint.

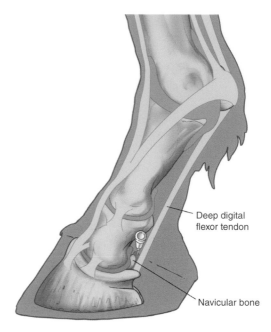

Deep digital flexor tendon

Navicular bone

Figure 1.115 Lateral (abaxial) approach to the navicular bursa that avoids penetrating the DDFT. The spinal needle is inserted just above the collateral cartilage and angled at approximately 45° to the horizontal plane to enter the bursa.

2) Excessive pressure when injecting – needle may be against the navicular bone.
3) Anesthesia of palmar soft tissues of the foot due to extravasation of anesthetic.

Calcaneal Bursa – Lateral Approach
- The lateral approach to the calcaneal bursa is usually performed with limb weight-bearing or with the tarsal slightly flexed.
- The calcaneal bursa is located between the SDFT and the caudal aspect of the calcaneus and when distended, the bursa has synovial outpouchings medial and lateral to the tendon both proximal and distal to the SDFT retinaculum. These can often be seen as four distinct pockets of fluid surrounding the point of the hock.
- Synovial aspiration is best performed using the lateral approach either above or below the SDFT retinaculum. The injection site is 1 cm dorsal to the SDFT and 1 cm distal or proximal to the lateral aspect of the SDFT retinaculum (Figure 1.116).

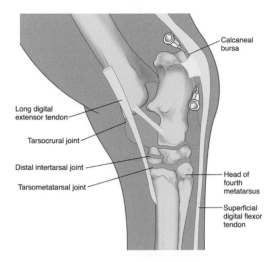

Figure 1.116 Injection sites for the calcaneal bursa are located either above or below the retinaculum of the SDFT. These injection sites can be difficult to find without effusion.

- A 1.5-inch, 20-gauge needle is angled slightly proximally or distally within these outpouchings to avoid the SDFT. 8–12 mL of anesthetic is recommended.

  Pitfalls:
  1) Contacting bone—needle usually hitting calcaneus.
  2) Excessive pressure when injecting – needle against or within the SDFT.
  3) Inability to obtain synovial fluid.

Bicipital Bursa – Distal Approach

- The distal approach to the bicipital bursa is performed with limb weight-bearing and ultrasound can be very helpful to guide the injection.
- The cranial prominence of the lateral tuberosity of the humerus is used as the landmark and the injection site is 2.5 inches (5–6 cm) distal and 3 inches (7–8 cm) caudal to this prominence.
- A 3-1/2-inch, 18- to 20-gauge spinal needle is directed proximomedially toward the intertuberal groove until it contacts the humerus. The depth of the needle depends on the size of the horse, but a 3-1/2-inch spinal needle

usually is inserted to the hub in most mature horses (Figure 1.117a). 20–30 mL of anesthetic is recommended.

- A variation of this approach uses the deltoid tuberosity of the humerus as a landmark, and the needle is inserted 1.5 inches proximal to the distal aspect of the deltoid tuberosity and directed proximomedially (toward the opposite ear) to a depth of 2 to 3 inches.
- **Pitfalls:**
1) Needle directed too superficially and does not enter bursa.
2) Inability to aspirate synovial fluid—not uncommon.
3) Difficulty palpating the deltoid tuberosity to determine correct needle placement.

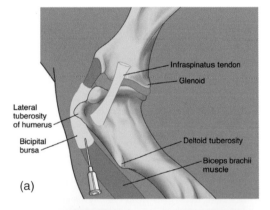

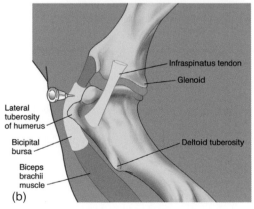

Figure 1.117 Distal (a) and proximal (b) approaches to the bicipital bursa from the lateral aspect of the limb in the standing horse.

Bicipital Bursa – Proximal Approach

- The proximal approach to the bicipital bursa is performed with limb weight-bearing and ultrasound can be very helpful to guide the injection.
- The proximal approach is performed in the intertuberal groove, which can be palpated medial to the edge of the cranial prominence of the lateral tuberosity of the humerus.
- A 1.5-inch, 20-gauge needle is inserted into the intertuberal groove in a plane parallel to the bearing surface of the foot at about a 45° angle to the sagittal axis of the horse until the needle strikes cartilage (Figure 1.117b).
- The primary advantages of the proximal approach compared with the distal approach are a slightly improved accuracy of entering the bursa and not needing a 3-1/2-inch spinal needle.
- **Pitfalls:**
1) Difficulty palpating the site of injection.
2) Inability to aspirate synovial fluid.

Trochanteric Bursa

- The approaches to the trochanteric bursa are performed with limb weight-bearing and ultrasound can be very helpful to guide the injection.
- The trochanteric bursa is located beneath the tendon of insertion of the middle gluteal muscle on the cranial aspect of the greater trochanter of the femur.
- The site for injection is between the tendon and the lateral surface of the greater trochanter at the most cranial aspect of the palpable greater trochanter. A 1.5-inch (3.8-cm), 18-gauge needle (may need longer needle in large horses) is inserted and directed horizontally at right angles to the sagittal plane until bone is encountered. 7–10 mL of anesthetic is recommended.
- An alternate approach is to direct the needle medially through the middle gluteal muscle directly over the bursa toward the trochanter. Positioning the limb caudally with the foot non-weight-bearing and on a Hickman block has been reported to facilitate centesis of the trochanteric bursa.
- **Pitfalls:**
1) Difficulty palpating landmarks for site of injection.
2) Inability to aspirate synovial fluid.

Bibliography

1 Adams SB, Moore GE, Elrashidy M, et al.: 2010. Effect of needle size and type, reuse of needles, insertion speed, and removal of hair on contamination of joints with tissue debris and hair after arthrocentesis. *Vet Surg* 39:667–673.
2 Arkell M, Archer RM, Guitian FJ, et al.: 2006. Evidence of bias affecting the interpretation of the results of local anesthetic nerve blocks when assessing lameness in horses. *Vet Rec* 159:346–349.
3 Armentrout AR, Beard WL, White BJ, et al.: 2012. A comparative study of proximal flexion in horses: 5 versus 60 seconds. *Equine Vet J* 44:420–424.
4 Back W, MacAllister CG, van Heel MCV, et al.: 2007. Vertical front limb ground reaction forces of sound and lame Warmbloods differ from those in Quarter horses. *J Equine Vet Sci* 27:123–129.
5 Baxter GM, Stashak TS: 2011. Examination for Lameness. *In*: Baxter GM (ed) *Adams and Stashak's Lameness in Horses*, *Sixth Edition*, Ames, IA, Wiley-Blackwell 109–150.
6 Baxter GM: 2020. Perineural and Intrasynovial Anesthesia. *In*: Baxter GM (ed) *Adams and Stashak's Lameness in Horses*, *Seventh Edition*, Ames, IA, Wiley-Blackwell 157–188.
7 Bell RP, Reed SK, Schoonover MJ, et al.: 2016. Associations of force plate and body-mounted inertial sensor measurements for identification of hind limb lameness in horses. *Am J Vet Res* 77:337–345.
8 Bidwell LA, Brown KE, Cordier A, et al.: 2004. Mepivacaine local anesthetic duration in equine palmar digital nerve blocks. *Equine Vet J* 36:723–726.

9 Buchner HH, Savelberg HH, Schamhardt HC, et al.: 1996. Limb movement adaptations in horses with experimentally induced fore- or hindlimb lameness. *Equine Vet J* 28:63–70.

10 Buchner HH, Savelberg HH, Schamhardt HC, et al.: 1996. Head and trunk movement adaptations in horses with experimentally induced fore - or hindlimb lameness. *Equine Vet J* 28:71–76.

11 Busschers E, van Weeren PR: 2001. Use of the flexion test of the distal forelimb in the sound horse: Repeatability and effect of age, gender, weight, height and fetlock joint range of motion. *J Vet Med A Physiol Pathol Clin Med* 48:413–427.

12 Carter GK, Hogan PM: 1996. Use of diagnostic nerve blocks in lameness evaluation. *Proc Am Assoc Equine Pract* 42:26–32.

13 Castro FA, Schumacher JS, Pauwels F, et al.: 2005. A new approach for perineural injection of the lateral palmar nerve in the horse. *Vet Surg* 34:539–542.

14 Churchill EA: 1979. The methodology of diagnosis of hind leg lameness. *Proc Am Assoc Equine Pract* 25:297–304.

15 Claunch KM, Eggleston RB, Baxter GM: 2014. Effects of approach and injection volume on diffusion of mepivacaine hydrochloride during local analgesia of the deep branch of the lateral plantar nerve in horses. *J Am Vet Med Assoc* 245:1153–1159.

16 Contino EK, King MR, Valdes-Martinez A, et al.: 2015. In vivo diffusion characteristics following perineural injection of the deep branch of the lateral plantar nerve with mepivacaine or iohexol in horses. *Equine vet J* 47:230–234.

17 Daniel AJ, Goodrich LR, Barrett MF, et al.: 2016. An optimized injection technique for the navicular bursa that avoids the deep digital flexor tendon. *Equine Vet J* 48:159–164.

18 David F, Rougier M, Alexander K, et al.: 2007. Ultrasound-guided coxofemoral arthrocentesis in horses. *Equine Vet J* 39:79–83

19 Denoix JM, Jacquet S: 2008. Ultrasound-guided injections of the sacroiliac area in horses. *Equine Vet Educ* 20:203–207.

20 Dyson S, Murray R: 2003. Pain associated with the sacroiliac joint region: A clinical study of 74 horses. *Equine Vet J* 35:240–245.

21 Dyson SJ, Arthur RM, Palmer SE, et al.: 1995. Suspensory ligament desmitis. *Vet Clin North Am Equine Pract* 11:177–215.

22 Dyson SJ, Romero JM: 1993. An investigation of injection techniques for local analgesia of the equine distal tarsus and proximal metatarsus. *Equine Vet J* 25:30–35.

23 Engeli E, Haussler KK, Erb HN: 2004. Development and validation of a periarticular injection technique of the sacroiliac joint in horses. *Equine Vet J* 36:324–330.

24 Fiske-Jacksonn A: 2015. Objective lameness assessment: can it really tell us anything different? *Livestock* 20:173–178.

25 Ford TS, Ross MW, Orsini PG: 1988. Communication and boundaries of the middle carpal and carpometacarpal joints in horses. *Am J Vet Res* 49:2161–2164.

26 Fuller CJ, Bladon BM, Driver AJ, et al.: 2006. The intra- and inter-assessor reliability of measurement of functional outcome by lameness scoring in horses. *Vet J* 171:281–286.

27 Galisteo AM, Cano MR, Morales JL, et al.: 1997. Kinematics in horses at the trot before and after induced forelimb supporting lameness. *Equine Vet J Suppl* 23:97–101.

28 Gayle JM, Redding WR: 2007. Comparison of diagnostic anaesthetic techniques of the proximal metatarsus in the horse. *Equine Vet Educ*:222–224.

29 Gough MR, Munroe GA, Mayhew G: 2002. Diffusion of mepivacaine between adjacent synovial structures in the horse. Part 2: tarsus and stifle. *Equine Vet J* 34:85–90.

30 Grant BD: 1996. Bursal Injections. *Proc Am Assoc Equine Pract* 42:64–68.

31 Greve L, Pfau T, Dyson S: 2017. Thoracolumbar movement in sound horses trotting in straight lines in hand and on the lunge and the relationship with hind limb symmetry or asymmetry. *Vet J* 220:95–104.

32 Hague BA, Honnas CM, Simpson RB, et al.: 1997. Evaluation of skin bacterial flora before and after aseptic preparation of clipped and nonclipped arthrocentesis sites in horses. *Vet Surg* 26:121–125.

33 Hammarberg M, Egenvall A, Pfau T, et al.: 2016. Rater agreement of visual lameness assessment in horses during lungeing. *Equine Vet J* 48:78–92.

34 Hassel DM, Stover SM, Yarbrough TB, et al.: 2000. Palmar-plantar axial sesamoidean approach to the digital flexor sheath in horses. *J Am Vet Med Assoc* 217:1343–1347.

35 Hendrickson DA, Nixon AJ: 1992. A lateral approach for synovial fluid aspiration and joint injection of the femoropatellar joint of the horse. *Equine Vet J* 24: 397–398.

36 Hewetson M, Christley RM, Hunt ID, et al.: 2006. Investigations of the reliability of observational gait analysis for the assessment of lameness in horses. *Vet Rec* 158:852–857.

37 Hoerdemann M, Smith RL, Hosgood G: 2017. Duration of action of mepivacaine and lidocaine in equine palmar digital perineural blocks in an experimental lameness model. *Vet Surg* 46:986–993.

38 Hughes TK, Eliashar E, Smith RK: 2007. In vitro evaluation of a single injection technique for diagnostic analgesia of the proximal suspensory ligament of the equine pelvic limb. *Vet Surg* 36:760–764.

39 Ingle-Fehr JE, Baxter GM: 1998. Endoscopy of the calcaneal bursa in horses. *Vet Surg* 27:561–567.

40 Ishihara A, Bertone AL, Rajala-Schultz PJ: 2005. Association between subjective lameness grade and kinetic gait parameters in horses with experimentally induced forelimb lameness. *Am J Vet Res* 66:1805–1815.

41 Jordana M, Martens A, Duchateau L, et al.: 2014. Distal limb desensitization following analgesia of the digital flexor tendon sheath in horses using four different techniques. *Equine Vet J* 46:488–493.

42 Just EM, Patan B, Licka TF: 2007. Dorsolateral approach for arthrocentesis of the centrodistal joint in horses. *Am J Vet Res* 68:946–952.

43 Kaido M, Kilborne AH, Sizemore JL, et al.: 2016. Effects of repetition within trials and frequency of trial session on quantitative parameters of vertical force peak in horses with naturally occurring lameness. *Am J Vet Res* 77:756–765.

44 Keegan KG, Dent EV, Wilson DA, et al.: 2010. Repeatability of subjective evaluation of lameness in horses. *Equine Vet J* 42:92–97.

45 Keegan KG, Kramer J, Yonezawa Y, et al. Assessment of repeatability of a wireless, inertial sensor-based lameness evaluation system for horses. *Am J Vet Res* 2011;72:1156–1163.

46 Keegan KG, MacAllister CG, Wilson DA, et al.: 2012. Comparison of an inertial sensor system with a stationary force plate for evaluation of horses with bilateral forelimb lameness. *Am J Vet Res* 73:368–374.

47 Keegan KG, Pai PF, Wilson DA, et al.: 2001. Signal decomposition method of evaluating head movement to measure induced forelimb lameness in horses trotting on a treadmill. *Equine Vet J* 33:446–451.

48 Keegan KG, Wilson DA, Kramer J, et al.: 2013. Comparison of a body-mounted inertial sensor system-based method with subjective evaluation for detection of lameness in horses. *Am J Vet Res* 74:17–24.

49 Keegan KG, Wilson DA, Kramer J: 2004. How to evaluate head and pelvic movement to determine lameness. *Proc Am Assoc Equine Pract* 50:206–211.

50 Keegan KG, Wilson DA, Smith BK, et al.: 2000. Changes in kinematic variables observed during pressure-induced forelimb lameness in adult horses trotting on a treadmill. *Am J Vet Res* 61:612–619.

51 Keegan KG, Yonezawa Y, Pai PF, et al.: 2004. Evaluation of a sensor-based system of equine motion analysis for the detection and quantification of forelimb and hindlimb lameness in horses. *Am J Vet Res* 65:665–670.

52 Keegan KG: 2007. Evidence-based lameness detection and quantification. *Vet Clin North Am Equine Pract* 23:403–423.

53 Keg PR, Barneveld A, Schamhardt HC, et al.: 1994. Clinical and force plate evaluation of the effect of a high plantar nerve block in lameness caused by induced mid-metatarsal tendinitis. *Vet Q* 16 Suppl 2:S70–75.

54 Keg PR, van Weeren PR, Back W, et al.: 1997. Influence of the force applied and its period of application on the outcome of the flexion test of the distal forelimb of the horse. *Vet Rec* 141:463–466.

55 Kramer J, Keegan KG, Wilson DA, et al.: 2000 Kinematics of the equine hindlimb in trotting horses after induced distal tarsal lameness and distal tarsal anesthesia. *Am J Vet Res* 61:1031–1036.

56 Lewis RD: 1996. Techniques for arthrocentesis of equine shoulder, elbow, stifle and hip joints. *Proc Am Assoc Equine Pract* 42:55–63.

57 Maliye S, Marshall JF: 2016. Objective assessment of the compensatory effect on clinical hind limb lameness in horses: 37 cases. *J Am Vet Med Assoc* 249:940–944.

58 Maliye S, Voute L, Lund D, et al.: 2013. An inertial sensor-based system can objectively assess diagnostic anaesthesia of the equine foot. *Equine Vet J Suppl* 45;26–30.

59 Marshall JF, Lund DG, Voute LC: 2012. Use of a wireless, inertial sensor-based system to objectively evaluate flexion tests in the horse. *Equine Vet J* 43:8–11.

60 Mattoon JS, Drost WT, Grguric MR, et al.; 2004. Technique for equine cervical articular process joint injection. *Vet Radiol Ultrasound* 45:238–240.

61 Miller SM, Stover SM: 1996. Palmaro-proximal approach for arthrocentesis of the proximal interphalangeal joint in the horse. *Equine Vet J* 28:376–380.

62 Misheff MM, Stover SM: 1991. A comparison of two techniques for arthrocentesis of the metacarpophalangeal joint. *Equine Vet J* 23:273–276.

63 Moorman VJ, Frisbie DD, Kawcak CE, et al.: 2017. Effects of sensor position on kinematic data obtained with an inertial sensor system during gait analysis of trotting horses. *J Am Vet Med Assoc* 250:548–553.

64 Moyer W, Schumacher J, Schumacher J: 2007. *A Guide to Equine Joint Injection and Regional Anesthesia.*PA, Learning Systems, Veterinary Yardley, 6–65.

65 Nagy A, Bodo G, Dyson SJ: 2012. Diffusion of contrast medium after four different techniques for analgesia of the proximal metacarpal region: an in vivo and in vitro study. *Equine Vet J* 44:668–673.

66 Nottrott K, De Guio C, Khairoun A, et al.: 2017. An ultrasound-guided, tendon sparing, lateral approach to injection of the navicular bursa. *Equine Vet J* 49:655–661.

67 Peham C, Licka T, Girtler D, et al.; 2001. Hindlimb lameness: Clinical judgement versus computerized symmetry measurement. *Vet Rec* 148:750–752.

68 Pfau T, Boultbee H, Davis H, et al.: 2016. Agreement between 2 inertial sensor systems for lameness examinations in horses. *Equine Vet Educ* 28:203–208.

69 Pfau T, Jennings C, Mitchell H, et al.: 2016. Lungeing on hard and soft surfaces: Movement symmetry of trotting horses considered sound by their owners. *Equine Vet J* 48:83–89.

70 Pfau T, Noordwijk K, Sepulveda Caviedes MR, et al.: 2018. Head, withers and pelvic movement asymmetry and their relative timing in trot in racing Thoroughbreds in training. *Equine Vet J* 50:117–124

71 Pfau T, Spicer-Jenkins C, Smith RK, et al.: 2014. Identifying optimal parameters for quantification of changes in pelvic movement asymmetry as a response to diagnostic analgesia in the hindlimbs of horses. *Equine Vet J* 46:759–763.

72 Pfau T, Sepulveda Caviedes, MF, McCarthy R, et al.: 2018. Comparison of visual lameness scores to gait asymmetry in racing Thoroughbreds during trot in-hand. *Equine Vet Educ* doi: 10.1111/eve.12914.

73 Piccot-Crezollet C, Cauvin ER, Lepage OM: 2005. Comparison of two techniques for injection of the podo-trochlear bursa in horses. *J Am Vet Med Assoc* 226: 1524–1527.

74 Poore LA, Lambert KL, Shaw DJ, et al.: 2011. Comparison of three methods of injecting the proximal interphalangeal joint in horses. *Vet Rec* 168:302.

75 Rhodin M, Roepstorff L, French A, et al.: 2016. Head and pelvic movement asymmetry during lungeing in horses with symmetrical movement on the straight. *Equine Vet J* 48:315–320.

76 Rocconi RA, Sampson SN: 2013. Comparison of basilar and axial sesamoidean approaches for digital flexor tendon sheath synoviocentesis and injection in horses. *J Am Vet Med Assoc* 243:869–873.

77 Ross MW: 2011. Manipulation and Movement. *In*: Ross MW, Dyson SJ (eds) *Diagnosis and Management of Lameness in the Horse*, St. Louis MO, Elsevier, 64–88.

78 Rungsri PK, Staecker W, Leelamankong P, et al.: 2014. Use of body-mounted inertial sensors to objectively evaluate the response to perineural analgesia of the distal limb and intra-articular analgesia of the distal interphalangeal joint in horses with forelimb lameness. *J Equine Vet Sci* 34:972–977.

79 Sack WO, Orsini PG: 1981. Distal intertarsal and tarsometatarsal joints in the horse: Communication and injection sites. *J Am Vet Med Assoc* 179:355–359.

80 Sams AE, Honnas CM, Sack WO, et al.: 1993. Communication of the ulnaris lateralis bursa with the equine elbow joint and evaluation of caudal arthrocentesis. *Equine Vet J* 25:130–133.

81 Schneeweiss W, Puggioni A, David F: 2012. Comparison of ultrasound-guided vs. 'blind' techniques for intra-synovial injections of the shoulder are in horses: Scapulohumeral joint, bicipital and infraspinatus bursae. *Equine Vet J* 44:674–678.

82 Schumacher J, de Graves F, Steiger R, et al.: 2001. A comparison of the effects of two volumes of local analgesic solution in the distal interphalangeal joint of horses with lameness caused by solar toe or solar heel pain. *Equine Vet J* 33:265–268.

83 Schumacher J, Livesey L, Brawner W, et al.: 2007. Comparison of 2 methods of centesis of the bursa of the biceps brachii tendon of horses. *Equine Vet J* 39: 356–359.

84 Schumacher J, Schramme MC, Schumacher J, et al.: 2003. A review of recent studies concerning diagnostic analgesia of the equine forefoot. *Proc Am Assoc Equine Pract* 49:312–316.

85 Schumacher J, Schumacher J, Schramme MC: 2004. Diagnostic analgesia of the equine forefoot. *Equine Vet Educ* 16:199–204.

86 Seabaugh KA, Selberg KT, Mueller POE, et al.: 2017. Clinical study evaluating the accuracy of injecting the distal tarsal joints in the horse. *Equine Vet J* 49:668–672.

87 Seabaugh KA, Selberg KT, Valdes-Martinez A, et al.: 2011. Assessment of the tissue diffusion of anesthetic agent following administration of a low palmar nerve block in horses. *J Am Vet Med Assoc* 239:1334–1340.

88 Southwood LL, Baxter GM, Fehr JE: 1997. How to perform arthrocentesis of the fetlock joint by using a distal palmar (plantar) approach. *Proc Am Assoc Equine Pract* 43:151–153.

89 Spoormakers TJ, Donker SH, Ensink JM: 2004. Diagnostic anaesthesia of the equine lower limb: A comparison of lidocaine and lidocaine with epinephrine. *Tijdschr Diergeneeskd* 129:548–551.

90 Stack JD. Bergamino C, Sanders R, et al.: 2016. Comparison of two ultrasound-guided injection techniques targeting the sacroiliac joint region in equine cadavers. *Vet Comp Orthop Traumatol* 29:386–393.

91 Starke SD, May SA, Pfau T: 2015. Understanding hind limb lameness signs in horses using simple rigid body mechanics. *J Biomech* 48:3323–3331.

92 Starke SD, Willems E, Head M, et al.: 2012. Proximal hindlimb flexion in the horse: Effect on movement symmetry and implications for defining soundness. *Equine Vet J* 44:657–663.

93 Steel CM, Pannirselvam RR, Anderson GA: 2013. Risk of septic arthritis after intra-articular medication: A study of 16,624 injections in Thoroughbred racehorses. *Aust Vet J* 91:268–273.

94 Swiderski CE, Linford R: 2005. How to inject the medial femorotibial joint: an alternate approach. *Proc Am Assoc Equine Pract* 51:476–480.

95 Toth F, Schumacher J, Schramme M, et al.: 2011. Evaluation of four techniques for injecting the trochanteric bursa of horses. *Vet Surg* 40:489–493.

96 Toth F, Schumacher J, Schramme MC, et al.: 2014. Effects of anesthetizing individual compartments of the stifle joint in horses with experimentally induced stifle lameness. *Am J Vet Res* 75:19–25.

97 Turner TA: 2006. How to subjectively and objectively examine the equine foot. *Proc Am Assoc Equine Pract* 52:531–537.

98 Vacek JR, Ford TS, Honnas CM: 1992. Communication between the femoropatellar and medial and lateral femorotibial joints in horses. *Am J Vet Res* 53: 1431–1434.

99 Vazquez de Mercado R, Stover SM, Taylor KT, et al.: 1998. Lateral approach for arthrocentesis of the distal interphalangeal joint in horses. *J Am Vet Med Assoc* 212:1413–1418.

100 Verschooten F, Verbeeck J: 1997. Flexion test of the metacarpophalangeal and interphalangeal joints and flexion angle of the metacarpophalangeal joint in sound horses. *Equine Vet J* 29:50–54.

101 Weishaupt MA: 2005. Compensatory load redistribution in forelimb and hind limb lameness. *Proc Am Assoc Equine Pract* 51: 141–148.

102 Weishaupt MA: 2008. Adaptation strategies of horses with lameness. *Vet Clin North Am Equine Pract* 24: 79–100.

Revised from Chapter 2, "Examination for Lameness" in *Adams and Stashak's Lameness in Horses, 7th Edition,* by Gary M. Baxter, Kevin G. Keegan, and Ted S. Stashak.

2

Common Conditions of the Foot

Navicular Region and Soft Tissue Injuries of the Foot

Navicular Disease/Syndrome

Overview

- Navicular disease or syndrome is estimated to be responsible for one-third of all chronic forelimb lameness in horses.
- Quarter horses, Thoroughbreds, and Warmbloods, particularly geldings, are at greatest risk, whereas it is rarely diagnosed in ponies or Arabians.
- The true definition of navicular disease/syndrome is variable as "navicular disease," "navicular syndrome," "palmar heel pain," or "palmar foot syndrome" are all terms that are used to describe horses that block to a low palmar digital (PD) nerve block.
- The disease/syndrome may be associated with pain arising from the navicular bone itself, collateral suspensory ligaments (CSLs) of the navicular bone, distal sesamoidean impar ligament (DSIL), navicular bursa, deep digital flexor tendon (DDFT), or any combination of these.
- A multitude of abnormalities within the foot can be desensitized with a PD block; therefore, a PD block is not specific for navicular disease/syndrome (Box 2.1).

Anatomy

- The palmar/plantar aspect of the foot is a complicated anatomic region that is intended to absorb many of the forces of weight-bearing.

- Important anatomic structures in this location include the heel bulbs, digital cushion, collateral (ungual) cartilages, navicular bone, navicular bursa, DDFT, distal phalanx, and DIP joint (Figure 2.1).
- The navicular bone itself is supported in position by three ligaments comprising the navicular suspensory apparatus – medial and lateral collateral sesamoidean ligaments proximally and the DSIL (Figures 2.1 and 2.2). Injuries to the navicular suspensory apparatus can occur concurrently in horses with navicular disease/syndrome.
- Innervation of the navicular region, heel bulbs, DIP joint, sole, and toe (essentially the entire foot) is from the PD nerve.
- Although a direct connection between the DIP joint and navicular bursa is rare, passive diffusion of injected dye, anesthetic, and medications can occur.

Imaging

- Radiography is usually the initial imaging tool, even though the lack of abnormalities in the navicular bone does not eliminate the bone as the site of the pain, and concurrent soft tissue injuries are common.
- A complete radiographic evaluation of the navicular bone requires a minimum of lateromedial, 60° dorsoproximal to palmarodistal oblique, and palmaroproximal to palmarodistal oblique (skyline) high-quality views. A 60° dorsoproximal to palmarodistal

Manual of Equine Lameness, Second Edition. Gary M. Baxter.
© 2022 John Wiley & Sons, Inc. Published 2022 by John Wiley & Sons, Inc.
Companion website: www.wiley.com/go/baxter/manual

Box 2.1   Abnormalities that may exist in horses classified as having navicular disease, navicular syndrome, palmar foot syndrome, or palmar heel pain

1) Navicular disease: radiographic, CT, or MRI abnormalities within the navicular bone
2) Desmitis/trauma of the podotrochlear apparatus
   a) CSLs of the navicular bone
   b) Desmitis of the DSIL
   c) Desmitis of the distal digital annular ligament
3) Tendonitis of the DDFT: usually at three locations

   a) The insertion
   b) Palmar to the navicular bone
   c) Proximal to the navicular bone
4) Desmitis of the collateral ligaments (CLs) of the DIP joint
5) Navicular bursitis
6) Synovitis/capsulitis/OA of the DIP joint
7) Primary hoof imbalances (improper trimming or shoeing)
8) Hoof capsule and/or heel distortions

---

oblique view of the distal phalanx and the weight-bearing dorsopalmar (DP) view are often included to completely evaluate all bony structures in the foot.

- Computed tomography (CT) is the best modality to detect and assess pathology within the cortex and trabeculae of the navicular bone but is less useful to detect soft tissue pathology. Intra-arterial contrast-enhanced CT has been shown to improve the imaging of soft tissue structures, and may be an alternative to using magnetic resonance imaging (MRI).
- MRI is currently the preferred imaging technique (recumbent or standing) after radiography to assess horses with navicular disease/syndrome. The different sequences permit accurate evaluation of soft tissues, cartilage, and bone within the digit in near anatomic detail.
- Ultrasonography and scintigraphy are usually not that beneficial in most horses with navicular disease/syndrome.

Etiology

- The two proposed causes of navicular disease are vascular compromise and biomechanical abnormalities leading to tissue degeneration. Wear and tear of the navicular apparatus from repetitive stress and biomechanical forces is considered the most likely cause.
- Excessive and repetitive force applied to the distal third of the navicular bone by the DDFT is a major contributor to the disease.
- Poor hoof conformation and balance, particularly the long-toe, low-heel hoof conformation accompanied by the broken-back hoof-pastern axis (HPA) is considered major risk factors (Figure 2.3).
- Factors such as excessive bodyweight, small feet, broken pastern angles, long toes, low heels, hoof imbalances, work on hard surfaces, etc., are likely to increase the forces/unit area of the navicular bone and podotrochlear apparatus (Figure 1.2).
- Pathologic changes to the navicular bone include cartilage erosion, subchondral bone sclerosis associated with thickening of the trabeculae, focal areas of lysis, edema, congestion, and fibrosis in the marrow spaces. Damage to the fibrocartilage together with DDFT fibrillation may predispose to adhesion formation between the tendon and the bone (Figure 2.4).
- Primary damage to the DDFT without damage to the navicular bone can also occur and

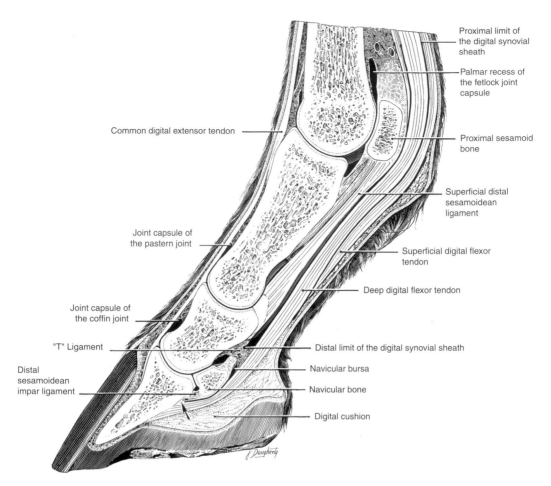

Figure 2.1 Sagittal section of equine fetlock and digit. *Source*: Courtesy of J Daugherty.

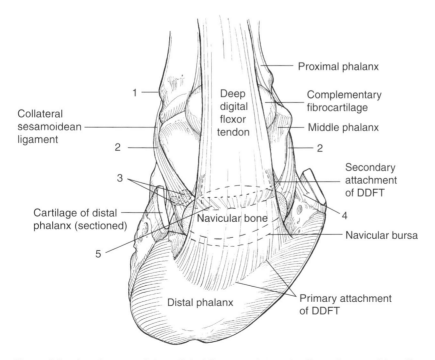

Figure 2.2 Attachments of deep digital flexor tendon and collateral sesamoidean ligaments (CSLs). (1) Attachment of CSL to proximal phalanx, (2) attachment of CSL to middle phalanx, (3) abaxial outpocketings of palmar pouch of the synovial cavity of the distal interphalangeal joint, (4) attachment of CSL to cartilage of the distal phalanx, and (5) attachment of medial and lateral CSLs to navicular bone.

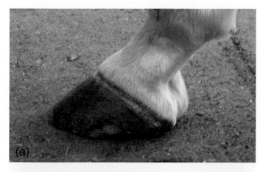

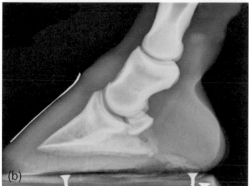

Figure 2.3 Front foot (a) and lateral radiograph (b) of a horse with a reverse or negative angle of P3 that is thought to predispose to problems in the palmar aspect of the foot.

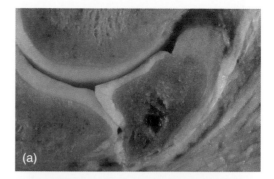

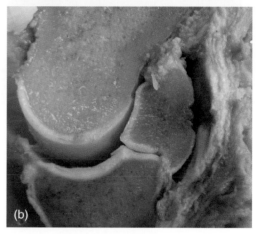

Figure 2.4 Cross sections of the navicular bone at necropsy demonstrating cyst-like lesions within the body of the navicular bone (a) and degeneration of the flexor cortex (b). The horse in (b) also had surface fibrillation of the DDFT.

concurrent soft tissue injuries to the podotrochlear apparatus (CSL, DSIL) are not uncommon.

- In most horses, lameness is due to a combination of bone and soft tissue injuries.

Clinical Signs

- The classic signalment is a middle-aged or older Quarter horse gelding with a history of a progressive, chronic, unilateral, or bilateral forelimb lameness.
- The history may include a gradual loss of performance, stiffness, shortening of the stride, loss of action, unwillingness to turn, and increased lameness when worked on hard surfaces.
- Unilateral lameness can be seen especially with lesions that involve the flexor surface of the navicular bone and/or the DDFT.

- Most horses will be more lame in one forelimb, both at a straight trot and when circled on a hard surface but will often demonstrate lameness on the opposite forelimb when circled with that limb on the inside. The lameness will often switch to the opposite (less lame limb) forelimb following a PD block of the lame forelimb.
- Common hoof problems seen in horses with navicular disease/syndrome include low, underrun heels, contracted or collapsed heels, medial to lateral imbalances, and long toes (Figure 1.2).
- At exercise, most horses will exhibit a mild-to-moderate lameness (2 to 3/5) that is worse on the inside limb when circled on a hard

surface. Horses with bilateral lameness tend to have a stiff, shuffling gait and often carry their head and neck rigidly.

- Most horses will demonstrate pain with hoof testers over the central and occasionally the cranial third of the frog. However, a negative response to hoof testers does not rule out navicular syndrome/disease. Horses with very thick soles and hard frogs may not respond to hoof tester pressure.
- Effusion of the DIP joint may be present in some horses but is not a consistent clinical feature.

Diagnosis

- Diagnosis begins with localizing the site of lameness to the foot or more specifically to the palmar aspect of the foot using a low PD block. The majority of horses will improve substantially (>80%) following a PD block and the lameness in the opposite forelimb will either worsen or become apparent if a unilateral lameness was initially present.
- Intrasynovial anesthesia of the DIP joint can be performed to further localize the site of pain but is not specific for the joint. The degree of improvement in lameness following DIP joint anesthesia is usually less than that following a PD block in most horses with navicular disease/syndrome.
- Anesthesia of the navicular bursa is probably the most specific nerve block that can be used to localize the site of pain to the navicular region but is not performed routinely by most clinicians.
- Radiography is usually the initial imaging tool, even though the lack of abnormalities in the navicular bone does not eliminate the bone as the site of the pain.
- The radiographic abnormalities that appear to be the most reliable indicators of navicular disease/syndrome are cyst-like lesions within the medullary cavity (Figure 2.5), sclerosis of the spongiosa with loss of demarcation of the flexor cortex and medulla (Figure 2.6a), and flexor cortex lesions (Figure 2.6).
- Other radiographic abnormalities that are usually present in lame horses include
  1) Large enthesophytes at the proximomedial and proximolateral aspect of the bone (Figure 2.7).

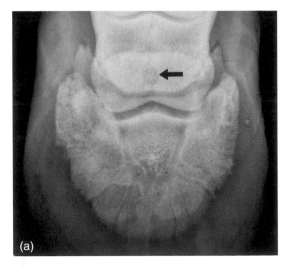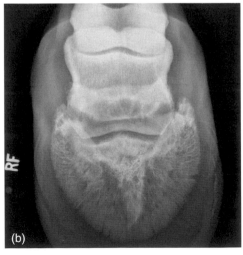

Figure 2.5 Single, large cystic lesion (a; arrow) and multiple cystic lesions (b; arrow) within the navicular bone demonstrated on oblique radiographs of two different horses (a and b) with signs of navicular syndrome.

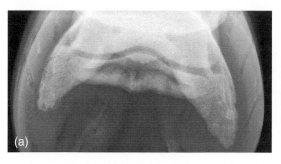 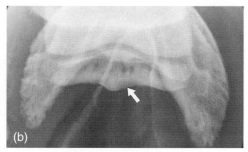

Figure 2.6 Skyline radiographs of the same horse as in Figure 2.9 (a) demonstrating sclerosis of the medullary cavity of the navicular bone and erosions along the flexor surface. (b) A single, large erosive lesion on the flexor surface of the navicular bone (arrow) in a horse with severe unilateral lameness.

2) Proximal or distal extension of the flexor border of the bone.
3) Distal border fragments (Figure 2.8).
4) Numerous (>7) large and variably shaped distal border radiolucent zones.
5) Discrete radiolucent areas in the spongiosa with or without detectable communication with the flexor cortex.
6) Increased thickness of the flexor cortex with or without defects or erosions.
7) New bone at the sagittal ridge.
8) Sclerosis of the spongiosa.
9) A bipartite bone.
10) Mineralization of the supporting ligaments of the navicular bone or the DDFT.

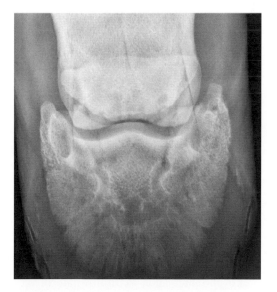

Figure 2.7 Multiple abnormalities within the navicular bone as seen on an oblique radiograph. Abnormalities include remodeling along the proximal border, multiple cystic lesions along the distal border, and enthesophytes on the wings of the navicular bone.

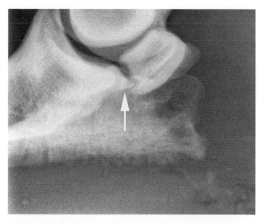

Figure 2.8 Fracture fragment from the distal border of the navicular bone (arrow) can be seen on this lateral radiograph. Their presence may be due to fracture from the distal border of the navicular, fracture of enthesophyte at the origin of the DSIL, or ectopic mineralization in the DSIL.

- Flexor cortex defects are seen in less than 1% of normal horses and represent lysis of subchondral bone and are linked to fibrocartilage degeneration and concurrent damage to the DDFT (Figures 2.6 and 2.9).
- The most common abnormalities found on MRI involve the navicular bone, CSL, DSIL, DDFT, navicular bursa, CL of the DIP joint, and the DIP joint (Figure 2.9). It is typical to find multiple abnormalities within the foot that may be contributing to the lameness.
- Injury to the DDFT is thought to be the most common soft tissue injury causing lameness in the horse's foot and is best diagnosed with an MRI.

Treatment

- The treatment plan is usually tailor-made for each individual horse based on the severity of lameness, intended use of the horse, wishes of the owner, results of diagnostics (or lack of diagnostics such as MRI), hoof conformation, previous treatments, and the most likely diagnosis.
- Horses with advanced radiographic abnormalities in the navicular bone and those with major injuries to the DDFT will be problematic regardless of the treatment employed.
- The goal is to manage the disease. The cornerstone of treatment is corrective trimming and shoeing. The goals of therapeutic shoeing are to:
  1) Restore normal foot balance.
  2) Correct foot problems such as underrun, contracted, and sheared heels and excessive toe length.
  3) Reduce biomechanical forces on the navicular region.
  4) Ease break-over at the toe.
  5) Support the heels and prevent heel descent during loading.
  6) Protect the injured areas of the foot.
- A variety of steel or aluminum shoes are thought to be effective in treating horses with heel pain and include the Tennessee navicular shoe, rolled or rockered toed shoes, egg-bar shoes, natural balance shoes, equine digital support system (EDSS), onion shoes, and full-bar support shoes.
- Nonsurgical treatments include rest and controlled exercise; NSAIDs; PSGAGs; bisphosphonates such as tiludronate or clodronate; and intrasynovial medications into the DIP joint, navicular bursa, or DFTS.
- Horses with DDFT injuries (primary or secondary) may benefit from intralesional biological therapies depending on the location of the lesion.

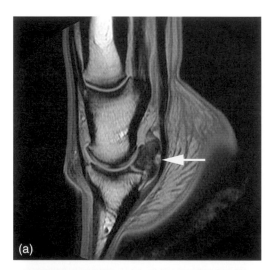

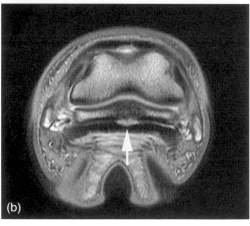

Figure 2.9 (a) Lateral STIR MR image demonstrating abnormal signal within the navicular bone (arrow) and (b) surface damage to the DDFT (arrow).

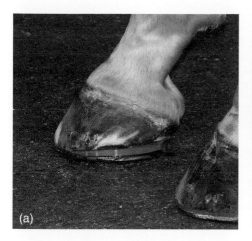 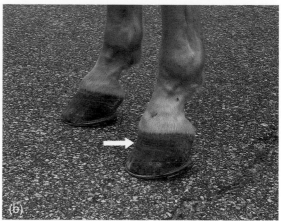

Figure 2.10 Heel elevation may be helpful in treating select horses with navicular disease/syndrome (a) and not in others (b). The horse in (a) was shod with wedge pads and dental impression material and improved after shoeing. The horse in (b) was shod with elevated heel shoes despite having a very upright hoof conformation on the LF, which likely contributed to the dorsal hoof wall concavity (arrow) and continued lameness.

- Surgical treatments include PD neurectomy, inferior check ligament desmotomy, and endoscopy of the navicular bursa in select cases. (The reader is referred to Chapter 4 in *Adams and Stashak's Lameness in Horses, 7th Edition*, for further details of treatment options.)

Prognosis
- In general, clinical resolution may occur in 40–50% of the horses but the optimal treatment and prognosis may differ depending on the specific pathologies that may be present (Figure 2.10).
- Horses with major radiographic abnormalities will most likely have a worse prognosis than horses with no radiographic changes or minor soft tissue pathology.
- Horses with navicular bone pathology demonstrated on radiographs or MRI together with concurrent DDFT lesions also tend to have a poor prognosis.
- Horses with primary soft tissue injuries of the DDFT have a guarded prognosis for return to full athletic function, and horses with major lesions in the navicular bone, *per se*, have a poor prognosis.

Fractures of the Navicular (Distal Sesamoid) Bone

Anatomy

- The navicular or distal sesamoid bone is a small wedge-shaped bone interposed between the DDFT and the palmar/plantar aspects of the distal and middle phalanges.
- The dorsal surface of the bone articulates with the DIP joint, and the palmar/plantar fibrocartilaginous flexor surface provides a gliding surface for the DDFT within the navicular bursa (Figures 2.1 and 2.11).
- The navicular bone itself is supported in position by the navicular suspensory apparatus (CSLs and DSIL) and serves as a major fulcrum within the foot.

Imaging

- Fractures of the navicular bone are usually detected with routine radiography of the region and advanced imaging is usually unnecessary.
- Most complete fractures are best identified on the skyline or 60° oblique views of the navicular bone and should be present on

(a)

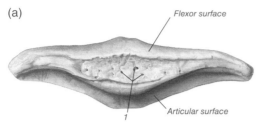

(b)

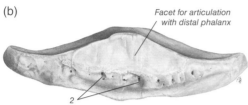

Figure 2.11   Distal sesamoid (navicular) bone. (a) Proximal view. (b) Distal view. (1) Foramina and (2) fossae.

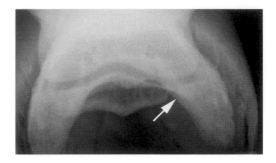

Figure 2.12   Bipartite navicular bone as seen on a skyline radiograph in a young horse with lameness isolated to the foot.

multiple views. Navicular bone fractures should be differentiated from congenital bipartite or tripartite separation.

Etiology

- Acute trauma (concussion) to the foot is the most likely cause of simple and comminuted complete navicular bone fractures.
- Severe navicular bone osteolysis associated with navicular disease or sepsis may predispose to pathologic fractures.
- Avulsion fractures occur along the distal border of the bone and are considered part of the pathologic changes associated with navicular disease. Their presence may be due to a fracture from the distal border of the navicular, fracture of an enthesophyte at the origin of the DSIL, or ectopic mineralization in the DSIL.
- Bipartite navicular bones are developmental abnormalities, are not a true fracture, and can be confused with a chronic fracture radiographically (Figure 2.12).

Clinical Signs

- Navicular bone fractures have been reported in many breeds and in horses with varied use.
- Complete fractures can occur in any limb, but avulsion fractures are most common in

the forelimb consistent with other signs of navicular disease/syndrome.

- Horses with complete navicular bone fractures typically have a history of an acute, severe unilateral lameness that improves with time. This is especially true for fractures in the hindlimb.
- Most horses with complete fractures have a painful response to hoof testers across the frog region and often have effusion within the DIP joint.
- A PD nerve block should improve the lameness in most cases but a high PD or abaxial sesamoid block may be required to completely eliminate the lameness.
- Intra-articular anesthesia of the DIP joint usually improves the lameness.

Diagnosis

- Radiography of the foot is required to confirm the diagnosis. Careful packing of the frog is necessary to avoid confusing the lines from the lateral sulci of the frog that may cross the navicular region and imitate a fracture. Complete simple fractures are typically located in the sagittal plane medial or lateral to the midline and are typically not displaced (Figure 2.13).
- Avulsion fractures can be difficult to identify on radiographs. Often, they are best seen on the 60° oblique view, but they also may be present at the distal aspect of the navicular bone on a lateromedial view (Figure 2.8) or within the medullary cavity of the navicular bone on the skyline view.

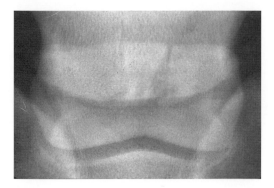

Figure 2.13 A wing fracture of the navicular bone (arrows) as seen on the oblique radiograph of the foot.

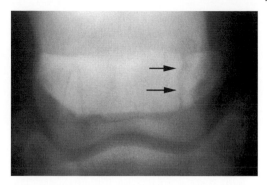

Figure 2.14 This oblique radiograph of the navicular bone was taken 23 months after the fracture occurred.

Treatment

- Horses with complete navicular bone fractures usually are treated nonsurgically by confinement alone, confinement and corrective shoeing (with heel elevation), or external coaptation aimed at reducing hoof expansion.
- Heel elevation is considered an important aspect of treatment in most horses.
- A minimum of four to six months of confinement may be necessary because these fractures are very slow to heal.
- Surgical repair of simple complete navicular bone fractures using a single cortical bone screw has been reported. Intraoperative imaging and specially designed aiming device are necessary to perform the procedure.
- PD neurectomy can be performed to relieve pain in cases that have not responded to conservative treatment but do not guarantee a sound horse.
- Chronic lameness may result from poor fracture healing and adhesions that develop between the DDFT and the navicular bone. A noncalcified fibrous union can still be evident years after the fracture occurred in many horses.
- There is no known specific treatment for avulsion fractures. Horses are treated similar to those with navicular disease/syndrome but often benefit from heel elevation (provided the heels are not already too long) to relieve tension on the DSIL and DDFT.

Prognosis

- The prognosis is considered guarded to poor for horses with complete navicular bone fractures to return to athletic performance.
- In general, horses with fractures in the hindlimb are considered to have a better chance to return to performance than those affected in the forelimbs.
- Complete radiographic healing seems to occur infrequently, even in horses that become sound (Figure 2.14).
- Horses with avulsion fractures and other radiographic signs of navicular disease have a fair to guarded prognosis to return to soundness.

Soft Tissue Injuries in the Foot (DDFT and Podotrochlear Apparatus)

Overview

- Soft tissue injuries of the foot have always been suspected in horses with foot pain without radiographic abnormalities, and advances in ultrasound, CT, and MRI techniques have enabled improved recognition of these potential problems.
- It is common for soft tissue and bony abnormalities to coexist in many lame horses with foot problems, and multiple abnormalities are often present.
- Primary tendinitis of the DDFT and other primary soft tissue injuries can be the cause of lameness in some horses with navicular disease/syndrome.

- Soft tissue structures within the foot that can be desensitized with a PD block include the heel bulbs, digital cushion, navicular bursa, collateral cartilages of the distal phalanx, podotrochlear apparatus, DDFT (may only partially improve with a PD block), and CLs of the DIP joint.
- The DDFT is the most commonly injured soft tissue structure in the foot. Lesions in the DDFT can occur in either lobe anywhere along its length, from the level of the PIP joint distally to its attachment on P3. The most common location of DDFT injuries is at the level of the navicular bone, and these can be true core lesions, sagittal splits, or dorsal abrasions (Figure 2.9).

Anatomy

- The DDFT lies along the palmar/plantar aspect of the pastern region and is enclosed within the DFTS distally to the level of the T-ligament (Figure 2.1).
- The DDFT is bound down by the distal digital annular ligament as it courses to its broad insertion on the flexor surface of the distal phalanx (Figure 2.2) and becomes bi-lobed within the foot.
- Within the hoof capsule, the DDFT passes over the navicular bursa, interposed between the tendon and the fibrocartilaginous distal scutum covering the flexor surface of the navicular bone.
- The podotrochlear apparatus holds the navicular bone in place both distally (DSIL) and proximally (CSLs) through attachments to the phalanges (Figure 1.2).

Imaging

- A definitive diagnosis of a soft tissue injury of the foot is best determined with MRI in either the recumbent or standing patient.
- Contrast-enhanced CT may also be used to document abnormalities in the DDFT but currently can only be performed in the recumbent patient.

- Certain aspects of both the DDFT and podotrochlear apparatus are inaccessible with ultrasound, suggesting that negative findings do not rule out the presence of a lesion. Currently, ultrasound is primarily being used to aid in the treatment of specific lesions that have been identified with other imaging modalities.

Etiology

- Similar biomechanical forces and repetitive trauma to the palmar aspect of the foot associated with navicular disease most likely contribute to these injuries.
- Horses that jump or have a low heel hoof conformation may be at risk for injuries to the DDFT.
- Acute onset or repetitive trauma is considered the most likely cause of most soft tissue injuries within the foot.
- Chronic repetitive trauma to the DDFT is often the most likely cause although single-event traumatic "tearing" of the DDFT causing a true tendinitis may also occur. Some suggest that chronic DDFT lesions may be a degenerative process due to vascular compromise rather than an inflammatory process from trauma.
- DDFT lesions can occur in single or multiple locations and can extend variable distances up or down the tendon (Figure 2.15).
- Abnormalities of the podotrochlear apparatus are often present in association with abnormalities of the navicular bone, although primary injuries do occur.

Clinical Signs

- In general, horses that have primary soft tissue injuries in the foot are more likely to have a history on an acute onset of lameness and be unilaterally lame compared with horses with navicular disease/syndrome.
- Often there is a history of an acute onset of moderate-to-severe lameness that may improve with rest and worsen with exercise.

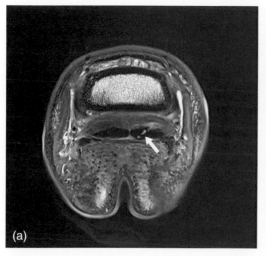 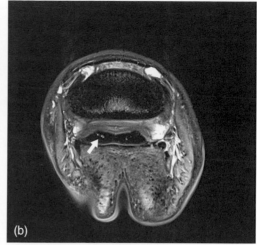

Figure 2.15 MRI images demonstrating a single, large DDFT lesion (a; arrow) and multiple, smaller DDFT lesions (b; arrow) at different locations along the DDFT in the same horse.

This may include a history of activity that caused excessive hyperextension of the foot such as working in soft ground and/or jumping.

- The lameness may be unilateral and may worsen in a circle or when exercised on soft ground.
- Pain may be elicited with deep palpation of the DDFT between the collateral cartilages of the heels. Increasing tension on the DDFT with the navicular wedge test may accentuate the lameness.
- The majority of horses will improve with a PD nerve block, but the lameness will not be completely abolished in many horses with lesions of the DDFT. Some lesions may improve with IA anesthesia of the DIP joint.
- The response to perineural anesthesia may depend on the location of the lesion(s) and whether concurrent problems exist in the foot.
- The clinical signs of horses with abnormalities of the podotrochlear apparatus may resemble those with navicular disease/syndrome because these injuries often occur concurrently with navicular bone pathology.

Diagnosis

- A definitive diagnosis of soft tissue injuries in the foot is best determined with an MRI. There is good correlation between MRI appearance of DDFT lesions and their pathological classification into core lesions, sagittal splits, insertional lesions, and dorsal surface erosions (Figures 2.16 and 2.17).
- Typically, horses with primary DDFT lesions will have minimal to no radiographic abnormalities.
- Ectopic mineralization may be seen in some horses with chronic DDFT lesions but is not necessarily correlated with active tendinitis of the DDFT.
- Enthesophytes involving the podotrochlear apparatus attachments to the navicular bone may suggest concurrent injury but a definitive diagnosis is best made with MRI (Figure 2.18).
- Erosive lesions of the flexor surface of the navicular bone seen on radiographs are often associated with dorsal abrasions of the DDFT, but navicular bursal endoscopy or MRI is usually needed for a definitive diagnosis (Figures 2.6 and 2.9).

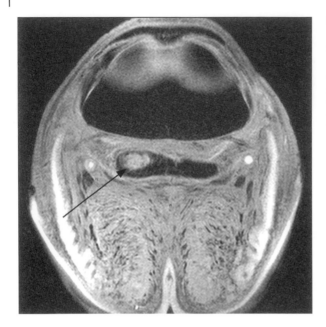

Figure 2.16 Transverse T1-weighted fast low angle shot (FLASH) image with fat saturation of the right front foot at the level of the middle phalanx of a horse with acute onset foot lameness. There is abnormal signal hyperintensity in a large core lesion of the medial lobe of the DDFT (arrow). *Source*: Courtesy of Michael Schramme.

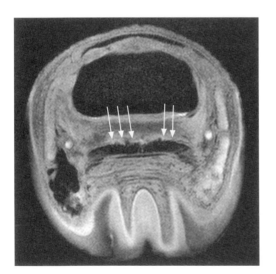

Figure 2.17 Transverse fast low angle shot (FLASH) image with fat saturation of the foot at the level of the middle phalanx of a horse with foot lameness. The dorsal surface of the DDFT is irregular due to the presence of fibrillations and short, incomplete sagittal splits disrupting the smooth dorsal contour of the tendon (arrows). *Source*: Courtesy of Michael Schramme.

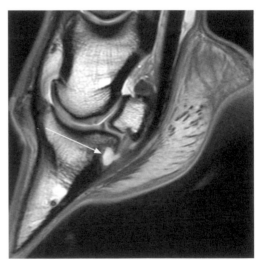

Figure 2.18 Sagittal proton density image of the central part of the foot of a horse with chronic foot lameness. There is localized signal hyperintensity in an osseous cyst-like lesion at the insertion of the distal sesamoidean impar ligament to the distal phalanx indicating chronic enthesopathy of this ligament (arrow). *Source*: Courtesy of Michael Schramme.

Treatment

- The most important aspects of treatment of soft tissue injuries of the foot are rest, rehabilitation, and corrective foot care to correct hoof imbalances.
- Rest and rehabilitation are usually performed over a minimum of six months for DDFT injuries and may be necessary for even longer depending on the lesion. In general, horses treated with an extended period of rest and rehabilitation are thought be able to return to use for a longer duration than horses without rest.
- Horses with injuries to the podotrochlear apparatus are usually treated similarly to horses with navicular disease.
- Types of shoes that may benefit horses with DDFT injuries include egg-bar shoes and shoes and/or pads to elevate the heels. Raised heel shoes may offer mixed results as they may paradoxically exacerbate lameness and may induce contracture of the DDFT during tendon healing even though many horses with DDFT lesions appear more comfortable when placed in elevated heel shoes.
- Intralesional or intrasynovial treatment with anti-inflammatories, platelet-rich plasma (PRP), stem cells, and other biologics may be performed if the lesion is accessible to this technique.
- Dorsal border lesions at the level of the navicular bone may benefit from endoscopy of the navicular bursa and debridement of torn tendon fibers although the benefit of this overconservative treatment has been questioned.

Prognosis

- The prognosis for horses with soft tissue injuries of the foot is considered guarded to poor for return to athletic performance.
- Horses with primary or secondary DDFT injuries have a poor prognosis for return to performance. The injury is often a career-ending with less than one-third of affected horses being able to return to performance.
- The overall prognosis of DDFT injuries is often dependent on lesion size, type, location, and severity and the presence of concurrent abnormalities within the navicular bone or other soft tissues (primary vs. secondary).
- Horses with dorsal border DDFT lesions tend to have a better prognosis than those with core or parasagittal split lesions.
- Horses with concurrent bone and soft tissue injuries (i.e. DDFT injury and concurrent navicular bone pathology) are particularly problematic.

Injuries to the CLs of the DIP Joint

Anatomy

- The distal articular surface of the middle phalanx, the articular surface of the distal phalanx, and the two articular surfaces of the navicular bone form the DIP joint.
- Short CLs of the joint arise from the distal end of the middle phalanx, pass distad deep to the cartilages of the distal phalanx, and terminate on either side of the extensor process and the dorsal part of each cartilage (Figure 2.19).
- Much of the CLs of the DIP are below the coronary band making access to diagnosis and treatment much more difficult.

Imaging

- A definitive diagnosis of an injury to the CL of the DIP joint is best determined with MRI in either the recumbent or standing patient.
- Ultrasound may also be helpful, but certain aspects of the CL of the DIP joint are inaccessible with ultrasound, suggesting that

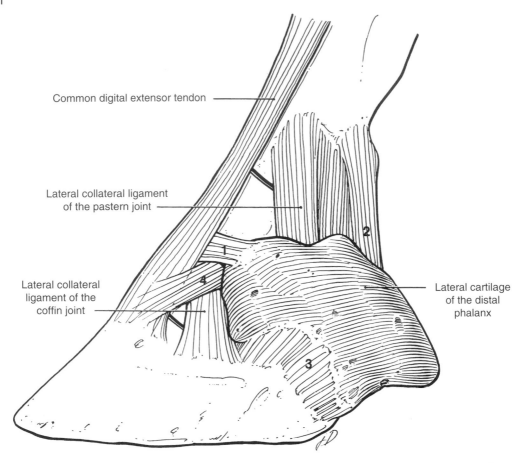

Common digital extensor tendon

Lateral collateral ligament of the pastern joint

Lateral collateral ligament of the coffin joint

Lateral cartilage of the distal phalanx

Figure 2.19 The medial and lateral collateral ligaments of the DIP joint arise from the distal end of the middle phalanx and terminate on either side of the extensor process of the distal phalanx. The numbered ligaments (1, 2, 3, and 4) serve to stabilize the cartilage of the distal phalanx. *Source*: Courtesy of J Daugherty.

negative findings do not rule out the presence of a lesion.

- Although concurrent osseous damage at the origin and insertion sites of the ligaments can be present in approximately 50% of these horses, scintigraphy is usually not recommended as an additional diagnostic tool because MRI can usually provide more specific information about the injury.

Etiology

- Desmitis of the CLs of the DIP joint is one of several soft tissue injuries that can occur

within the foot and it can occur alone or together with other injuries.

- Acute onset or repetitive trauma is considered the most likely cause.
- Asymmetrical foot placement or foot imbalances may cause sliding and rotation of the distal phalanx relative to the middle phalanx, contributing to these injuries.
- Lesions within the CL of the DIP joint have been reported to be a primary degenerative process rather than inflammatory and may explain the poor response to conservative treatment in many horses with desmitis of the CL of the DIP joint.

- There are no known predisposing factors, but a recent study reported a correlation between a reduced palmar angle of the foot detected with radiography and alterations in the CLs of the DIP joint with MRI.

Clinical Signs

- Horses that have primary soft tissue injuries in the foot such as injuries to the CLs of the DIP joint are more likely to have a history of an acute onset of lameness and be unilaterally lame compared with horses with other foot-related lameness.
- Often, there are few localizing clinical signs in horses with injuries to the CL of the DIP joint.
- The medial CL of the forelimb is the most common site of the injury.
- Horses often have a history of a chronic forelimb lameness of variable severity that is worse in the circle. Phalangeal flexion usually is positive.
- Palpable swelling and pain of the ligament at its proximal attachment to the P2 may be present above the coronary band in severe cases.
- Effusion of the DIP joint is not a consistent clinical finding.
- Most horses improve with a PD nerve block but may not be completely sound until a more proximal block is performed, and less than half of horses will improve with IA anesthesia of the DIP joint.

Diagnosis

- Lesions within the CLs of the DIP joint on MRI are identified by the alteration in size and signal intensity (Figure 2.20). In addition, some horses may have abnormal mineralization and fluid within the distal phalanx at the insertion of the ligament.
- Ultrasound may be able to detect abnormalities in the proximal aspect of the CL, but negative findings do not rule out the presence of a lesion.
- Bone exostosis, lysis, or sclerosis seen with radiography at the insertion sites of the CLs

may be suggestive of desmitis but are not commonly identified (Figure 2.21).

Treatment

- The most important aspects of treating any soft tissue injury of the foot are rest, rehabilitation, and corrective foot care. Foot imbalances that may have contributed to their occurrence such as low heels, long toes, mediolateral imbalance, reverse angle of the distal phalanx, etc., should be corrected if possible.
- Horses should be shod to decrease tension on the side of the injury by increasing the width to the branch of the shoe on the affected side and beveling the shoe on the opposite (unaffected side).
- Ultrasound-guided intralesional therapy with stem cells, PRP, and other biological products may also be used, especially if the injury is accessible above the hoof.
- Additional treatments include extracorporeal shock wave therapy, application of a half-limb or foot cast, and medication of the DIP joint.

Prognosis

- The reported prognosis of affected horses is variable although generally they have a poor prognosis for future performance.
- Reported rates of returning to previous performance in several studies have ranged from 27 to 60% depending on the type of treatment and extent of initial injuries.
- Horses with multiple soft tissue and osseous injuries within the hoof capsule typically do substantially worse.

Coffin Joint and Distal Phalanx

Osteoarthritis (OA) of the DIP Joint

Anatomy

- The distal articular surface of the middle phalanx, the articular surface of the distal phalanx, and the two articular surfaces of the navicular bone form the DIP joint.

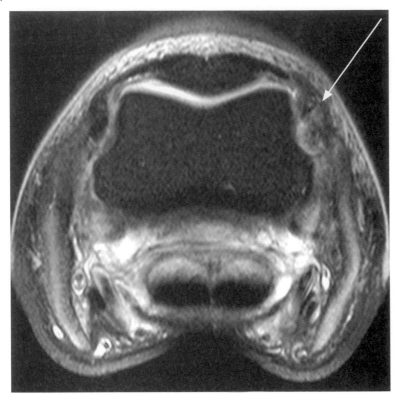

Figure 2.20 Transverse proton density image with fat saturation oriented parallel with the solar surface of the foot of a horse with collateral ligament injury of the distal interphalangeal joint. The affected collateral ligament is enlarged, and its margins are irregular (arrow). There is loss or architecture and irregular areas of signal hyperintensity are dispersed throughout the cross section of the ligament (arrow). *Source*: Courtesy of Michael Schramme.

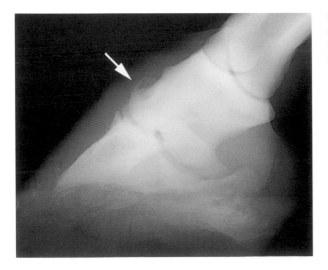

Figure 2.21 Bony proliferation on the dorsomedial aspect of P2 on this oblique radiograph (arrow) is suggestive of an injury to the CL of the DIP joint.

- A complex array of ligaments within the foot helps in stabilizing the collateral cartilages of the distal phalanx as well as the DIP joint itself (Figure 2.19).
- Short CLs of the joint arise from the distal end of the middle phalanx and terminate on either side of the extensor process (Figure 2.19).
- The common (or long) digital extensor tendon courses over the dorsal aspect of the DIP joint and attaches to the extensor process of the distal phalanx.

Imaging

- A complete radiographic study of the foot can often confirm or at least suggest the presence of OA within the joint. However, the lack of radiographic abnormalities does not rule out a problem within the joint.
- Oblique views can aid in detecting periarticular new bone formation of the distal aspect of the middle phalanx.
- Additional diagnostics that may be used particularly if the radiographs are nondiagnostic, include ultrasound, MRI, and diagnostic arthroscopy.
- Since many horses with DIP OA will have other abnormalities within the foot, MRI is usually the next imaging modality recommended after radiography.

Etiology

- OA/synovitis of the DIP joint often is referred to as "low ringbone" and may occur as a primary problem or secondary to other injuries within the foot.
- Primary OA can be due to acute or repetitive trauma to the joint comparable to any articulation in the horse. Horses with a broken pastern axis (forward or backward) and other types of hoof imbalances appear particularly prone to this type of trauma.
- Excessive strain of the attachments of the long or common digital extensor tendon to the extensor process may contribute to

periostitis and enthesophyte formation along the dorsal aspect of the joint.
- Secondary OA can occur from other lameness conditions that involve the DIP joint either directly or indirectly such as navicular disease, navicular bone fractures, articular fractures of the distal phalanx, subchondral cystic lesions (SCL) of the distal phalanx, osteochondral fragmentation within the joint, and desmopathy of the CLs of the DIP joint.

Clinical Signs

- Effusion of the DIP joint is usually present in most horses with OA or synovitis/capsulitis of the DIP joint. Most times, significant effusion of the DIP joint can be seen as a slight bulging just above the coronary band (Figure 2.22).
- With chronic or advanced disease, the joint capsule may become thickened, resulting in a firm swelling just above the dorsal aspect of the coronary band.
- The joint may be painful to flexion and rotation, but this is uncommon unless the OA is advanced or secondary to another problem in the joint.
- The lameness is variable depending on the severity of the disease, and is often worse on hard ground, when circled, and after distal limb or phalangeal flexion.
- The lameness often is greatly improved and sometimes eliminated with a PD nerve block, but a basisesamoid block may be required for complete resolution of the lameness.
- IA anesthesia of the DIP joint is not specific for problems within the joint but using a small volume of anesthetic (6 mL or less) and observing for a change in lameness very soon after the injection (within 10 minutes) can improve the specificity of the IA block.
- Most horses with DIP joint pain improve rapidly and substantially after IA anesthesia.

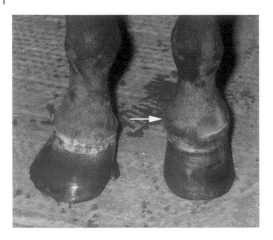

Figure 2.22 Effusion within the DIP joint can be seen and palpated as swelling just above the coronary band.

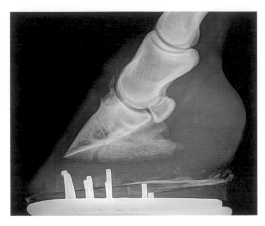

Figure 2.23 The calcification of the extensor tendon seen on this lateral radiograph was not clinically significant in this horse following removal of an extensor process fracture.

Diagnosis

- Close inspection of the extensor process, palmar/plantar aspect of distal P2, and dorsoproximal aspect of the navicular bone for osteophyte and enthesophyte formation are important when evaluating radiographs of the DIP joint.
- Joint space narrowing is difficult to assess on radiographs because limb positioning is known to affect joint space width.
- In general, the radiographic abnormalities surrounding the DIP joint should not be overinterpreted because there is much variation in the shape of the extensor process among horses and enthesophytes may not be associated with lameness (Figure 2.23).
- MRI is the most comprehensive imaging modality that can detect articular cartilage, subchondral bone, and soft tissue abnormalities of the DIP joint if present.

Treatment

- Horses with primary OA or synovitis/capsulitis of the DIP joint are usually treated with a combination of intra-articular medication and corrective shoeing. Correcting hoof imbalances and moving the break-over

farther palmarly often helps these horses and using a rim pad may alleviate concussion to the joint.
- Direct medication of the DIP joint usually is more effective than systemic medications to reduce the inflammatory response within the joint. Corticosteroids alone or corticosteroids combined with hyaluronan are used most frequently.
- Chondroprotective agents such as PSGAGs or biologics may also be used if desired.
- Treatment of horses with secondary OA of the DIP joint usually focuses on the underlying contributing problem to prevent worsening of the problems within the DIP joint. For instance, horses with navicular disease should be shod appropriately to minimize progression of OA within the DIP joint and articular distal phalanx fractures should either be removed or stabilized to minimize secondary joint issues.

Prognosis

- Horses with synovitis/capsulitis of the DIP joint usually have a very good prognosis to return to performance if the predisposing hoof imbalances can be corrected and maintained. However, one study indicated that only 30% of horses responded to treatment.

- The prognosis often is related to the severity of the radiographic or MRI abnormalities. Horses with advanced OA often respond less to any form of treatment or the lameness recurs more quickly.
- Horses with secondary OA of the DIP joint have a variable prognosis depending on the underlying problem.
- The development of radiographic signs of OA within the DIP joint does not preclude athletic performance. It is possible that the radiographic abnormalities within the DIP are over-interpreted as to their influence on lameness.

Fractures of the Distal Phalanx (P3, Coffin Bone)

Overview

- Fractures of the distal phalanx can occur in any foot in a variety of different configurations and are classified according to their location within the bone (Figure 2.24).
- Type I fractures are nonarticular oblique palmar/plantar process (wing) fractures.
- Type II fractures are articular oblique palmar or plantar process (wing) fractures.

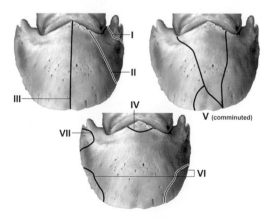

Figure 2.24 Classification of P3 fractures in horses. *Source*: Reprinted with permission from Dr. Alicia Bertone, Equine Fracture Repair, Nixon AL, ed. Reproduced with permission from John Wiley & Sons.

- Type III fractures are sagittal articular fractures that roughly divide the distal phalanx into two separate halves.
- Type IV fractures are articular fractures involving the extensor process.
- Type V fractures are comminuted articular or nonarticular fractures and can be a variety of configurations.
- Type VI fractures are nonarticular solar margin fractures of the distal phalanx.
- Type VII fractures are nonarticular fractures of the palmar or plantar process of the distal phalanx in foals. These fractures begin and end at the solar margin and are usually triangular or oblong in shape.
- In racehorses, P3 fractures commonly affect the lateral aspect of the left forelimb and the medial aspect of the right forelimb (Type I and II articular "wing" fractures).

Anatomy

- The distal phalanx is a triangular-shaped bone located within the hoof capsule that serves as a major insertion site for the flexor tendons palmarly/plantarly and the extensor tendons dorsally (Figure 2.1).
- It is attached to the hoof wall dorsally through a complicated network of epidermal and dermal laminae and protected distally by the digital cushion, sole, heels, and frog.
- The distal phalanx, together with the hoof, must absorb tremendous forces during weight-bearing of the limb.

Imaging

- Most P3 fractures are readily apparent on routine radiographic projections.
- Scintigraphy, CT, or MRI can be used to help identify radiographically occult fractures and CT can be useful to determine the exact fracture configuration of comminuted fractures.

Etiology

- Single-event trauma such as kicking a solid object appears to be the predominant cause of P3 fractures in non-racehorses.
- Repetitive trauma leading the stress-related bone injury is the likely cause of P3 fractures in racehorses (Figure 2.25).
- Type VI fractures may be related to the shape and location of the solar margin within the hoof and the tremendous forces the distal phalanx undergoes during weight-bearing. These fractures may also occur concurrently with laminitis and septic pedal osteitis (PO) due to resorption of P3.
- Type VII fractures in foals are thought to occur from compression either on the solar or dorsal cortex of the distal phalanx during weight-bearing or from tension forces generated by the DDFT and may be related to hoof conformation.
- Type IV extensor process fractures may occur due to excessive tension on the common digital extensor tendon, overextension of the DIP joint, or they may be developmental in origin (osteochondrosis lesion; Figure 2.26).

Clinical Signs

- There is usually a history of an acute onset of a moderate-to-severe lameness (grade 4 to 5/5). Exceptions to this are solar margin fractures, Type VII fractures in foals, and developmental Type IV fractures of the extensor process. These horses are usually much less lame.
- If the fracture is chronic, the signs of lameness are usually diminished, and the lameness must be differentiated from the many other potential problems within the foot.
- An increased digital pulse may be palpable and heat in the affected foot may be appreciated in the acute stage.
- DIP joint effusion often is present if the fracture is articular and swelling and edema may also be present above the hoof wall in horses with acute fractures.
- Hoof tester examination usually reveals pain over the sole region and focal pressure over the fracture site usually induces a marked response. A negative hoof tester response does not rule out the presence of a chronic P3 fracture.
- Perineural anesthesia of the PD nerves or IA anesthesia of the DIP joint may aid in localizing the lameness to the foot region but are often only necessary in horses with chronic fractures.
- Horses with large chronic extensor process fractures may have enlargement of the dorsal aspect of the coronary band and abnor-

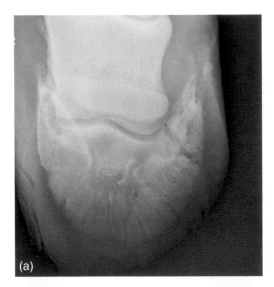

(a)

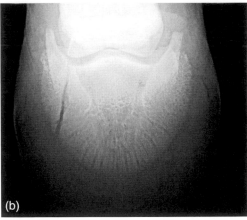

(b)

Figure 2.25 Two variable sized Type II "wing" fractures of the P3. These are the most common type of P3 fracture.

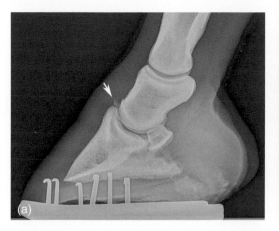
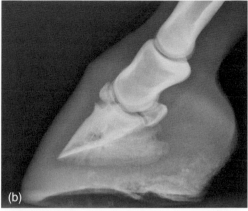

Figure 2.26 Small (a) and large (b) Type IV P3 fractures involving the extensor process.

mal growth of the dorsal hoof wall (it develops a "V" or triangular shape called a "buttress foot").

Diagnosis

- Radiography is usually reliable to confirm the diagnosis and document the type and location of the fracture (Figure 2.25). Solar margin fractures are most easily identified on the 60° dorsoproximal-palmarodistal view. Extensor process fractures are usually identified on the lateral view (Figure 2.26).

- Some non-displaced or stress-related fractures in racehorses may not be apparent on the initial radiographs. Radiographs should be repeated in one to two weeks, or scintigraphy, CT, or MRI can be used to help identify the fracture.

- CT can be used to document occult fractures in the palmar/plantar processes or to confirm the fracture configuration in comminuted P3 fractures (Figure 2.27).

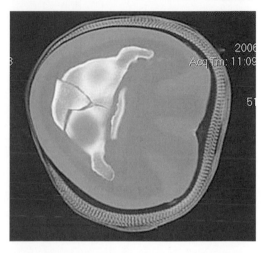

Figure 2.27 CT image of a Type V, comminuted fracture of P3. Fracture lines were present on both the lateral and dorsoplantar radiographs.

Treatment

- In general, the majority of horses with P3 fractures are treated with confinement and corrective shoeing aimed at immobilizing the fracture and preventing expansion of the hoof wall (Table 2.1).

- The need to immobilize the foot with shoeing or casting in these horses is debatable since the outcome did not appear to be influenced by whether the foot was immobilized in a large series of horses with P3 fractures.

- Type I fractures are best treated with confinement and methods to prevent hoof expansion, but horses also may respond to confinement and rest alone.

- Type II fractures in foals less than six months of age should be treated with stall confinement for at least six to eight weeks. Most adult

Table 2.1 Types of distal phalanx fractures and their recommended treatment.

Fracture type	Location	Articular	Recommended treatment	Prognosis
I	Palmar/plantar process	No	Confinement ± shoeing (foot cast instead of shoe)	Very good to excellent
II	Oblique fractures of palmar/plantar process ("wing" fractures)	Yes	Confinement ± shoeing (foot cast instead of shoe) lag screw repair of large Type II fractures	Fair to good
III	Midsagittal fracture	Yes	Confinement ± shoeing (foot cast instead of shoe) best candidate for lag screw repair	Unpredictable; guarded?
IV	Extensor process(variable size)	Yes	Removal in most cases regardless of size: arthroscopy/arthrotomy	Small: excellent Large: good
V	Comminuted	Yes or no	Confinement + shoeing (foot cast instead of shoe) removal if secondary to infection	Dependent on fracture configuration
VI	Solar margin	No	Confinement + protective shoeing (wide-web shoes or shoes with full or rim pads)	Very good
VII	Palmar/plantar process—begins and ends at solar margin	No	Primarily in foals; confinement alone; no shoeing	Very good to excellent

horses are treated with confinement and methods to restrict hoof expansion (foot cast or shoe). Screw placement is often only considered in horses with large wing fractures.

- Type III fractures can be treated similarly to Type II fractures although Acute Type III fractures in adult horses are usually the best candidates for surgical repair using lag screw fixation. The primary advantages are less risk of secondary OA developing in the DIP joint and faster healing of the fracture due to surgical compression.
- Type IV fractures are usually treated with surgical removal of the fracture/fragment in chronic fractures or OCD lesions (Figure 2.26). Very large fractures may not warrant treatment and are best managed conservatively.
- Type V fractures are best treated with confinement and methods to prevent hoof expansion (foot cast or shoe).
- Type VI, solar margin, fractures are usually treated with corrective shoeing (wide-web shoes, shoes and full pads, or shoes with rim pads) and stall or paddock rest for several months.
- Type VII fractures in foals are usually treated satisfactorily with confinement alone for six to eight weeks. Application of restrictive external coaptation (e.g. bar shoe or acrylic) to the hoof is not recommended.

Prognosis

- In general, horses with hindlimb P3 fractures have a better prognosis for performance than those in the forelimb.
- The prognosis usually is very good for all ages of horses for nonarticular P3 fractures (Types I, V, VI, and VII).
- Foals with Type VII P3 fractures have an excellent prognosis for return to performance and fracture healing is expected in about eight weeks.
- A range from 50 to 70% return to soundness has been reported for horses with Type II wing fractures treated conservatively.

- Conservative management of horses with Type III fractures was reported to have a 74% success rate and it remains unknown if horses treated with lag screw fixation have an improved prognosis over confinement and corrective shoeing.
- The prognosis for small extensor process fractures treated by arthroscopic removal usually is excellent. Removal of large, chronic extensor process fragments is also thought to result in a reasonably good prognosis (Figure 2.28).
- OA of the DIP joint can be sequel to any articular P3 fracture but may not preclude athletic soundness, and refracture of the bone can occur especially in horses with Type II and III fractures.

Ossification of the Collateral Cartilage of the Distal Phalanx (Sidebone)

Overview

- Ossification of the collateral cartilages (i.e. sidebone) of the distal phalanx is relativity common in larger breeds such as draft horses, Warmbloods, Finnhorses, and Brazilian jumpers.

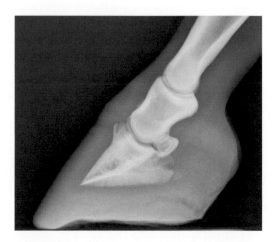

Figure 2.28 Lateral radiograph of the same horse in Figure 2.26b following arthroscopic removal of a large extensor process fracture.

- The fore feet appear to be more commonly involved than the hind feet, females more than males, and the lateral cartilage often ossifies more than the medial cartilage.
- The clinical significance of the condition remains questionable.

Anatomy

- The "collateral" cartilages of the distal phalanx (often "lateral cartilages"; most correctly ungual cartilages) lie deep to the hoof and the skin, covered on their abaxial surfaces by the coronary venous plexus.
- They extend from each palmar process of the bone and project proximad to the coronary band of the hoof where they may be palpated (Figure 2.19).
- The cartilages are concave on their axial surfaces, convex on their abaxial surfaces, and thicker distally where they attach to the bone.
- Several ligaments stabilize each ungual cartilage within the hoof (Figure 2.19).

Imaging

- Radiographic examination of the foot usually reveals the extent of the ossification of the cartilage or cartilages (Figure 2.29).
- The mere presence of an ossified cartilage is not diagnostic that the ossification is clinically relevant.
- Scintigraphy and MRI may help determine whether the abnormalities within the cartilage may be contributing to the lameness.

Etiology

- The specific cause(s) of sidebones is/are not clear and it is considered partly hereditary in certain horse breeds in Australia, Finland, and Sweden.
- Hoof concussion causing trauma to the cartilage, poor conformation, particularly base narrow, and poor trimming and shoeing have been proposed as inciting causes.

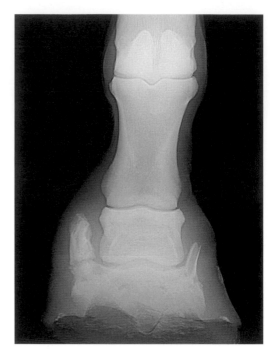

Figure 2.29 Standing dorsopalmar radiograph demonstrating a large uniaxial sidebone that was thought to be contributing to lameness.

- It has been suggested that prolonged exercise and/or racing may have some preventative influence on ossification of the collateral cartilages.
- The amount of weight placed on the foot may also be contributory because primarily larger breed horses develop sidebone.

Clinical Signs

- Lameness due to sidebone is considered rare and the clinical significance of radiographic apparent ossification is questionable.
- A large sidebone may be visually apparent as an enlargement of the lateral and medial dimensions of the pastern region. Palpation may reveal firmness to the cartilage and pain with digital pressure suggests that the sidebone may be contributing to the lameness or may be associated with a secondary fracture of the distal phalanx.
- Sidebone may accompany other lameness conditions of the palmar heel region (e.g.

navicular syndrome) and may be mistaken for the cause.

Diagnosis

- Multiple radiographic views of the foot may help reveal the extent of the ossification of the cartilage or cartilages, but the standing horizontal beam view permits direct comparison of the medial and lateral cartilages (Figure 2.29).
- A fracture of the ossified cartilage can occur and large sidebones have been seen in horses with Type II distal phalanx fractures that were thought to potentially contribute to the fracture (Figure 2.30).
- Documenting that sidebone is the cause of lameness can be difficult. Asymmetrical swelling of pastern region, pain on palpation of the collateral cartilage, and improvement of the lameness with a uniaxial PD nerve block would be suggestive of a problem in this region.
- Currently, the clinical relevance of ossification of the collateral cartilages has not been docu-

mented but should be considered when clinical abnormalities associated with sidebones are found in lame horses.

Treatment

- If sidebone is suspected as the cause of lameness, conservative treatment with confinement, topical 1% diclofenac sodium cream (Surpass®), and oral administration of NSAIDs is recommended. Any contributing foot problems should be addressed.
- Surgical removal of a suspected fractured sidebone is not recommended.
- If the lameness persists and sidebone is considered the cause of the lameness, a PD neurectomy can be performed.
- Horses with sidebone and a secondary distal phalanx fracture are treated similarly to horses with a Type II P3 fracture alone (see P3 fractures).

Prognosis

- The prognosis is difficult to predict because this condition is thought to rarely cause overt lameness.

Miscellaneous Conditions of the Foot

Sole Bruises, Corns, and Abscesses

Overview

- A bruise results from the rupture of blood vessels in the dermis (corium or sensitive tissue) beneath the sole, frog, or hoof wall. With time, the hemorrhage spreads into the deep layers of the epidermis and becomes visible as the hoof grows.
- A corn is a bruise that involves the tissues of the sole at the angle formed by the wall and the bar. Corns occur most frequently on the inner angle of the front feet and are rarely found in the hind feet.
- Abscesses can develop almost anywhere in the foot but are commonly associated with

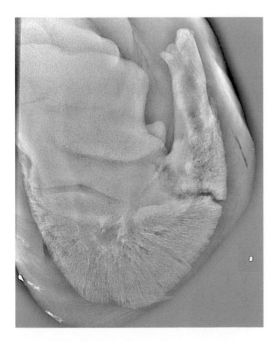

Figure 2.30 Type II articular fracture that was associated with a large sidebone of P3.

the white line region close to the toe and the heel bulbs. For example, ascending infection of the white line occurs when an opening at the sole–wall junction that permits infection to invade the laminae, which follows the path of least resistance to break open and drain at the coronary band.

Anatomy

- Bruises, corns, and abscesses often occur on the solar surface of the foot and heel bulbs (Figure 2.31).
- The digital cushion lies beneath the sole, frog, and heel bulbs and is often involved concurrently with these conditions (Figure 2.1).

Imaging

- Imaging is usually unnecessary to identify bruises, corns, and abscesses within the foot.
- Radiography may be able to help confirm a subsolar abscess as a visible gas pocket within the sole. However, most cannot be seen identified and the lack of radiographic abnormalities does not rule out an abscess.
- Radiography is important to identify contributing factors that may be associated with subsolar abscesses.

Etiology

- Trauma to the sole is the cause of most sole bruising. Horses with flat feet, thin soles,

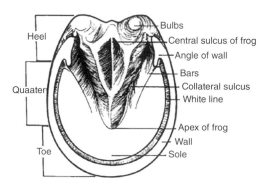

Figure 2.31 Normal solar surface of the forefoot showing anatomic structures.

and soft soles appear to be predisposed to sole bruising. Any form of shoeing that concentrates weight-bearing on the sole is likely to cause bruising.
- Corns are usually caused by pressure from horseshoes or when a stone becomes wedged between the shoe and sole. Corns are rare among horses that are not shod. Bending the inside branch of the shoe toward the frog to prevent pulling or stepping off the shoe can result in direct pressure to the sole leading to bruising.
- Abscesses within the foot can develop from a variety of causes but are usually associated with bacteria entering a defect in the sole/wall junction, penetrating injuries into the foot, or occur secondary to other problems within the hoof (i.e. laminitis, keratoma, necrosis of the collateral cartilage, sole bruises, etc.).

Clinical Signs

- Most sole bruises occur at the toe or quarter regions and corns occur at the angle of the wall and bar.
- The degree of lameness can be variable depending upon the severity and type of the bruise or corn. If the bruise is acute, the hoof may appear warmer, and an increased digital pulse may be present. Hoof tester application often identifies a focal site of pain at the site of the bruise or corn.
- Horses with foot abscesses are typically very lame and often non-weight-bearing. Increased heat is often palpable in the foot and distal limb, and an increased digital pulse is commonly found. Hoof tester pain is typically severe and simple digital pressure at the site of the abscess may cause a painful response in some cases.
- Increased swelling at the coronary band (especially at one heel bulb) may be present if the abscess has migrated up along the hoof wall.

Diagnosis

- A tentative diagnosis often can be made based on the history and clinical signs.

- If pain is localized to the foot without obvious external abnormalities, the shoe should be removed, and the sole explored.
- Acute sole bruises may not be readily apparent, because the hemorrhage has not migrated far enough distally. Chronic bruises are usually visible as a "stippled" reddened region.
- Sole abscesses may have a small defect in the sole where the abscess is trying to break through. Removing a small area of sole around this defect or inserting a large bore needle through the soft sole may reveal purulent material, confirming a subsolar abscess (Figure 2.32).
- Chronic sole bruising may be associated with osteopenia of the distal phalanx.
- Chronic abscessation may lead to osteolysis or sequestrum formation of the distal phalanx.

Treatment

- Many bruises often resolve without treatment if the source of the trauma is removed. The horse should be removed from heavy work and the environment changed so that the horse is not worked on rough ground.
- If the horse must be used, the sole can be protected with a full pad applied under the shoe. The pad should be placed to avoid pressure to the bruised site. Wide-web shoes also may be beneficial to relieve pressure on the sole. Additionally, light paring of the sole overlying the bruise often relieves the pressure and makes the horse more comfortable.
- Drainage is the key to treating suppurative bruises and other subsolar abscesses. Only a small amount of sole overlying the abscess should be removed to permit ventral drainage. The foot can then be soaked in antiseptic solution if desired, and the foot bandaged. Once the abscess has resolved, the sole can be protected with protective boots or shoes until the defect has completely keratinized.
- In cases in which shoeing is contributing to the bruising, removal of the shoe may be all that is necessary. To prevent shoes from causing corns, the heels of the shoe should extend well back on the buttresses and should fit full on the wall at the quarters and heels.

Prognosis

- The prognosis is usually very good for horses suffering from a single traumatic episode and in horses with good foot conformation.
- The prognosis is reduced in horses with poor hoof conformation that are continually worked on hard ground because recurrence is common.
- Horses with routine foot abscesses also have a very good prognosis provided the infection does not involve deeper structures in the foot.
- It should always be remembered that subsolar abscesses can be associated with other conditions of the foot such as keratomas, chronic laminitis, and septic PO (Figure 2.33).

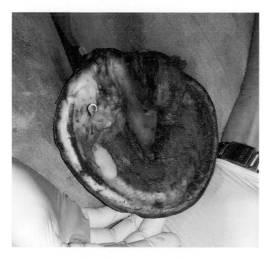

Figure 2.32 This horse was non-weight-bearing lame with no evidence of a hoof abscess or fracture. Focal pain was detected near the lateral heel and insertion of a 16-gauge needle confirmed the suspicion of an abscess.

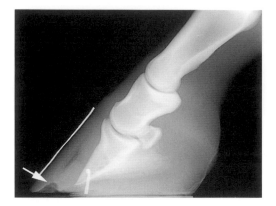

Figure 2.33 This horse had what was thought to be a routine abscess at the toe, but a lateral radiograph revealed chronic laminitis.

Septic Pedal Osteitis (PO)

Anatomy

- The distal phalanx is a triangular-shaped bone located within the hoof capsule that serves as a major insertion site for the flexor tendons palmarly/plantarly and the extensor tendons dorsally (Figure 2.1).
- The distal phalanx is protected dorsally by the hoof wall and distally by the sole, digital cushion, frog, and heel bulbs (Figures 2.1 and 2.31).

Imaging

- Radiography is usually the imaging modality of choice to detect potential abnormalities within the distal phalanx or hoof itself.
- Cross-sectional imaging (CT and MRI) may be necessary in select cases of septic PO, but these are unusual.

Etiology

- Septic PO refers to bacterial infection within the distal phalanx usually as an extension of a subsolar abscess, secondary to penetrating injuries or from hematogenous spread in foals.
- Other causes include chronic severe laminitis, subsolar abscesses, solar margin fractures (Figure 2.34), deep hoof wall cracks, and avulsion hoof injuries.

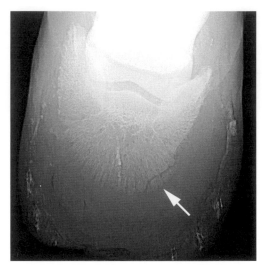

Figure 2.34 Type VI fractures are also referred to as solar margin fractures of P3 (arrow) and can be secondary to osteopenia and predispose to septic pedal osteitis.

- Septic PO in foals should be considered as a potential site for hematogenous spread of infection associated with the septic arthritis/joint ill syndrome.
- A sequestrum may develop in the distal phalanx as the osseous infection progresses.

Clinical Signs

- Septic PO occurs most commonly in the forelimbs in adult horses and in the hindlimbs in foals.
- The severity of lameness in horses with septic PO is usually severe (in one study, over 50% of the horses were grade 4 of 5 lame), and the lameness may be chronic.
- Increased hoof temperature, prominent digital pulses, and localized hoof tester pain are common in the affected limb.
- Perineural anesthesia of the PD nerves may not eliminate the lameness in all horses with septic PO.

Diagnosis

- Radiographic signs suggestive of septic PO are usually straightforward and are consistent with areas of bone infection (Figure 2.35).

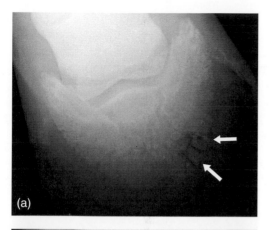

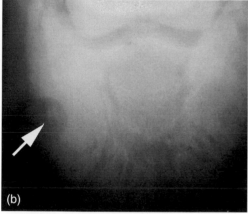

Figure 2.35 Dorsopalmar radiographs of the distal phalanx in two adult horses with severe lameness. (a) Osteolysis of the solar margin (arrows) is evident consistent with infection and (b) lysis and a sequestrum can be seen along the solar surface of P3 (arrow).

- Radiographic signs of septic PO may include focal osteolysis, decrease in bone density, and sequestration (Figure 2.34).
- In foals with septic PO, evidence of localized lysis or focal loss of bone density were observed at the toe (14/22 cases), extensor process (5/22 cases), or the palmar/plantar process (3/22 cases) of the distal phalanx.
- CT or MRI examination of the foot can often provide more detailed information but is usually unnecessary to make a diagnosis.

Treatment

- Treatment of septic PO usually involves systemic and local antimicrobials (regional limb perfusion) and surgical debridement of the infected bone.
- In most cases, the site of infection is approached through the draining tract, which is usually located on the sole. One study suggested that up to 24% of the distal phalanx could be removed without long-term adverse effects.

Prognosis

- The prognosis for horses with septic PO appears very good to excellent if the infection can be controlled. All 33 affected horses returned to their intended use in one study.
- Foals with septic PO also usually have a good prognosis; 86% survival in one study.

Penetrating Injuries of the Foot

Anatomy

- The distal phalanx is a triangular-shaped bone located within the hoof capsule that serves as a major insertion site for the flexor tendons palmarly/plantarly and the extensor tendons dorsally (Figure 2.1).
- The distal phalanx is protected dorsally by the hoof wall and distally by the sole, digital cushion, frog, and heel bulbs (Figures 2.1 and 2.31).
- The navicular bursa, DIP joint, and DFTS are synovial cavities that can be involved with penetrating injuries of the foot.

Imaging

- Radiography is usually the imaging modality of choice to aid diagnosis of penetrating injuries to the foot.
- Ultrasound may be advantageous for injuries along the coronary band especially those involving nonmetallic foreign material (i.e. wood; Figure 2.36).

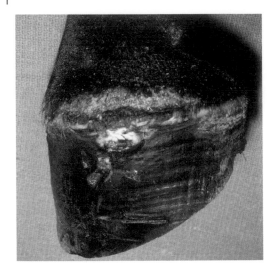

Figure 2.36 This horse had a draining tract at the dorsal coronet, but no abnormalities could be found on the solar surface of the foot. Exploration of the tract revealed a small piece of wood.

- Cross-sectional imaging (CT and MRI) may be necessary in select cases when radiography is inconclusive.

Etiology

- Penetrating injuries of the foot are usually caused by the horse stepping on (bottom of the foot) or contacting (coronary band, heel bulbs, and pastern region) a sharp object.
- Structures at risk with injuries to the central third of the frog include the navicular bursa, navicular bone, DDFT, or distal phalanx (Figure 2.37).
- Coronary band injuries may involve the DIP joint, distal phalanx, and collateral cartilages of the distal phalanx.
- Injuries to the heel bulb region are most likely to damage the DDFT, DFTS, or palmar/plantar aspect of the DIP joint.
- Injuries elsewhere on the bottom of the foot will most likely only damage the digital cushion or the solar surface of the distal phalanx and are usually less problematic.

Clinical Signs

- The clinical signs vary depending on the depth (superficial vs. deep), location (sole vs.

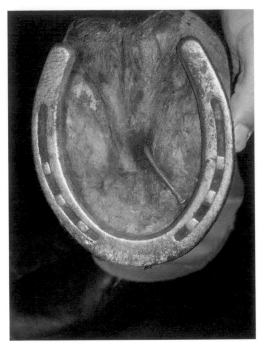

Figure 2.37 This horse presented for an acute onset hindlimb lameness. A nail was found protruding from the apex of the frog. Based on the location, entry into the navicular bursa would be unlikely.

coronary band), and duration (acute vs. chronic) of the injury.
- Minor injuries that only penetrate the cornified layer of the sole into the digital cushion may not cause clinical signs unless an abscess develops.
- Deep injuries that completely penetrate through the hoof wall and contact a bone, tendon, or synovial cavity typically cause severe and acute lameness.
- Increased heat and a prominent digital pulse usually can be palpated.
- If a foreign body such as a nail is present in the bottom of the foot, it is ideal to take a radiograph to determine the exact depth and direction of the nail's path before it is removed (Figures 2.37 and 2.38). However, this is rarely possible as owners will typically remove the foreign object.
- If a wound is not obvious, careful application of hoof testers may help identify focal pain which may indicate the site of penetration.

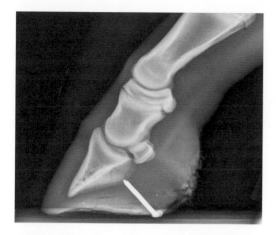

Figure 2.38 Taking radiographs of the foot prior to removing the foreign body can help identify the direction and depth of the puncture.

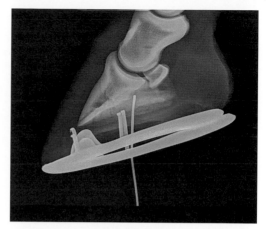

Figure 2.39 This horse had a history of stepping on a farriery nail with its hind foot 24 hours previously. Exploration of the tract revealed that it had penetrated through the digital cushion to the solar surface of the third phalanx.

- Wounds that penetrate the frog can be particularly difficult to locate because the softer and more elastic tissues of the frog tend to collapse and fill in the tract. Probing of the tract can help identify both the depth and direction of the injury. A radiograph can be taken with the probe placed into the tract to further verify its location (Figure 2.39).
- A penetrating wound of the coronary band can be overlooked if the hair is long or if local swelling and wound drainage are not present.
- Perineural anesthesia usually is not needed to localize the site of lameness but is very beneficial to facilitate close examination of the injury site and removal of the frog or sole if necessary.

Diagnosis
- Additional diagnostics that can be performed to confirm the location and depth of a penetrating injury include distention of a synovial cavity with saline to detect leakage from the wound, plain radiographs, radiographs with a metallic probe inserted in the wound, or contrast radiography (fistulogram; Figure 2.40).
- Ultrasound may be helpful to document injuries to the DDFT and involvement of the

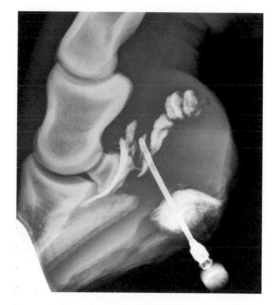

Figure 2.40 Lateromedial (LM) projection of the distal limb after injection of iodinated contrast material into an externally draining tract demonstrating filling of the navicular bursa with contrast material consistent and a communication between the draining tract and the bursa.

DFTS in the palmar/plantar aspect of the foot and for coronary band injuries.
- Synovial fluid analysis (increased WBC count total protein concentration) usually

can be used to help confirm the diagnosis of infectious synovitis.

- Cross-sectional imaging (CT and MRI) can also be very helpful to confirm both the location and the presence of infection if other diagnostics are equivocal.

Treatment

- Treatment of superficial penetrating wounds that do not involve vital structures (bone, tendon, or synovial cavities) is aimed at providing adequate drainage, removing infected and necrotic tissue, and protecting the site from further contamination. An antiseptic dressing is recommended, and the foot is protected to minimize further contamination.
- Penetrating injuries that involve bone, tendon, or synovial cavities require more aggressive treatment depending on the deeper structure that is involved. Typical treatments include both systemic (IV) and local (IV regional perfusion and intrasynovial) antimicrobials; NSAIDs; local debridement of the wound; and lavage, endoscopy, or arthroscopy if a synovial cavity is involved. Involvement of the navicular bursa is best treated with endoscopy or lavage and local debridement of the defect in the frog (reader is referred to Chapter 7 for more details of therapy).
- Wounds that penetrate the distal phalanx should be enlarged and the distal phalanx curettaged to prevent further progression of the infection into the bone.
- Soaking the foot to lavage deep wounds of the foot is generally not recommended.

Prognosis

- Horses with penetrating injuries that do not involve bone, tendon, or a synovial cavity typically do very well. Horses with deep penetrating injuries outside the frog or frog sulci also do well (>90% in two separate studies).
- Horses with synovial involvement following solar foot penetration have a poor prognosis (36 and 29% in two recent studies) for return to preinjury athletic function.

- In general, prompt treatment of any penetrating injury to the foot regardless of the structure(s) involved improves the chance of a successful outcome.

Keratoma

Overview

- A keratoma is a non-neoplastic condition of the hoof that is characterized by keratin-containing tissue growing between the hoof wall and the distal phalanx.
- The growth usually begins near the coronary band, but it may extend to the solar surface anywhere along the white line.
- A visible deviation of the coronary band and/or hoof wall is often present, and the most commonly affected areas of the foot are the toe and quarter.
- Keratomas have been observed in horses ranging from two to 20 years of age and should be differentiated from other growths that can occur in the hoof such as squamous cell carcinoma, canker, and melanoma.

Anatomy

- The distal phalanx is attached to the hoof wall through a complicated network of epidermal and dermal laminae that is thought to become disturbed in horses that develop keratomas.
- The hoof wall is composed of three layers: stratum externum, stratum medium, and stratum internum, and growth of the hoof wall is primarily from the coronary epidermis toward the ground (Figure 2.41).
- Nearly the entire hoof is composed of a thick layer of anucleate squamous keratinocytes, and the keratinaceous tissues are devoid of nerves endings.

Imaging

- A definitive diagnosis of keratoma can usually made based on the characteristic radiographic features within the distal phalanx.

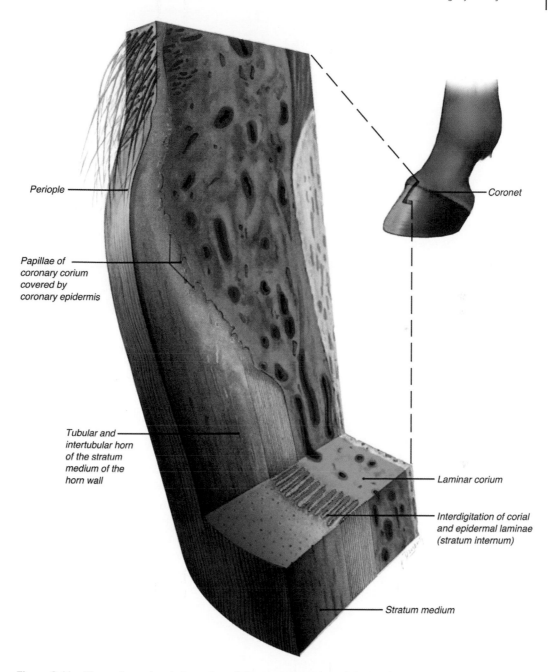

Periople

Papillae of
coronary corium
covered by
coronary epidermis

Tubular and
intertubular horn
of the stratum
medium of the
horn wall

Coronet

Laminar corium

Interdigitation of corial
and epidermal laminae
(stratum internum)

Stratum medium

Figure 2.41 Three-dimensional dissection of the coronary region of the hoof wall.

- Cross-sectional imaging (CT or MRI) is currently the preferred technique to both definitively diagnose and accurately localize keratomas within the hoof wall.

Etiology

- Trauma and chronic irritation in the form of sole abscesses or direct hoof injuries are the cause in the majority of cases.

- Keratomas can develop without a history of previous injury and the initiating cause often cannot be determined.
- Lameness and the radiographic changes are thought to arise from the growth of the keratoma and the subsequent pressure that it applies to the sensitive lamina and distal phalanx.

Clinical Signs

- A history of a slow onset of intermittent lameness is common. Moderate-to-severe lameness is commonly observed at presentation.
- The lameness is often seen before the distortion at the coronary band and hoof wall becomes obvious. The coronary band and hoof wall may or may not be abnormally shaped and close examination of the foot may be required to identify any abnormality.
- A slight bulge in the hoof wall and a deviation in the white line toward the center of the foot may be all that is seen.
- Common clinical signs of keratomas in one study were lameness and the presence of a subsolar abscess.
- Hoof tester examination often elicits a painful response when pressure is applied over the lesion.
- A PD nerve block often improves the lameness, but a basisesamoid or abaxial sesamoid block may be required to completely eliminate the lameness.

Diagnosis

- A discrete semicircular defect in the distal phalanx is often seen on routine radiographs (Figure 5.33). The radiographic signs of a keratoma can usually be differentiated from lysis from infection because of the smooth borders and lack of a sclerotic margin.
- Ultrasonographic imaging of a keratoma has been reported as a hypoechoic, well-delineated soft tissue mass under the hoof wall (Figure 2.42).
- The use of CT to accurately localize keratomas was recently reported to minimize the

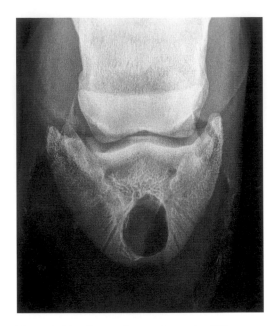

Figure 2.42 Dorsopalmar radiograph of P3 demonstrating a smooth margined lytic defect within the bone that is characteristic of a keratoma. *Source*: Courtesy of Scott Katzman.

amount of hoof wall that needed to be removed and reduced postoperative complications in operated horses (Figure 2.43).

Treatment

- Treatment involves complete surgical removal of the abnormal growth. Incomplete removal of the keratoma is thought to result in recurrence of the growth.
- Partial hoof wall resection directly over the location of the keratoma is the preferred technique. Windows within the hoof wall can be made with a motorized burr, a cast cutting saw, oscillating saw, or an osteotome (Figure 2.44).
- The overall goal of surgery is to remove as little hoof wall as possible to facilitate complete removal of the keratoma.

Prognosis

- The prognosis is generally very good for return to performance if the abnormal tissue is completely removed. 25/26 and 28/31

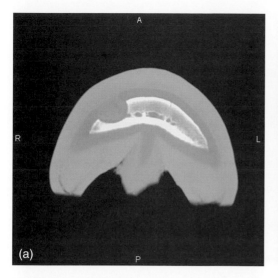
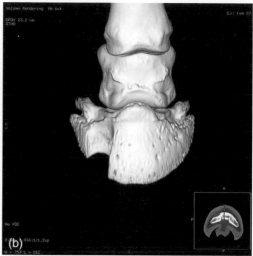

Figure 2.43 Single CT image of a foot (a) demonstrating a defect within the distal phalanx consistent with a keratoma, and CT reconstruction of the CT images (b) that illustrates the exact location of the keratoma within the distal phalanx. *Source*: Courtesy of Scott Katzman.

horses returned to their previous exercise level after surgery in two separate studies.

- Using cross-sectional imaging (CT or MRI) is thought to facilitate more accurate localization of the keratoma, enabling a smaller hoof wall resection and an improved prognosis.

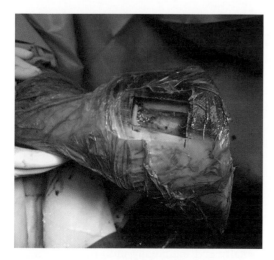

Figure 2.44 Hoof wall removal directly over the keratoma that was located with CT. *Source*: Courtesy of Scott Katzman.

- Adequate stabilization of the hoof defect and complete removal of the lesion are important for a successful outcome.

White Line Disease

Overview

- White line disease (WLD) is a keratolytic process on the solar surface of the hoof and is characterized by progressive separation of the inner zone of the hoof wall.
- WLD differs from laminitis because it does not involve the sensitive tissue beneath the hoof wall. The separation occurs in the nonpigmented horn between the stratum medium and stratum internum.
- The separation, which can originate at the toe, the quarter, and/or the heel, appears to be invaded by opportunistic bacteria/fungi leading to infection that can progress to varying heights and configurations proximally toward the coronet.
- WLD does not invade the coronet and the disease process nearly always occurs secondary to hoof wall separation.

Anatomy and Imaging (Please refer to previous section on "Keratoma")

Etiology

- WLD can affect a horse of any age, sex, or breed.
- Proposed causes include mechanical stress on the hoof wall associated with long toes and hoof capsule distortions, environmental conditions such as excessive moisture or dryness that affects the inner hoof-wall attachment, toxicity associated with selenium, and infection of the white line with bacteria and/or fungi.
- The fact that WLD can be resolved with debridement alone further detracts from infection as a primary cause.

Clinical Signs

- Horses with WLD may have variable to no lameness, and the condition is often only found during routine trimming.
- In the early stages, the only noticeable change on the solar surface of the foot is a small separation containing powdery material located at the inner part of the hoof wall adjacent to the sole/wall junction (white line). Other early signs may include sole pain with hoof testers, occasional heat, and increasingly flat soles.
- As the separation becomes more extensive and extends into a quarter, a concavity (dish) may form along one side of the hoof and a bulge is present on the opposite side directly above the affected area at the coronary band (Figure 2.45).
- Any significant loss of epidermal lamellae from hoof wall separation may permit the distal phalanx to shift toward the side with the separation.
- Other clinical signs may include slow hoof wall growth, poor consistency of hoof wall, and a hollow sound noted when the outer hoof wall over the separation is tapped with a hammer.

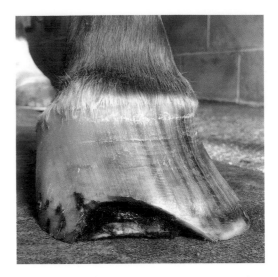

Figure 2.45 Extensive separation under lateral hoof wall causing a shift of the distal phalanx in the hoof capsule. Note the concavity in the medial wall and the soft tissue enlargement above the coronet on the lateral side. *Source*: Courtesy of Stephen O'Grady.

Diagnosis

- A tentative diagnosis is usually made on the basis of clinical findings. The sole/wall junction will usually be wider than normal and further examination may reveal a hoof concavity that contains white/gray powdery material.
- Radiographs are always recommended to determine the extent of the hoof wall separation and whether rotation of the distal phalanx within the hoof capsule has occurred. A gas line along the dorsal hoof wall may be seen with both WLD and chronic laminitis.

Treatment

- Treatment for WLD is directed toward protecting and unloading the damaged section of the foot with therapeutic farriery combined with resection of the hoof capsule overlying the affected area(s).
- The debridement should be continued proximally and marginally until there is a solid attachment between the hoof wall and external lamellae (Figure 2.46).

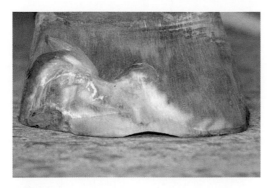

Figure 2.46 Dorsal hoof wall resection to treat a horse with WLD. Note the solid margins around the periphery of the resection. *Source*: Courtesy of Stephen O'Grady.

- The type of therapeutic shoe and its method of attachment are dictated by the extent of the damaged hoof wall that must be removed.
- After thorough hoof wall resection, the affected area is left to grow out with debridement performed at frequent intervals.
- The feet should be kept as dry as possible and the hoof wall defects cleaned with a wire brush by the owners as often as necessary.
- The duration of treatment depends on the amount of wall removed, but most horses can return to work when the surface of the defect has cornified.

Prognosis
- Most horses with WLD have a very good prognosis with local debridement and appropriate farriery.
- Displacement of the distal phalanx secondary to WLD will likely have a reduced prognosis.
- There is no known medical treatment, and the condition is unlikely to improve unless the affected, undermined hoof wall is removed.

Thrush

Overview
- Thrush is a degenerative condition that affects the body and base of the frog generally caused by a bacterial infection.

- The disease begins when bacteria penetrate the outer horn or epidermis of the frog and is characterized by deterioration of the frog and the presence of black necrotic exudate with a foul odor.
- Severe cases of thrush must be differentiated from canker, which is a proliferative disease where abnormal frog tissue increases in comparison to thrush, which is a degenerative disease where the horn of the frog deteriorates (Figure 2.47a and b).

Anatomy
- The frog (cuneus ungulae) is a wedge-shaped mass of keratinized stratified squamous epithelium rendered softer than other parts of the hoof by increased water content.
- The ground surface of the frog presents a pointed apex and central sulcus enclosed by two crura (Figure 2.48).
- Paracuneal (collateral) sulci separate the crura of the frog from the bars and the sole and the palmar aspect of the frog blends into the bulbs of the heels.
- Compression of the frog during weight-bearing serves to transfer forces to the heels and assists with circulation within the foot and distal limb.

Imaging
- There are no specific imaging techniques that can aid in the diagnosis of conditions that affect the frog.

Etiology
- The health of the frog is an important cause of thrush. An unhealthy frog is markedly smaller in size and recessed below the level of the ground surface of the hoof, which creates an environment conducive to accumulation of debris and bacterial growth.
- Although no specific organism has been identified as the cause, two anaerobic bacteria species, *Bacteroides sp.* and *Fusobacterium*

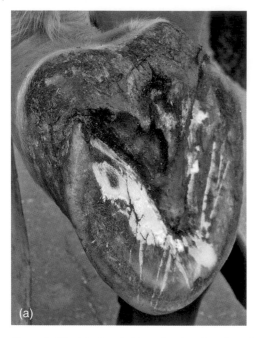
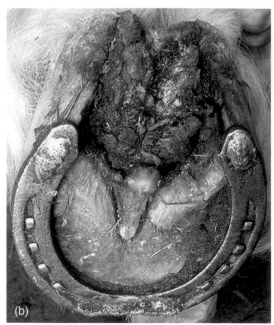

Figure 2.47 A is thrush. Note the deterioration of the frog that is recessed below ground surface of foot. B is severe canker. Note the proliferation of the diseased horn. *Source*: Courtesy of Stephen O'Grady.

necrophorum, are commonly isolated from the bottom of the horse's foot.
- Contributing factors are wet, unhygienic stable conditions, especially when horses stand in urine- and manure-soiled bedding, neglect of daily foot care, and lack of exercise.
- Inadequate or improper trimming and shoeing, which promote long contracted heels and deep sulci, also contributes to the risk of infection.

Clinical Signs
- The hindlimbs are most frequently involved.
- There is usually an increased amount of moisture on the bottom of the foot and a black, odiferous discharge in the sulci of the frog. The affected sulci of the frog are often deeper than usual, and the frog may be undermined and detached from the underlying tissue.
- Lameness is usually present in severe cases that involve the dermis and swelling of the distal limb may be seen.

Diagnosis
- The diagnosis is usually based the presence of black, odiferous discharge in the sulci of the frog together with the loss of the frog.
- The frog will generally be small, recessed within the hoof capsule, lack a solid firm consistency, and have a necrotic appearance.

Treatment
- Treatment for thrush begins with improving the hoof capsule, the conformation of the palmar/foot, and the health of the frog. Thrush is unlikely to resolve as long as the frog remains recessed below the ground surface of the foot.
- Ideally the shoes should be removed, the heels trimmed to the same plane as the frog, the perimeter of the hoof wall rounded, and the horse left barefoot.
- Mild cases usually respond to debridement of the diseased tissue, soaking, and topical application of an astringent.
- Topical antiseptics/astringents including 2% iodine, Merthiolate, chlorohexidine, and

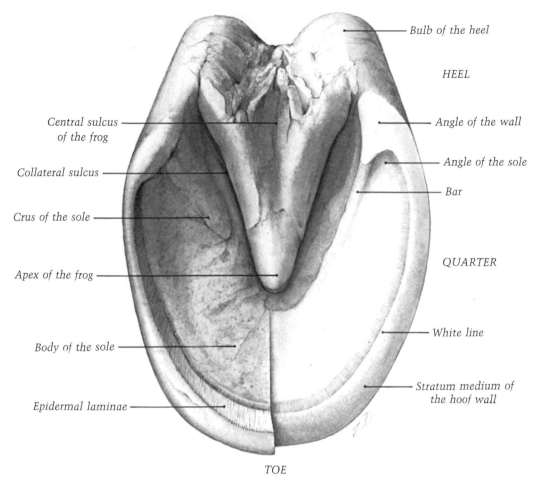

Bulb of the heel

HEEL

Central sulcus of the frog

Angle of the wall

Angle of the sole

Collateral sulcus

Bar

Crus of the sole

Apex of the frog

QUARTER

Body of the sole

White line

Stratum medium of the hoof wall

Epidermal laminae

TOE

Figure 2.48 Topography of the solar surface of the hoof. The right half has been trimmed to emphasize the region of the white line.

various copper sulfate solutions can be applied on a daily basis until the infection is controlled.

- The horse should be kept in a dry, clean stall or in a dry yard and have its feet cleaned and the frogs brushed vigorously with a stiff brush daily.
- Severe cases of thrush are treated in a similar manner as above except debridement of the diseased undermined tissue is more extensive and often must be repeated.
- Prevention is superior to treatment and emphasis should be placed on good farriery as the primary means for preventing this disease.

Prognosis
- The prognosis is good if the disease is diagnosed early before the foot has suffered extensive damage, and the health of the frog can be restored.
- The prognosis is less favorable if the infection and frog deterioration are extensive, hoof distortions are severe, and corrective farriery is not maintained.

Canker

Overview
- Equine canker is described as an infectious process that results in the development of

chronic hypertrophy of the horn-producing tissues. It also has been described as a chronic hypertrophic, moist pododermatitis of the epidermal tissues of the foot.

- The infection is thought to cause abnormal keratin production or dyskeratosis, which is seen as filamentous fronds of hypertrophic horn.
- The disease is considered to be especially common in draft horses but can be seen in any breed, and one or multiple feet can be affected.
- Canker can be misdiagnosed as "thrush," particularly in the early course of the disease (Figure 2.47).

Anatomy and Imaging (see above section on "Thrush")

Etiology
- Affected horses often have a history of being housed on moist pastures or in wet, unhygienic conditions.
- Horses standing in urine-, feces-, or mud-soaked bedding appear to be at risk, although it can be seen in horses that are well cared for that receive regular hoof care.
- The causative anaerobic Gram-negative organisms are thought to be *Fusobacterium Necrophorum* and one or more *Bacteroides* spp.

Clinical Signs
- Lameness usually is not present in early stages of the disease because the superficial epidermis is primarily involved.
- Early stages of canker may present as a focal area of granulation tissue in the frog that bleeds easily when abraded.
- Examination of the foot usually reveals a fetid odor, and the frog, which may appear intact, has a ragged proliferative filamentous appearance.
- Canker is characterized by numerous, small, finger-like papillae of soft off-white material that resembles a cauliflower-like appearance (Figure 2.49).

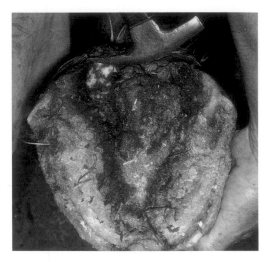

Figure 2.49 Small, pale, demarcated growth along the caudal aspect of the frog that could be consistent with early canker.

- The epidermal tissue of the frog is usually friable, bleeds easily when abraded, may be painful when touched, and is usually covered with a caseous white exudate that resembles cottage cheese.
- It generally remains focal within the frog but has the capacity to invade the adjacent sole, bars, and hoof wall.

Diagnosis
- Often a presumptive diagnosis can be made based on the physical findings of a moist exudative pododermatitis with characteristic hypertrophic filamentous fronds involving the frog together with a fetid odor.
- It can be confirmed with a biopsy, but this is seldom done - usually interpreted as a chronic hypertrophic moist, pododermatitis of the frog.
- Bacterial cultures are rarely beneficial.

Treatment
- Treatment consists of thorough, careful debridement of the affected tissue followed by a regimen of topical therapy applied daily until the disease has resolved.
- It is important to trim the foot appropriately prior to surgery.

- The debridement of the cankerous tissue can be performed standing under local anesthesia or under general anesthesia if considered necessary.
- Cryotherapy of the debrided area is recommended to remove residual bacteria from the surface in a double freeze-thaw pattern.
- There are a variety of topical preparations that can be used but the astringents appear to play the most important role.
- Topical treatments include 10% benzoyl peroxide in acetone combined with metronidazole powder, solution of tricide/gentocin/lincomycin, or an oxytetracycline and metronidazole paste.
- Oral prednisolone at a dose of 1 mg/kg q24h for seven days, 0.5 mg/kg q24h for seven days, and then 0.25 mg/kg q24h for seven days has been reported to improve the success of treatment.
- Topical medications usually are applied directly to the debrided area; direct contact of the medication to the defect is important for success.
- Keeping the wound clean and dry with bandages or by other means and maintaining the horse in a dry environment are critical aspects of aftercare.
- The duration of treatment may be several weeks to months depending on the severity of the disease.

Prognosis

- The prognosis is favorable for complete resolution of canker if the lesion is small, and treatment is instituted early in the course of the disease.
- Advanced cases of canker that invade the sole, bars, and hoof wall, and those that involve multiple limbs, remain very difficult to treat.

Laminitis

Overview

- Equine laminitis is a structural failure of the lamellae between the distal phalanx and hoof wall resulting in displacement of the distal phalanx within the hoof capsule.
- When either the structural integrity of the lamellar epidermal cells or the adhesion of these cells to the underlying dermis is compromised, the resulting loss of structural strength of the digital lamellae, combined with the forces on the distal limb, leads to displacement of the distal phalanx.
- Three types of displacement of the distal phalanx can take place:
  1) Symmetrical distal displacement or "sinking" of the phalanx (Figure 2.50).

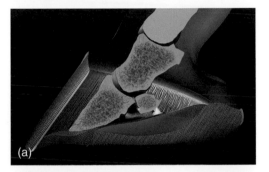

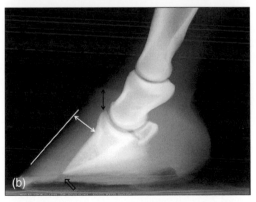

Figure 2.50 In symmetrical distal displacement, the distal phalanx descends within the hoof capsule (a). Therefore, the distal phalanx retains its alignment with the more proximal phalanges and the hoof capsule (b), but the distance between the parietal surface of the distal phalanx and the hoof wall increases (white arrow) and the distance between the proximal extensor process and the proximal border of hoof wall (black double arrow) and the distance between the distal phalanx and the sole and ground decrease (open arrow). *Source:* Courtesy of James Belknap and Andy Parks.

2) Asymmetric distal displacement of the phalanx (either medial or lateral; Figure 2.51).
3) Dorsal rotation in which the dorsodistal tip of the distal phalanx displaces in a palmarodistal direction away from the dorsal hoof wall (Figure 2.52).
4) A combination of distal displacement and rotation can occur in many horses.

- Laminitis occurs as a sequela to other diseases and three different types of laminitis have been categorized based on these predisposing factors:
1) Systemic sepsis/endotoxemia (sepsis-related laminitis [SRL]).
2) Systemic endocrinopathies (endocrinopathic laminitis).
3) Disease or injury to one limb that necessitates preferential weight-bearing on the opposite limb (supporting limb laminitis [SLL]).

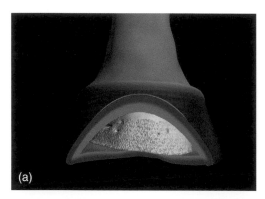
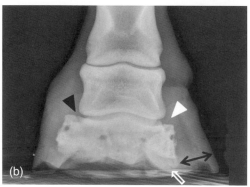

Figure 2.51 In medial or lateral asymmetrical displacement (a), one side of the distal phalanx descends (white open arrow in (b)). The distance between the wall and the distal phalanx increases (black double arrow), and the distance between the distal phalanx and the sole and ground decreases on the affected side (white open arrow). Additionally, the DIP joint becomes asymmetrical when viewed on a DP radiograph; the joint space is increased on the affected side (white arrowhead) and decreased on the unaffected side (black arrowhead). *Source*: Courtesy of James Belknap and Andy Parks.

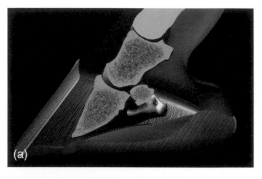
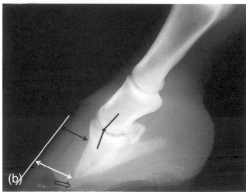

Figure 2.52 (a and b) In horses with early chronic laminitis, the surface of the hoof wall is unchanged, but the distal phalanx rotates about the DIP joint (the joint flexes, black lines in b); consequently, the normal alignment of the distal phalanx with the other phalanges is changed (phalangeal rotation). Additionally, the distance between the dorsal distal parietal surface of the distal phalanx and hoof capsule increases (white double arrow) while it remains close to normal proximally (black double arrow); (i.e. there is divergence of the surfaces [capsular rotation]). Also, the distance between the dorsal margin of the distal phalanx and the sole and ground is decreased (open arrow). *Source*: Courtesy of James Belknap and Andy Parks.

- Laminitis is often classified into three different stages: developmental (before clinical signs), acute (presence of clinical signs but no movement of the distal phalanx), and chronic (movement of the distal phalanx has occurred).

Anatomy

- The distal phalanx of the equine digit is surrounded by the hoof consisting of the deeper dermal tissues and more superficial epidermal tissues.
- Similar to the skin, the epidermal component of the hoof contains both keratinized nonviable components externally and live epidermal cells internally (Figure 2.41).

- The outer hoof wall (stratum externum and stratum medium) provides both protection to the digit and supports the weight of the horse during weight-bearing.
- The epidermal lamellae, part of the stratum internum of the hoof wall, extend vertically from the coronary groove of the proximal hoof wall distad to merge with the sole and around the entire periphery of the distal phalanx.
- The epidermal lamellae interdigitating with the same number of dermal lamellae (Figures 2.41 and 2.53).
- Numerous secondary epidermal lamellae emanate from each primary epidermal lamella, interdigitating with secondary dermal lamellae (Figure 2.53).

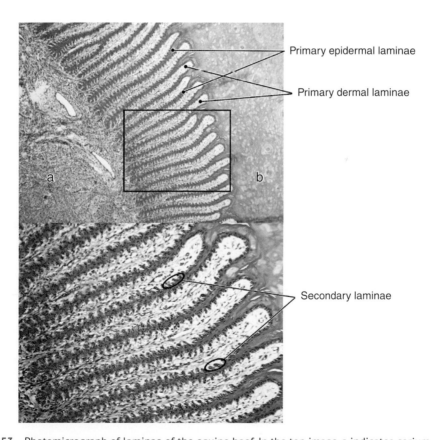

Primary epidermal laminae

Primary dermal laminae

Secondary laminae

Figure 2.53 Photomicrograph of laminae of the equine hoof. In the top image, a indicates corium; b is the epidermis (hoof wall). Laminae extending from the corium (primary dermal laminae) are the so-called "sensitive laminae." Laminae extending from the epidermal portions of the hoof (primary epidermal laminae) are the "insensitive laminae." The box indicates the region enlarged in the lower image. Here, smaller interdigitating projections, the secondary laminae, can be seen arising perpendicular to the primary laminae. *Source*: Courtesy of Anna Fails.

- The secondary epidermal lamellae are made up of two types of live epithelial cells and failure of these cells is thought to contribute to separation of the epidermal and dermal lamellae leading to laminitis.

Imaging

- Radiography is the imaging technique of choice to evaluate horses with laminitis.
- Radiographs should be taken at the first sign of acute laminitis to serve as a baseline for subsequent radiographic comparisons and to determine if radiographic changes suggestive of previous laminitis are present.
- Radiography is critical as a diagnostic tool to determine the presence of the disease and to monitor progress of the disease and guide treatment.

Etiology

- In SRL, a profound inflammatory response is thought to occur within the lamellar tissue causing lamellar epithelial cell dysregulation and dysadhesion with subsequent lamellar failure.
- In endocrinopathic laminitis, including both metabolic syndrome and pituitary pars intermedia dysfunction (PPID), both clinical and experimental studies indicate that hyperinsulinemia (commonly termed insulin dysregulation) is the primary factor inducing lamellar failure.
- In SLL laminitis, a decrease in lamellar blood flow due to a lack of movement is thought to contribute to tissue hypoxia and subsequent breakdown of the lamellar epithelial structure.
- Regardless of the type of laminitis, the final stage of the disease process is thought to involve the induction of growth factor-related signaling that leads to lamellar failure through disruption of epithelial cell cytoskeletal dynamics and adhesion to the underlying matrix.
- Malfunction of the epithelial cells may lead to both stretching of the epidermal lamellae

and the loss of attachment (dysadhesion) between the lamellar basal epithelial cells and the basement membrane. The end result is separation of the epidermal and dermal lamellae and displacement of the distal phalanx.
- The severity of the lamellae damage will most likely correlate with how fast and how much the distal phalanx moves within the hoof wall.
- Predisposing factors include diseases causing sepsis/toxemia (grain overload, retained placenta, colitis, etc.), equine metabolic syndrome, PPID, excessive weight-bearing, eating lush pasture, exercise on hard surfaces, and potentially the use of corticosteroids.
- The reader is referred to Chapter 4 in *Adams and Stashak's Lameness in Horses, 7th Edition*, for further information.

Clinical Signs

- Laminitis is seen most commonly in both front feet but all four feet, both hind feet, or only a single foot (with support limb laminitis) may be affected.
- The clinical signs in horses with SRL are commonly observed 24–72 hours following the onset of a septic process.
- The onset of disease in endocrinopathic laminitis is extremely variable; insidious displacement of the distal phalanx may occur over months to years in horses with EMS while pasture-associated laminitis may cause an acute and severe onset similar to SRL.
- In SLL, disease progression is extremely inconsistent between animals; clinical signs may occur days, weeks, or months after the onset of excessive weight-bearing.
- Clinical signs of acute laminitis include lameness, an increase in the temperature of one or more hooves, increased digital pulses, and elicitation of a painful withdrawal response to hoof-testers over the toe.
- The characteristic stance of a laminitic horse with both fore feet affected is placement of

the fore feet well in front of the normal position and anterior placement of the hind feet in order to shift more weight to the hindlimbs.

- Horses with chronic laminitis may have different degrees of hoof capsule deformation and lameness. These include a dorsal concavity to the hoof wall, abnormal growth rings which are more widely spaced in the heel than the toe, and a flat or convexity to the sole dorsal to the apex of the frog.
- In cases of distal displacement of the third phalanx, there may be a palpable (and sometimes visible) groove at the junction of the skin of the pastern and the coronary band.
- The severity of lameness can vary from being barely detectable to complete recumbency.

Diagnosis

- The diagnosis of acute laminitis is often made based on the history, the characteristic stance, and the digital exam (pulse, heat, and hoof testers).
- Horses with acute laminitis may not improve with a PD block but usually respond to an abaxial sesamoid block. In some severely painful cases, the lameness may not block out entirely with local perineural anesthesia.
- Horses with chronic laminitis often improve with a PD block because a significant part of the lameness is often due to sole pain instead of lamellar pain.
- Radiographs may or may not be useful in the acute stage but are usually diagnostic in horses with chronic laminitis. The most important views are the lateral and horizontal beam DP views. It is important that the foot is placed on a block and that the X-ray beam is centered as close as possible to the solar margin of the distal phalanx (approximately 1.5 cm proximal to the surface of the block).
- The types of movement of the distal phalanx that should be assessed using radiography include capsular vs. phalangeal rotation, symmetrical distal displacement, asymmetrical or uniaxial distal displacement of the distal phalanx, or any combination of these (Figures 2.51, 2.54, 2.55).

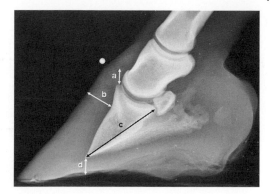

Figure 2.54 Several measurements obtained from lateral radiographs of the digit can be used to assess horses with distal displacement of the distal phalanx. a = distance from the proximal extensor process to the proximal aspect of the hoof wall (immediately distal to coronary band), b = the distance from the dorsal parietal surface of the distal phalanx to the dorsal surface of the hoof capsule, b/c = the ratio of the distance from the dorsal parietal surface of the distal phalanx to the dorsal surface of the hoof capsule (b) to the length of the palmar cortex of the distal phalanx (c), and d = the distance from the dorsodistal tip of the distal phalanx to the ground surface of the sole. *Source*: Courtesy of James Belknap.

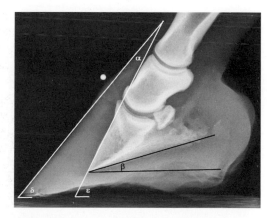

Figure 2.55 For assessment of rotation of the distal phalanx, the clinician can assess the degree of capsular rotation (angle α) at the intersection of the dorsal capsular and dorsal phalangeal lines, or can measure the difference between the dorsal angles δ and ε. The relationship of the solar margin of the distal phalanx to the ground surface of the foot can be assessed by measuring angle β. *Source*: Courtesy of James Belknap.

- The reader is referred to Chapter 4 in *Adams and Stashak's Lameness in Horses, 7th Edition*, for further information.

Treatment

- The initial goal of treatment of acute laminitis is to stabilize the digit regardless of the degree of displacement, which in turn will limit the structural failure of the lamellae.
- Concurrent treatment of the inciting cause in horses with SRL and endocrinopathic laminitis is especially important.
- Anti-inflammatory therapy is considered mandatory in acute laminitis and most often includes the use of NSAIDs, and local cryotherapy of the affected digit(s).
- Digital hypothermia can also be used as a prophylactic therapy in the "at risk" patient.
- Flunixin meglumine, phenylbutazone, ketoprofen, and firocoxib (COX-2 selective) are NSAIDs that can be used in the horse.
- Pentafusion (CRI of ketamine, morphine, lidocaine, detomidine, and acepromazine) can be used to supplement NSAIDs in horses that are extremely painful.
- An epidural can also be used to help control pain if the hind feet are involved.
- Anticoagulant therapy (aspirin, heparin, pentoxifylline) and drugs thought to promote digital blood flow (acepromazine, nitroglycerin, isoxsuprine) appear to be ineffective in most cases of laminitis.
- The two main objectives of hoof care are to redistribute the force of weight-bearing away from the wall and decrease the extensor moment of the DIP joint (Figure 2.56).
- Methods to recruit the sole, frog, and bars for weight-bearing include removing the shoes and placing the horse in sand, shavings, or peat, or applying rolled gauze, Lilly pads, silicone putty, Styrofoam insulation board, closed cell foam, or commercial pad systems such as the Soft-Ride boots (Soft-Ride, Inc., Vermillion, OH) to the affected feet.
- Methods to decrease the extensor moment or torque around the DIP joint include elevating the heels and/or moving the break-over more palmar/plantar usually by shortening the toe (Figure 2.56). Commercial plastic cuff and pad combinations conveniently combine a wedged heel and cased break-over (NANRIC Ultimate, NANRIC Co., Lawrenceburg, KY).
- The goals of treating horses with chronic laminitis include maintaining stability of the distal phalanx, controlling pain, and restoring the relationship between the hoof capsule and the distal phalanx.

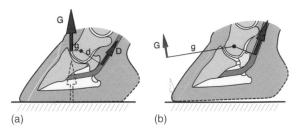

(a) (b)

Figure 2.56 (a) At rest, the foot is stable with respect to the ground. The ground reaction force is approximately vertical and positioned approximately in the center of the foot, slightly in front of the center of rotation of the distal interphalangeal joint. The product of the magnitude of the GRF (G, large red arrow) and the length of its moment arm (g) is the extensor moment, which is opposed by the flexor moment, which is the product of the force in the deep digital flexor tendon (D, small red arrow) multiplied by the length of its moment arm (d). (b) At break-over, the position of the foot is dynamic, and the magnitude of the ground reaction force (G, small red arrow) is decreased as the horse moves off the leg, but the length of the moment arm (g) is increased because the GRF is positioned at the toe. To cause the foot to move from the stable position at rest to the dynamic state, the flexor moment exceeds the extensor moment. *Source*: Courtesy of Andy Parks.

- The mainstay of treatment is usually hoof care (trimming with or without shoeing) and will vary with the type of displacement, severity of lameness, the way in which the horse moves, and stability of the distal phalanx.
- Several shoe types can be used in horses with chronic laminitis including regular keg shoes, egg-bar shoes, reverse shoes, heart-bar shoes, four-point rail shoes, and wooden shoes/clog (Figure 2.57).
- The choice of shoe is largely based on personal preference and experience and should be titrated to the specific symptoms of the individual horse.
- There is no perceived benefit to elevating the heels in horses with symmetrical distal displacement and the wooden shoe/clog is the shoeing method of choice to treat horses with distal displacement in the forelimbs.
- The goal of shoeing horses with unilateral distal displacement should be to redirect the load to the opposite side of the foot in conjunction with ground surface support. This can be accomplished by either placing a 4- to 8-mm extension (concentrating ground support on the extended side; Figure 2.57) or placing a thin wedge on the side of the foot opposite the displacement.

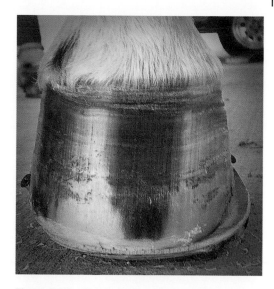

Figure 2.57 This horse has medial asymmetrical distal displacement, evidenced by disparate growth of the medial and lateral walls. A wooden shoe has been positioned to act as a lateral extension to increase weight-bearing by the healthier lateral side of the foot to decrease pain from compression of the sole and tension in the laminae medially. *Source*: Courtesy of Andy Parks.

A DDFT tenotomy, usually performed in the mid-metacarpus, can be used in select refractory cases (Figure 2.58). The surgery is primarily indicated in horses with:

1) Early chronic laminitis that continues to rotate despite all other measures taken.

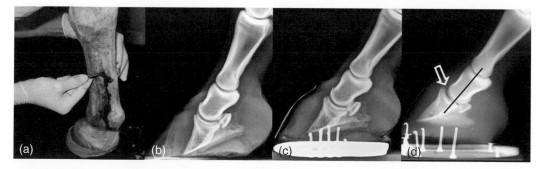

Figure 2.58 Tenotomy of the DDFT is most commonly performed while standing at the mid-cannon region using a guarded bistoury (a). The tenotomy allows realignment of the rotated distal phalanx (b) with the ground surface (note realignment of the foot in (c) after six weeks). Subluxation of the DIP can occur following the procedure (d), characterized by dorsal displacement of the extensor process of the distal phalanx away from middle phalanx (arrow), and by caudal displacement of the distal articular surface of the middle phalanx so that a line bisecting the middle and proximal phalanges does not bisect the middle of the articular surface of the distal phalanx (black line). *Source*: Courtesy of James Belknap.

2) Intractable pain originating from the dorsal sole and wall despite stabilization and shoeing.

3) Secondary flexural deformities.

- Sole abscesses, distal phalanx osteopenia, and solar margin fractures are sequelae of chronic laminitis. Digital sepsis is most common and can be very difficult to manage.

Prognosis

- The three most important factors that affect the prognosis are the severity of the original pathology, the type of displacement, and the severity of the clinical signs.
- Horses with rotation are considered to have a more favorable prognosis than those with either symmetrical or asymmetrical distal displacement.
- The prognosis following distal displacement is always considered guarded to poor although it may be slightly be better for asymmetrical vs. symmetrical displacement.
- Capsular rotation greater than 11.5° and a coronet-to-extensor-process distance of greater than 15.2 mm ("founder" distance) have both been associated with poor outcomes, although these studies are dated and should probably be reassessed.
- The thickness of the sole, and the angle that the solar margin of the distal phalanx subtends with the ground, may help assess prognosis; thinner soles and greater angles of the solar margin are anecdotally associated with a reduced prognosis.

Foot Care and Farriery

Basic Foot Care

Overview

- The structures of the hoof complex comprise the hoof capsule, sole, frog, digital cushion, ungual cartilages, and DDFT.
- The equine foot has several functions:
  1) Supports the weight of the horse.

2) Dissipates the energy of impact as the foot strikes the ground.

3) Protects the structures contained within the hoof capsule.

4) Provides traction during motion.

- A good, ideal, healthy, or functional foot has been described to comprising the following features:
  1) Thick hoof wall
  2) Adequate sole depth (thickness)
  3) Solid heel base
  4) Growth rings of equal size at the toe and heel
  5) Acceptable foot conformation
- Farriery assumes a dominant role in maintaining the health of the foot and preserving the integrity of both the internal and external structures of the hoof capsule.

Static Observation

- With the horse standing and viewed from the lateral side, the HPA should form a relatively straight line and the dorsal hoof wall should be parallel to the dorsal surface of the pastern (Figure 2.59a).
- Ideally, an imaginary line that bisects the third metacarpus (MC3) should intersect the ground at or near the most palmar aspect of the weight-bearing surface of the heels (Figure 2.59a).
- When viewed from the front, a line drawn between two comparable points on the coronet should be parallel to the ground, and a vertical line bisecting the third metacarpal bone should be perpendicular to this line (Figure 1.7).
- When viewing the hoof from the palmar aspect, the height of the inside and outside heel should be similar and ideally similar in conformation to the contralateral limb.
- Viewed from the ground surface of the foot, a line drawn across the widest part of the foot, a line from the widest part of the foot to the base of the frog at the heels and a line from the widest part of the foot to the toe should approximate each other (Figure 2.59b).

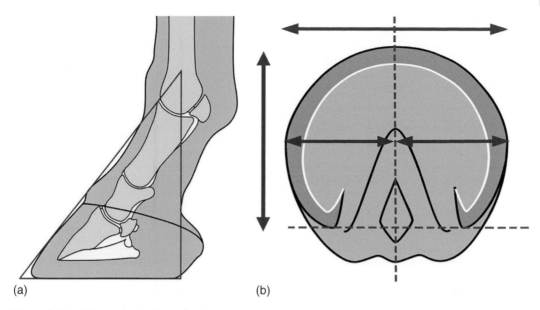

(a)   (b)

Figure 2.59   Schematic drawings showing the ideal hoof-pastern axis (a), extent of weight-bearing surface and ideal proportions for the solar surface of the foot (b). *Source*: Courtesy of Stephen O'Grady.

- The width of the frog should be 67% of the frog length and the weight-bearing surface of the heels should extend to or coincide with the base of the frog.

Dynamic Observation

- The strike pattern of the foot should be viewed from the side, and ideally the horse should either land slightly heel first or flat, with the toe and heel contacting the ground simultaneously.
- Excessive toe-first or heel-first landing are usually considered to be abnormal.
- Mediolateral orientation of the heels as they strike the ground is usually best viewed from the front or from the rear. Ideally, both heels should contact the ground simultaneously.
- Abnormal mediolateral hoof wall strike can be conformation-related and should be differentiated from other causes such as hoof imbalances, sheared heels, and faulty farriery.
- With the horse standing and viewed from the lateral side, the HPA should form a relatively straight line and the dorsal hoof wall should be parallel to the dorsal surface of the pastern (Figure 2.59a).

Hoof Imbalances

- The term hoof balance is often used to describe a theoretical "ideal" geometrical shape or conformation of a foot, the position of the hoof relative to the limb above, or how the foot should be trimmed.
- In reality, no single method of balance will achieve optimum foot conformation for every horse and the term "hoof balance" is often an ambiguous term.
- A more effective approach is to use a set of biomechanical principles or hoof parameters that can be used as guidelines to evaluate and trim every horse. These include:
  1) HPA
  2) The center of rotation
  3) Heels of the hoof capsule extending to the base of the frog
- The guidelines can help standardize the communication between the farriery and veterinarian and be used to modify existing

hoof conformation and improve hoof capsule distortions that affect the landing patterns of the foot.

Guidelines for Trimming

- Hoof conformation embraces the shape and function of the foot in relation to the ground and is extremely important because of its relationship to the foot's biomechanical function.
- The soft tissue structures that form the palmar/plantar section of the foot are often the limiting factor when trying to achieve and maintain good hoof conformation or shape.
- **The first guideline considered when trimming the foot is the HPA (Figure 2.59).**
  1) It is assumed that the straight alignment of the phalanges places the solar surface of the distal phalanx in the correct alignment relative to the ground surface of the hoof capsule/ground.
  2) The correct DP orientation of the distal phalanx within the hoof capsule helps prevent disproportionate load concentration on the solar surface of the hoof capsule.

3) Changes in the HPA are usually associated with two common hoof capsule distortions: low or underrun heels (+/− long toe) or upright or clubfeet.
4) The low heel is generally correlated with a lack of soft tissue mass in the palmar/plantar aspect of the foot.

- **The second guideline or landmark used for trimming the foot is the center of rotation (COR).**
  1) A vertical line drawn on a lateral radiograph from the center of the lateral condyle of the distal middle phalanx to the ground should bisect the bearing surface just palmar/plantar to the middle of the foot (Figure 2.60a).
  2) This line demarcates the biomechanical center of rotation of the DIP joint and should be in close proximity with a line drawn across the solar surface of the foot through the middle one-third of the frog or the widest part of the foot (Figure 2.60b).
  3) The widest part of the foot is the one point on the solar surface of the foot that remains relatively constant regardless of

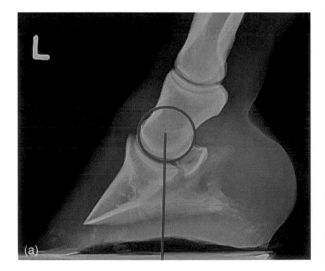
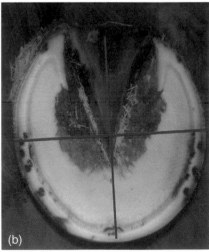

Figure 2.60 (a) Lateral radiograph demonstrating the center of rotation that should approximately bisect the weight-bearing surface of the foot (red line). (b) Solar surface of the foot showing the middle or widest part of the foot, which should approximate the center of rotation. Note that the foot is basically as wide as it is long. *Source*: Courtesy of Stephen O'Grady.

the shape or length of the ground surface that is dorsal or palmar to this point.

4) Following the trim, the ground surface of the ideal foot should be as wide as it is long and the ground surface of the hoof capsule at the heels should not project dorsal to the base of the frog.

- **The third guideline for trimming is that the heels of the hoof capsule should extend to the base of the frog.**

  1) The soft tissue structures in the palmar/plantar aspect of the foot are thought to absorb concussion during load bearing and help dissipate the energy of impact.

  2) For effective physiologic functioning of the foot, the osseous and soft tissue structures should be located on the same plane within the hoof capsule, and this is accomplished by having the heels of the hoof capsule extend to or approximate the base of the frog (Figure 2.61).

  3) Variations in hoof conformation, farrier training, empiric considerations, and owner pressure not to trim the heels often dictate how the heels are trimmed.

  4) Lack of a healthy and robust frog will complicate the trim and the length of the frog far exceeding its width often suggests a chronic foot problem.

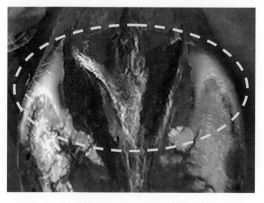

Figure 2.61 Heels of the hoof capsule trimmed to the base of the frog. Note that the hoof wall at the heels and the frog are on the same horizontal plane (yellow circle). *Source*: Courtesy of Stephen O'Grady.

5) When the frog is recessed between the heels, the heels of the hoof capsule should be trimmed to the point where all structures located on the ground surface of the foot are on the same horizontal plane.

6) Radiographs are helpful to locate or confirm the guidelines for trimming and to identify other hoof abnormalities that may influence the trimming process.

Hoof Capsule Distortions/Abnormal Conformation

Overview

- Hoof capsule distortions or abnormal hoof conformation can occur in both lame and non-lame horses.
- Abnormal weight distribution on the foot or disproportionate forces placed on a section of the hoof wall over time will cause it to assume an abnormal shape.
- The abnormal hoof conformations/distortions can often lead to hoof imbalances in either a DP or medial-lateral (ML) direction.
- Three of the most common types of abnormal hoof conformation include: the long-toe and/or low heel, the club foot, and the sheared heel.
- Hoof distortions can be a primary cause of lameness or secondary to other conditions in the foot such as navicular disease/syndrome, laminitis, flexural deformity of the DIP joint, hoof cracks, etc.

Anatomy

- The hoof capsule is comprised of the hoof wall, sole, frog, and bulbs of the heels and forms a casing on the ground surface of the limb that affords protection to the soft tissue and osseous structures enclosed within the capsule (Figures 2.41 and 2.48).
- The hoof wall is a viscoelastic structure that has the ability to temporarily deform under load and then return to its original shape when the load or weight is removed.

- The responses of the foot to stress and differing patterns of weight-bearing are threefold; change in position of the coronary band, change in hoof growth rate, and deviation(s) of the hoof wall.

Imaging

- Radiography is considered to be the main imaging tool to help assess hoof wall distortions and abnormal conformation.
- Considerable information can be obtained from the image regarding the overall shape and mass of the hoof capsule, the soft tissue structures, and the position of the distal phalanx within the hoof capsule.
- Lateral to medial and DP 0° horizontal views of the foot can be used as a precise guide to implement basic or therapeutic trimming and shoeing (Figure 2.62).

Etiology

- Increased stress or weight-bearing placed on a section of the hoof capsule may originate from a single source or from multiple contributing factors such as weight of the horse, abnormal limb conformation, strike pattern of the foot, amount of work, type of footing, and inappropriate farrier practices.
- Increased load or weight-bearing by a portion of the wall has three potential consequences: (i) deviation of the wall outward (flares) or inward (under running) from its normal position; (ii) movement of the wall proximally; or (iii) decreased hoof wall growth.
- A reduction in load or weight-bearing as is seen with chronic lameness will generally have the opposite effects.
- The increased or decreased load on the foot changes the center of pressure (CoP) which determines how the hoof will respond to either increased or decreased load.
- Conformational defects in the upper limb and hereditary factors may also contribute to hoof capsule distortions and abnormal hoof conformation.

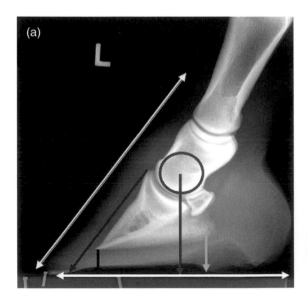 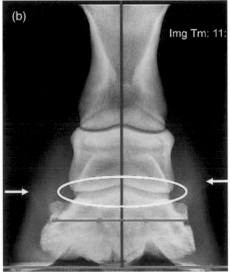

Figure 2.62 (a) Lateral radiograph that illustrates hoof-pastern axis (yellow), center of rotation (red), sole depth (black) and palmar angle of distal phalanx (green), break-over (blue), and the proportions of the ground surface (white). (b) DP radiograph that illustrates the axial alignment of the digit (red), position of the foramina in the distal phalanx relative to the ground (blue), alignment of the joint space (yellow), and position of the coronary band at the heel bulbs (white). *Source*: Courtesy of Stephen O'Grady.

Clinical Signs

- Closer visual examination of the hoof will usually reveal most hoof wall distortions and abnormal hoof conformation. For example, a low or underrun heel conformation is defined as the angle of the heels being considerably less than the angle of the dorsal hoof wall.
- Signs include disparity in heel length, disparity in wall length and angle, outward hoof wall flares, inward hoof wall running, low heels +/− long toes, concavity of the dorsal hoof wall, hoof wall cracks, broken back HPA, broken forward HPA, and displacement of the coronary band and/or heel bulbs (Figures 1.2, 1.3, 2.3, and 2.63).
- The foot strike may be abnormal both in a ML (lands on the longer side first and then rolls to the opposite side of the hoof) and/or DP direction (excessive toe first or heel first landing).
- Three of the most common types of abnormal hoof conformations that often occur in lame horses are those with a low heel accompanied by a long toe (Figures 2.3 and 2.63), the upright or club foot (Figure 2.64), and those with sheared heels (Figure 2.65).

- With sheared heels, the heel bulb and/or quarter on the affected side are visually higher, the hoof wall is straighter, and there is an abnormal flare to the hoof wall on the opposite unaffected side (Figure 2.65).
- The lameness can be variable and depends on the severity of the hoof capsule distortion and whether the distortion is primary or secondary to another condition.
- Pain across the heels and frog or area of the hoof distortion is often found with hoof testers regardless of the type of abnormal conformation. This is especially true in horses with the low heel accompanied by long toe conformation.
- A PD nerve block usually eliminates the lameness regardless of the type of hoof capsule distortion/abnormal conformation.

Diagnosis

- Most hoof capsule distortions/abnormal conformations can be diagnosed by visual inspection of the hoof combined with standing lateral and horizontal DP radiographs of the feet (Figure 2.62).
- Many hoof distortions/abnormal conformations are secondary to a musculoskele-

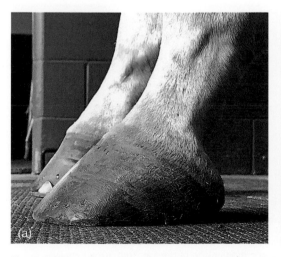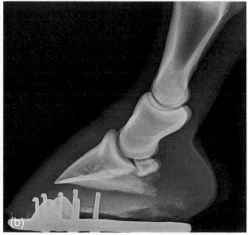

Figure 2.63 Long-toe low heel foot conformation. Note the broken back hoof-pastern axis and the acute angle of the coronet (a). Lateral radiograph revealing the angle of the solar border of the distal phalanx is negative (b). Note the lack of mass under the palmar process of the distal phalanx and the "knob" shape of the heel. *Source*: Courtesy of Stephen O'Grady.

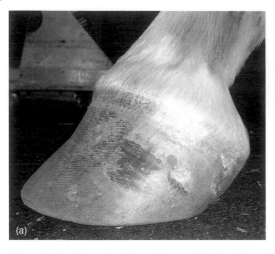
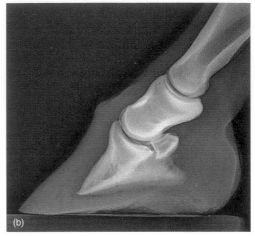

Figure 2.64 Example of a moderate club foot. Note the disparity of the growth rings and the broken forward hoof-pastern axis (a). Radiograph of the clubfoot on the left (b). Note the flexural deformity of the DIP joint and the concavity in the dorsal hoof wall. *Source*: Courtesy of Stephen O'Grady.

tal problem in the foot, which should be determined and treated appropriately to prevent recurrence of the abnormal hoof conformation.

- Complete radiographic examination of the foot and other imaging such as MRI may be needed to determine the primary musculo-skeletal abnormality.

- Primary hoof capsule distortions do occur, but other contributing factors should be ruled out before focusing only on the hoof capsule distortion/abnormal conformation.

Treatment

- Treatment is directed at correcting the cap-sule distortion/abnormal conformation with

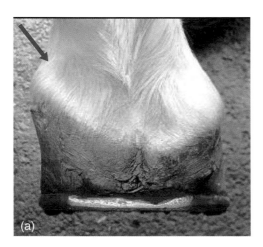
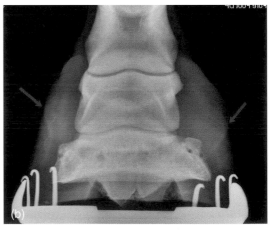

Figure 2.65 (a) Dorsopalmar view of a foot with sheared heels. Note the disparity between the length of the two heels and the deformation of the structures on the medial side of the foot (red arrow). (b) DP radiograph of a horse with sheared heels. Note the disparity in the height of the coronary bands (red arrows) yet the plane of the distal phalanx remains parallel with the ground. *Source*: Courtesy of Stephen O'Grady.

corrective trimming and/or shoeing and treating the primary lameness condition.

- Farriery is often the mainstay of therapy and mild cases of hoof capsule distortion usually respond to trimming alone.
- Most horses will require therapeutic shoeing to address both the hoof capsule distortion/abnormal conformation as well as the primary lameness problem.
- **Horses with low-heel foot conformation:**
  1) This type of hoof conformation alters the structural mass of the foot as the compromised heels lose the ability to accept weight and dissipate the energy of impact.
  2) It can be perpetuated by not continually trimming the hoof wall at the heels to the same plane as the frog.
  3) Allowing the horse to remain barefoot for a period of time with controlled exercise can markedly improve the heel structures.
  4) Farriery should be directed at improving the heel structures, utilizing the entire palmar foot to share the load, and heel elevation when possible.
  5) Farriery is often problematic and usually requires a trial-and-error process using a combination of various methods.
- **Horses with club foot conformation:**
  1) Flexural deformities of the DIP joint (club foot) cause more hoof wall growth at the heel than at the toe, and the frog generally recedes below the ground surface of the hoof wall due to the excessive heel height.
  2) The hoof wall assumes more energy of impact often resulting in thin flat soles, poor dorsal hoof wall consistency, toe cracks, and hoof wall separations.
  3) In most horses, the heels should be trimmed, the toe shortened, the concavity removed from the dorsal hoof wall with a rasp, and a shoe placed that extends 1–2 cm beyond the end of the heel.
  4) With a more advanced clubfoot, the heels should still be trimmed to load the heels and unload the toe, but heel elevation must be added to compensate for the shortening of the musculotendinous unit of the DDFT.
  5) Severe flexural deformities in young horses or those that result in chronic lameness in adults can be treated by performing a desmotomy of the accessory ligament of the DDFT combined with the appropriate farriery (Figure 2.66).
- **Horses with sheared heel conformation:**
  1) When the weight of the horse is not distributed uniformly over the entire hoof during weight-bearing, one focal area of the foot, usually a heel or heel and accompanying quarter, receives a disproportionate amount of the total load during impact, and displaces proximally.
  2) The continual increased compressive stresses on one quarter/heel predisposes the foot to subsolar bruising, corns, quarter/heel cracks, fracture of the bar, and deep fissures within the base of the frog that are susceptible to thrush.
  3) Proper trimming of the foot and leaving the horse barefoot for a brief period may permit the displaced heel to descend, the compressed area between the coronet and middle phalanx to widen, and the palmar section of the foot to assume a more relaxed position.
  4) In more severe cases, the foot is trimmed, and a wide-web steel or aluminum straight-bar shoe is used. Before applying the shoe, a second trim is performed under the proximally displaced quarter heel creating a wedge-shaped space between the shoe and the hoof wall permitting the displaced heel to descend distally into a more acceptable configuration (Figure 2.67).

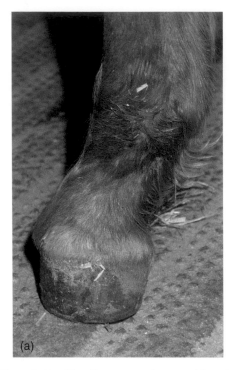

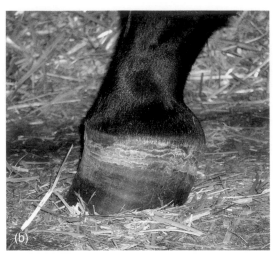

Figure 2.66 Weanling quarter horses with typical club foot appearances. The dorsal hoof wall was vertical to the ground (a) with a concavity of the hoof wall (b). The deformities were corrected in both with an inferior check ligament desmotomy.

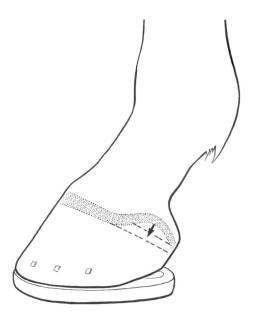

Figure 2.67 Corrective trimming and shoeing of a horse affected with sheared heels. The affected side is trimmed from the heel through the quarter to create a space between the hoof wall and the full-bar shoe. The stippled area indicates the level of the coronary band. The arrow is pointing to where the coronary band should be.

Prognosis

- The prognosis is considered very good for mildly affected horses regardless of the type of hoof capsule distortion and for horses without a primary lameness condition.
- Horses with severe hoof capsule distortions/abnormal conformation will usually require several shoe resets to correct the problem, and many will require long-term management.
- Horses with hoof distortions/abnormal conformations secondary to a primary musculoskeletal problem must have the lameness problem treated concurrently.
- Horses with a low heel accompanied by a long toe conformation can be problematic because expanding the structural mass of the palmar aspect of the foot is difficult.
- Horses with club foot conformation usually have a very good prognosis provided that therapeutic farriery can be maintained.

- Horses with sheared heel conformation also have a very good prognosis with appropriate corrective shoeing.
- A lateral radiograph of the foot is necessary to document whether a flexural deformity of the DIP joint is present.
- Diagnostic nerve blocks and other imaging may be required to document other musculoskeletal abnormalities if a concurrent lameness is present.

Toe Cracks, Quarter Cracks, Heel Cracks

Overview

- Hoof wall cracks represent a focal wall failure, and as such, they can occur anywhere on the hoof wall and can be parallel or horizontal to the horn tubules.
- Hoof wall cracks are generally described by their location (toe, quarter, or heel), length along the hoof wall, depth (partial or full thickness), and the presence or absence of hemorrhage or infection (Figures 2.68 and 2.69).
- Vertical hoof wall cracks can either originate at the ground surface and extend proximally or begin at the coronet and extend distally.
- Quarter cracks and heel cracks are usually the most severe because they often involve the sensitive laminae.

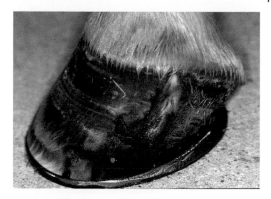

Figure 2.69 A full-thickness quarter crack just after debridement down to the sensitive laminae.

Anatomy and Imaging (Please refer to previous section on "Hoof Capsule Distortions")

Etiology

- Contributing factors include direct hoof wall trauma, overloading of the hoof, and hoof capsule distortions.
- Direct trauma to the coronet can contribute to a horizontal crack and/or cause a weak and deformed hoof wall that grows distally.
- Drying of the hoof and thin walls contribute to weakening of the wall and cracking.
- Chronic laminitis, WLD, club foot conformation, and excessive toe length may contribute to central toe cracks (Figure 2.68).
- Heel and quarter cracks are frequently associated with underrun heels and long toes and placing the shoe too far forward also contributes to quarter cracks.
- Secondary infection can develop in any full thickness crack from environmental bacteria.

Clinical Signs

- The presence of the defect in the hoof wall is usually obvious. However, not all hoof cracks are clinically significant and contribute to lameness.
- Lameness may not be present with partial thickness cracks but is usually obvious with deep cracks because they "pinch" the sensitive tissues beneath the hoof wall.

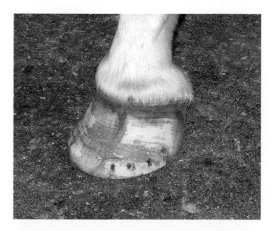

Figure 2.68 A partial-thickness toe crack that developed in a horse with a concavity of the dorsal hoof wall.

- If secondary infection is present, lameness may be severe and purulent exudate may be seen within the hoof crack.
- The hoof wall around the crack is usually very sensitive to hoof testers when the crack is infected and in those that are contributing to lameness.
- Perineural anesthesia can be used to determine if the hoof crack is contributing to the lameness and nearly all will improve with PD block.

Diagnosis

- The diagnosis is based on the presence of the crack and can be classified according to its location and depth. Blood or purulent exudate is usually only present with full-thickness hoof cracks.
- Radiographs of the feet are advisable in many cases but especially in horses with central toe cracks to determine if there is an underlying cause.
- A true quarter crack is a full-thickness defect that originates at the coronary band and travels distally leading to instability, inflammation, and/or infection (Figure 2.70).
- Toe cracks may be partial or full-thickness dorsal hoof wall extending from the coronet distally but rarely reach the ground surface.
- Heel cracks are the least common type of crack and are often associated with poor palmar foot conformation.

Treatment

- The type of treatment often depends on the location and depth of the crack. Initial treatment of partial thickness cracks is often to apply the necessary farriery to change the abnormal forces on the section of the foot with the defect.
- Any hoof capsule distortions or abnormal hoof conformation that may be contributing the crack should be corrected if possible.
- **Horses with a full-thickness quarter crack**:
  1) When possible, the horse should be removed from work and the foot trimmed to address the hoof capsule distortion, rather than to repair the crack.
  2) Most horses should be placed in a bar shoe with the affected quarter below the crack unloaded until the crack has grown at least half-way down the hoof wall (Figure 2.71).
  3) A variety of bar shoes such as a straight-bar, egg bar, or heart-bar can be used since they all effectively increase the ground surface of the foot on the affected side, provide palmar support, and decrease the independent vertical movement at the bulbs of the heels.
  4) If greater stability of the crack is necessary, the crack itself can be repaired with stainless steel wires placed across the defect from dorsal to palmar/plantar (Figure 2.72).

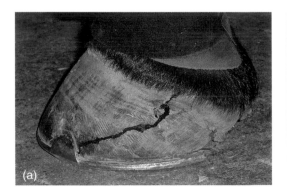 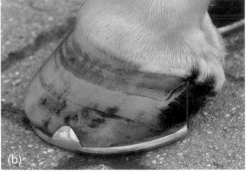

Figure 2.70 (a) Acute quarter crack with hemorrhage. Note the tightly packed growth rings distal to the coronet as a result of chronic overload. (b) Chronic quarter crack. The origin of crack coincides with the end of shoe that is too small (arrow), and the coronet is displaced proximally. *Source*: Courtesy of Stephen O'Grady.

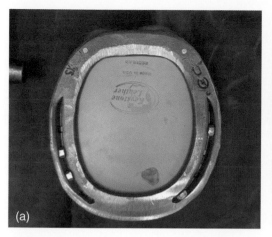

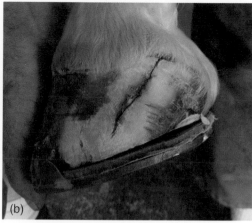

Figure 2.71 Straight-bar shoe (a) with the medial heel unloaded (b). Note the quarter crack which is often present with a sheared heel (b). *Source*: Courtesy of Stephen O'Grady.

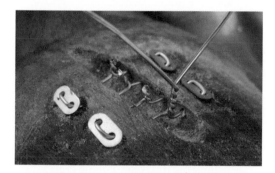

Figure 2.72 Placement of wires for a quarter crack repair. *Source*: Courtesy of Stephen O'Grady.

- **Horses with a full-thickness toe crack:**
  1) Full-thickness toe cracks are usually movable, opening when load is removed and closing when load is applied. This movement can contribute to pain and prevent healing.
  2) Farriery is directed toward improving hoof conformation, decreasing the toe length, and shifting the weight-bearing function in a palmar direction to unload the toe.
  3) An appropriate trim and application of a shoe in a manner that unloads the toe is often sufficient to stop the movement of the defect and promote healing.

  4) If further stabilization of the crack is needed, a metal or brass band can be fabricated and attached to the dorsal hoof wall with screws.
- **Horses with a full-thickness heel crack:**
  1) This type of crack is not as common as a toe or quarter crack but can be difficult to treat and resolve.
  2) Some type of bar shoe with or without a "spider" plate is recommended to increase the ground surface in the palmar foot, redistribute the weight-bearing on the solar surface, and unload the affected heel.
  3) The horn in this section of the foot is generally too thin to accept an implant, and therefore the hoof wall palmar to the defect is either removed or the heel can be rebuilt using an appropriate composite material.
  4) If infection is present, the crack should be opened, debrided, and bandaged with a suitable disinfectant before any type of surgical stabilization is considered. (The reader is referred to Chapter 11 in *Adams and Stashak's Lameness in Horses, 7th. Edition*, for further details of treatment options).

Prognosis

- Partial thickness cracks at any location often do not contribute to lameness and usually can be successfully managed with farriery alone.
- Full-thickness quarter cracks can be problematic, especially if infection is present and can contribute to continued lameness until the crack grows out completely.
- Factors contributing to the hoof cracks must be addressed to both facilitate healing and to prevent recurrence of the crack in the future.

Bibliography

1 Adams SB, Santschi EM: 2000. Management of congenital and acquired flexural limb deformities. *Proc Am Assoc Eq Pract* 46:117–125.

2 Bach O, Butler D, White K, et al.: 1995. Hoof balance and lameness: Improper toe length, hoof angle, and mediolateral balance. *Compend Contin Educ Pract Vet* 17:1275–1282.

3 Barber MJ, Sampson SN, Schneider RK, et al.: 2006. Use of magnetic resonance imaging to diagnose distal sesamoid bone injury in a horse. *J Am Vet Med Assoc* 229:717–720.

4 Barr ARS: 1993. Internal fixation of fractures of the third phalanx in 4 horses. *Equine Vet Educ* 5: 308–312.

5 Barrett MF, Frisbie DD, King MR, et al.: 2017. A review of how magnetic resonance imaging can aid in the case management of common pathological conditions of the equine foot. *Equine Vet Educ* 29:683–692.

6 Baxter GM, Ingle JE, Trotter GW: 1995. Complete navicular bone fractures in horses. *Proc Am Assoc Equine Pract* 41:243–244.

7 Baxter GM, Morrison S: 2008. Complications of unilateral weight bearing. *Vet Clin North Am Equine Pract* 24:621–642.

8 Baxter GM: 1986. Equine laminitis caused by distal displacement of the distal phalanx—12 cases (1976–1985). *J Am Vet Med Assoc* 189:326–329.

9 Baxter GM: 2005. Treatment of wounds involving synovial structures. *Clin Tech Equine Pract* 3:204–214.

10 Baxter GM, Stashak TS: 2011. The Foot. *In*: Baxter GM (ed) *Adams and Stashak's Lameness in Horses, Sixth Edition*. Ames, IA, Wiley-Blackwell, 475–535.

11 Belknap JK, Moore JN, Crouser EC: 2009. Sepsis—From human organ failure to laminar failure. *Vet Immunol Immunopathol* 129:155–157.

12 Biggi M, Dyson SJ: 2012. Distal border fragments and shape of the navicular bone: radiological evaluation in lame horses and horses free from lameness. *Equine Vet J* 44:325–331.

13 Boyce M, Malone ED, Anderson LB, et al.: 2010. Evaluation of diffusion of triamcinolone acetonide from the distal interphalangeal joint into the navicular bursa in horses. *Am J Vet Res* 71:169–175.

14 Bras RJ: 2011. How to use foot casts to manage horses with laminitis and distal displacement secondary to systemic disease. *Proc Am Assoc Equine Pract* 57:415–423.

15 Blunden A, Dyson S, Murray R, et al.: 2006. Histopathology in horses with chronic palmar foot pain and age-matched controls. Part 1: Navicular bone and related structures. *Equine Vet J* 38:15–22.

16 Blunden A, Dyson S, Murray R, et al.: 2006. Histopathology in horses with chronic palmar foot pain and age-matched controls. Part 2: The deep digital flexor tendon. *Equine Vet J* 38:23–27.

17 Blunden A, Murray R, Dyson S: 2009. Lesions of the deep digital flexor tendon in the digit: A correlative MRI and postmortem study in control and lame horses. *Equine Vet J* 41:25–33.

18 Bosch G, van Schie MJ, Back W. 2004. Retrospective evaluation of surgical versus conservative treatment of keratomas in

41 lame horses (1995–2001). *Tijdschr Diergeneeskd* 129:700–705.

19 Boys Smith SJ, Clegg PD, Hughes I, et al.: 2006. Complete and partial hoof wall resection for keratoma removal: Postoperative complications and final outcome in 26 horses (1994–2004). *Equine Vet J* 38:127–133.

20 Bowker RM, Linder K, Van Wulfen KK, et al.: 1997. An anatomical study of the distal interphalangeal joint in the horse: Its relationship to the navicular suspensory ligaments sensory nerves and neurovascular bundle. *Equine Vet J* 29:126.

21 Busoni V, Heimann M, Trenteseaux J, et al.: 2005. Magnetic resonance imaging findings in the equine deep digital flexor tendon and distal sesamoid bone in advanced navicular disease—an ex vivo study. *Vet Radiol Ultrasound* 46:279–286.

22 Cauvin ER, Munroe GA: 1998. Septic osteitis of the distal phalanx: Findings and surgical treatment in 18 cases. *Equine Vet J* 30:512–519.

23 Cillan-Garcia E, Milner PI, Talbot A, et al.: 2013. Deep digital flexor tendon injury within the hoof capsule; does lesion type and location predict prognosis? *Vet Rec* 173:70. doi:10.1136/vr.101512.

24 Compagnie E, Ter Braake F, de Heer N, et al.: 2016. Arthroscopic removal of large extensor process fragments in 18 Friesian horses: Long-term clinical outcome and radiological follow-up of the distal interphalangeal joint. *Vet Surg* 45:536–541.

25 Cripps PJ, Eustace RA: 1999. Factors involved in the prognosis of equine laminitis in the UK. *Equine Vet J* 31:433–442.

26 Crowe OM, Hepburn RJ, Kold SE, et al.: 2010. Long-term outcome after arthroscopic debridement of distal phalanx extensor process fragmentation in 13 horses. *Vet Surg* 39:107–114.

27 Dabareiner RM, Carter GK: 2003. Diagnosis, treatment, and farriery for horses with chronic heel pain. *Vet Clin North Am Equine Pract* 19:417–441.

28 Dabareiner RM, Carter GK, Honnas CM: 2003. Injection of corticosteroids, hyaluronate, and amikacin into the navicular bursa in horses with signs of navicular area pain unresponsive to other treatments: 25 cases (1999–2002). *J Am Vet Med Assoc* 223:1469–1474.

29 Denoix JM, Thibaud D, Riccio B: 2003. Tiludronate as a new therapeutic agent in the treatment of navicular disease: A double-blind placebo-controlled clinical trial. *Equine Vet J* 35:407–413.

30 Dorner C, Fueyo P, Olave R: 2017. Relationship between the distal phalanx angle and radiographic changes in the navicular bone of horses: a radiological study. *Global J Med Res.* 17:7–13.

31 Dyce KM, Sack WO, Wensing CJG: 2002. *Textbook of Veterinary Anatomy.* Philadelphia, PA, Elsevier Science.

32 Dyson S, Murray R: 2007. Use of concurrent scintigraphic and magnetic resonance imaging evaluation to improve understanding of the pathogenesis of injury of the podotrochlear apparatus. *Equine Vet J* 39: 365–369.

33 Dyson S, Murray R, Schramme M, et al.: 2003. Lameness in 46 horses associated with deep digital flexor tendonitis in the digit: Diagnosis confirmed with magnetic resonance imaging. *Equine Vet J* 35: 681–690.

34 Dyson SJ, Murray R, Schramme MC: 2005. Lameness associated with foot pain: Results of magnetic resonance imaging in 199 horses (January 2001-December 2003) and response to treatment. *Equine Vet J* 37: 113–121.

35 Dyson SJ, Murray R: 2007. Magnetic resonance imaging evaluation of 264 horses with foot pain: The podotrochlear apparatus, deep digital flexor tendon and collateral ligaments of the distal interphalangeal joint. *Equine Vet J* 39:340–343.

36 Dyson SJ, Murray RC, Schramme M, et al.: 2004. Collateral desmitis of the distal interphalangeal joint in 18 horses (2001–2002). *Equine Vet J* 36:160–166.

37 Dyson SJ, Marks D: 2003. Foot pain and the elusive diagnosis. *Vet Clin North Am Equine Pract* 19:531–565.

38 Dyson SJ: 2011. Primary Lesions of the Deep Digital Flexor Tendon within the Hoof Capsule. *In*: Ross MW, Dyson SJ (eds) *Diagnosis and Management of Lameness in the Horse*. St. Louis, MO, Elsevier Saunders, 344–348.

39 Dyson SJ: 2011. Radiological interpretation of the navicular bone. *Equine Vet Educ* 23:73–87.

40 Dyson SJ, Murray R, Schramme M, et al.: 2011. Current concepts of navicular disease. *Equine Vet Ed* 23:27–39.

41 Dyson SJ, Blunden T, Murray R: 2012. Comparison between magnetic resonance imaging and histological findings in the navicular bone of horses with foot pain. *Equine Vet J* 44:692–698.

42 Dyson SJ, Brown V, Collins S, et al.: 2010. Is there an association between ossification of the cartilages of the foot and collateral desmopathy of the distal interphalangeal joint or distal phalanx injury? *Equine Vet J* 42:504–511.

43 Eggleston RB: 2012. Equine imaging: The framework for applying therapeutic farriery. *Vet Clin North Am Equine* 28:293–312.

44 Faramarzi B, Dobson H: 2015. Palmar process fractures of the distal phalanx in foals: A review. *Equine Vet Educ* 29:577–580.

45 Faramarzi B, McMicking H, Halland S, et al.: 2015. Incidence of palmar process fractures of the distal phalanx and association with front hoof conformation in foals. *Equine Vet J* 47:675–679.

46 Findley JA, Pinchbeck GL, Milner PI, et al.: 2014. Outcome of horses with synovial structure involvement following solar foot penetrations in four UK veterinary hospitals: 95 cases. *Equine Vet J* 46:352–357.

47 Fitzgerald BW, Honnas CM: 2008. Management of Wounds in the Foot. *In*: Robinson NE (ed) *Current Therapy in Equine Medicine, Sixth Edition*. Philadelphia, WB Saunders, 535–540.

48 Frevel M, King BL, Kolb DS, et al.: 2017. Clodronate disodium for treatment of clinical signs of navicular disease—a double-blinded placebo-controlled clinical trial. *Pferdeheilkunde* 33:271–279.

49 Furst AE, Lischer CJ: 2012. Fractures of the Distal Sesamoid Bone. *In*: Auer JA, Stick JA (eds) *Equine Surgery*. St. Louis, MO, Elsevier Saunders, 1286–1288.

50 Gaughan EM, Rendano VT, Ducharme NG: 1989. Surgical treatment of septic pedal osteitis in horses: Nine cases (1980–1987). *J Am Vet Med Assoc* 195:1131–1134.

51 Geor R, Frank N: 2009. Metabolic syndrome—From human organ disease to laminar failure in equids. *Vet Immunol Immunopathol* 129:151–154.

52 Gutierrez-Nibeyro SD, White NA, Werpy NM, et al.: 2009. Magnetic resonance imaging findings of desmopathy of the collateral ligaments of the equine distal interphalangeal joint. *Vet Radiol Ultrasound* 50: 21–31.

53 Gutierrez-Nibeyro SD, Werpy NM, White NA, et al.: 2015. Outcome of palmar/plantar digital neurectomy in horses with foot pain evaluated with magnetic resonance imaging: 50 cases (2005-2011). *Equine Vet J* 47:160–164.

54 Honnas CM, Dabareiner RM, McCauley BH: 2003. Hoof wall surgery in the horse: Approaches to and underlying disorders. *Vet Clin North Am Equine Pract* 19:479–499.

55 Jansson N, Sonnichsen HV: 1995. Acquired flexural deformity of the distal interphalangeal joint in horses: Treatment by desmotomy of the accessory ligament of the deep digital flexor tendon. A retrospective study. *J Equine Vet Sci* 15:353–356.

56 Johnson SA, Barrett M, Frisbie DD: 2018. Additional palmaroproximal-palmarodistal oblique radiographic projections improve accuracy of detection and characterization of equine flexor cortical lysis. *Vet Radiol Ultrasound* 59:387–395.

57 Kaneps AJ, O'Brien TR, Redden RF, et al.: 1993. Characterization of osseous bodies of the distal phalanx of foals. *Equine Vet J* 25:285–292.

58 Katzman SA, Spriet M, Galuppo LD: 2019. Outcome following computed tomographic imaging and subsequent surgical removal of keratomas in equids: 32 cases (2005–2016). *J Am Vet Med Assoc* 254:266–274.

59 Keegan KG, Twardock AR, Losonsky JM, et al.: 1993. Scintigraphic evaluation of fractures of the distal phalanx in horses: 27 cases (1979–1988). *J Am Vet Med Assoc* 202:1993–1997.

60 Kilcoyne I, Dechant JE, Kass PH, et al.: 2011. Penetrating injuries to the frog (cuneus ungulae) and collateral sulci of the foot in equids: 63 cases (1998–2008). *J Am Vet Med Assoc* 239:1104–1109.

61 Kristiansen KK, Kold SE: 2007. Multivariable analysis of factors influencing outcome of 2 treatment protocols in 128 cases of horses responding positively to intraarticular analgesia of the distal interphalangeal joint. *Equine Vet J* 39:150–156.

62 Kullmann A, Holcombe SJ, Hurcombe SD, et al.: 2014. Prophylactic digital cryotherapy is associated with decreased incidence of laminitis in horses diagnosed with colitis. *Equine Vet J* 46:554–559

63 Lillich JD, Ruggles AJ, Gabel AA, et al.: 1995. Fracture of the distal sesamoid bone in horses: 17 cases (1982– 1992). *J Am Vet Med Assoc* 207:924–927.

64 Lindford S, Embertson R, Bramlage L: 1994. Septic osteitis of the third phalanx: A review of 63 cases. *Proc Am Assoc Equine Pract* 40:103.

65 Loftus JP, Black SJ, Pettigrew A, et al.: 2007. Early laminar events involving endothelial activation in horses with black walnut-induced laminitis. *Am J Vet Res* 68: 1205–1211.

66 Loftus JP, Johnson PJ, Belknap JK, et al.: 2009. Leukocyte-derived and endogenous matrix metalloproteinases in the lamellae of horses with naturally acquired and experimentally induced laminitis. *Vet Immunol Immunopathol* 129:221–230.

67 Maher O, Davis DM, Drake C, et al.: 2008. Pull-through technique for palmar digital neurectomy: Forty-one horses (1998–2004). *Vet Surg* 37:87–93.

68 Marsh CA, Schneider RK, Sampson SN, et al.: 2012. Response to injection of the navicular bursa with corticosteroid and hyaluronan following high-field magnetic resonance imaging in horses with signs of navicular syndrome: 101 cases (2000–2008). *J Am Vet Med Assoc* 241:1353–1364.

69 McIlwraith CW: 2005. Diagnostic and Surgical Arthroscopy of the Phalangeal Joints. *In*: McIlwraith CW, Nixon AJ, Wright IM, et al. (eds) *Diagnostic and Surgical Arthroscopy in the Horse*. Philadelphia, Elsevier, 347–364.

70 Melo e Silva SR, Vulcano LC: 2002. Collateral cartilage ossification of the distal phalanx in the Brazilian Jumper horse. *Vet Radiol Ultrasound* 43:461–463.

71 Miller SM, Bohanon TC: 1994. Arthroscopic surgery for the treatment of extensor process fractures of the distal phalanx in the horse. *Vet Comp Orthop Traumat* 7:2–6.

72 Mitchell A, Wright G, Sampson SN, et al.: 2018. Clodronate improves lameness in horses without changing bone turnover markers. *Equine Vet J August.* doi:10.1111/evj.13011.

73 Moyer W: 2003. Hoof wall defects: chronic hoof wall separations and hoof wall cracks. *Vet Clin North Am Equine Pract* 19:463–477.

74 Murray RC, Schramme MC, Dyson SJ, et al.: 2006. Magnetic resonance imaging characteristics of the foot in horses with palmar foot pain and control horses. *Vet Radiol Ultrasound* 47:1–16.

75 Nagy A, Dyson SJ, Murray RM: 2008. Radiographic, scintigraphic and magnetic resonance imaging findings in the palmar processes of the distal phalanx. *Equine Vet J* 40:57–63.

76 Nemeth F, Dik KJ: 1985. Lag screw fixation of sagittal navicular bone fractures in five horses. *Equine Vet J* 17:137–139.

77 Neil KM, Axon JE, Todhunter PG, et al.: 2007. Septic osteitis of the distal phalanx in foals: 22 cases (1995–2002). *J Am Vet Med Assoc* 230:1683–1690.

78 Neil KM, Axon JE, Begg AP, et al.: 2010. Retrospective study of 108 foals with septic osteomyelitis. *Aust Vet J* 88:4–12.

79 O'Grady SE, Madison JB: 2004. How to treat equine canker. *Proc Am Assoc Equine Pract* 50:202–205.

80 O'Grady SE: 2006. How to manage white line disease. *Proc Am Assoc Equine Pract* 52:520–525.

81 O'Grady SE, Parks AH: 2008. Farriery options for acute and chronic laminitis. *Proc Am Assoc Eq Pract* 54: 354–363.

82 O'Grady SE, Poupard, DE: 2003. Proper physiologic horseshoeing. *Vet Clin North Am Equine Pract.* 19:2:333–344.

83 O'Grady SE: 2006. Strategies for shoeing the horse with palmar foot pain. *Proc Am Assoc Equine Pract* 52:209–214.

84 O'Grady SE: 2008. Basic farriery for the performance horse. *Vet Clin North Am Equine Pract* 24:1:203–218.

85 O'Grady SE: 2005. How to manage sheared heels. *Proc Am Assoc Equine Pract* 51:451–456.

86 O'Grady SE: 2001. Quarter crack repair—an overview. *Equine Vet Educ* 3:280–282.

87 O'Grady SE: 2012. Flexural deformities of the distal interphalangeal joint (clubfeet): A review. *Equine Vet Educ* 24:260–268.

88 Ohlsson J, Jansson N: 2005. Conservative treatment of intra-articular distal phalanx fractures in horses not used for racing. *Aust Vet J* 83:221–223.

89 Orsini JA, Parsons CS, Capewell L, et al.: 2010. Prognostic indicators of poor outcome in horses with laminitis at a tertiary care hospital. *Can Vet J* 51:623–628.

90 O'Sullivan CB, Dart AJ, Malikides N, et al.: 1999. Nonsurgical management of type II

fractures of the distal phalanx in 48 Standardbred horses. *Aust Vet J* 77:501–503.

91 Parks A: 1998. Foot Bruises: Diagnosis and Treatment. *In*: White NA, Moore JN (eds) *Current Techniques in Equine Surgery and Lameness, Second Edition.* Philadelphia, WB. Saunders Co., 528–529.

92 Parks AH: 2012. Therapeutic farriery – one veterinarians perspective. *Vet Clin North Am Equine Pract* 28:333–350.

93 Parks AH: 2003. Form and function of the equine digit. *Vet Clin North Am Equine Pract* 19:285–296.

94 Parkes RS, Newton RJ, Dyson SJ: 2015. Is there an association between clinical features, response to diagnostic analgesia and radiological findings in horses with a magnetic resonance imaging diagnosis of navicular disease or other injuries of the podotrochlear apparatus? *Vet J* 204:40–46.

95 Pauwels FE, Schumacher J, Castro FA, et al.: 2008. Evaluation of the diffusion of corticosteroids between the distal interphalangeal joint and navicular bursa in horses. *Am J Vet Res* 69:611–616.

96 Pollitt CC: 1996. Basement membrane pathology: A feature of acute equine laminitis. *Equine Vet J* 28:38–46.

97 Pool RR, Meagher DM, Stover SM: 1989. Pathophysiology of navicular syndrome. *Vet Clin North Am Equine Pract* 5:109–112.

98 Pulchalski SM: 2012. Advances in equine computed tomography and use of contrast media. *Vet Clin Equine* 28:563–581.

99 Puchalski SM, Galuppo LD, Hornof WJ, et al.: 2007. Intra-arterial contrast-enhanced computed tomography of the equine distal extremity. *Vet Radiol Ultrasound* 48:21–29.

100 Rabuffo TS, Ross MW: 2002. Fractures of the distal phalanx in 72 racehorses: 1990–2001. *Proc Am Assoc Equine Pract* 48:375–377.

101 Redding WR, O'Grady SE: 2012. Septic diseases associated with the hoof complex: Abscesses and punctures wounds. *Vet Clin North Am Equine Pract* 28:423–440.

102 Riijkenhuizen AB, de Graaf K, Hak A, et al.: 2012. Management and outcome of fractures of the distal phalanx: A retrospective study of 285 horses with a long-term outcome in 223 cases. *Vet J* 192:176–182.

103 Rovel T, Audigie F, Coudry V, et al.: 2019. Evaluation of standing low-field magnetic resonance imaging for diagnosis of advanced distal interphalangeal primary degenerative joint disease in horses: 12 cases (2010–2014). *J Am Vet Med Assoc* 254:257–265.

104 Ruohoniemi M, Ryhanen V, Tulamo RM: 1998. Radiographic appearance of the navicular bone and distal interphalangeal joint and their relationship with ossification of the collateral cartilages of the distal phalanx in Finn horse cadaver forefeet. *Vet Rad and Ultrasound* 39:125–132.

105 Ruohonieme M, Raekallio M, Tulamo RM, et al.: 1997. Relationship between ossification of the cartilages of the foot and conformation and radiographic measurements of the front feet in Finn horses. *Equine Vet J* 29:44–48.

106 Sack WO, Habel RE: 1977. *Rooney's Guide to the Dissection of the Horse*. Ithaca, NY, Veterinary Textbooks.

107 Sampson SN, Schneider RK, Gavin PR, et al.: 2009. Magnetic resonance imaging findings in horses with recent onset navicular syndrome but without radiographic abnormalities. *Vet Radiol Ultrasound* 50:339–346.

108 Schoonover MJ, Jann HW, Blaik MA: 2005. Quantitative comparison of three commonly used treatments for navicular syndrome in horses. *Am J Vet Res* 66:1247–1251.

109 Schramme MC: 2008.Treatment of deep digital flexor tendonitis in the foot. *Equine Vet Educ* 20:389–391.

110 Schramme MC: 2018. Treatment of tendinopathy in the foot—what have we learned so far? *Equine Vet Educ* 30:545–548.

111 Schumacher J, Schramme MC, Schumacher J. et al.: 2013. Diagnostic analgesia of the equine digit. *Equine Vet Educ* 225:408–421.

112 Schumacher J, Stashak TS: 2017. Management of Wounds of the Distal Extremities. *In*: Theoret C, Schmacher J (eds) *Equine Wound Management, Third Edition*. Ames, IA, Wiley-Blackwell, 312–351.

113 Seabaugh KA, Baxter GM: 2017. Diagnosis and Management of Wounds Involving Synovial Structures in Horses. *In*: Theoret CL, Schmacher J (eds) *Equine Wound Management, Third Edition*. Ames, IA, Wiley-Blackwell, 385–402.

114 Selberg K, Werpy N: 2011. Fractures of the distal phalanx and associated soft tissue and osseous abnormalities in 22 horses with ossified sclerotic ungual cartilages diagnosed with magnetic resonance imaging. *Vet Radiol Ultrasound* 52:394–401.

115 Sherlock C, Mair T, Blunden T: 2008. Deep erosions of the palmar aspect of the navicular bone diagnosed by standing magnetic resonance imaging. *Equine Vet J* 40:684–692.

116 Smith MR, Wright IM: 2012. Endoscopic evaluation of the navicular bursa: Observations, treatment and outcome in 92 cases with identified pathology. *Equine Vet J* 44:339–345.

117 Smith MR, Wright IM, Smith RK: 2007. Endoscopic assessment and treatment of lesions of the deep digital flexor tendon in the navicular bursae of 20 lame horses. *Equine Vet J* 39:18–24.

118 Steward ML: 2003. How to construct and apply atraumatic therapeutic shoes to treat acute or chronic laminitis in the horse. *Proc Am Assoc Eq Pract* 49: 337–346.

119 Turner TA: 1997. How to treat navicular bone fractures. *Proc Am Assoc Equine Pract* 43:370–371.

120 Turner TA: 1986. Shoeing principles for the management of navicular disease in horses. *J Am Vet Med Assoc* 189:298–301.

121 Vanel M, Olive J, Gold S, et al.: 2012. Clinical significance and prognosis of deep digital flexor tendinopathy assess over time using MRI. *Vet Radiol Ultrasound* 53:621–627.

122 van Eps AW, Pollitt CC: 2004. Equine laminitis: Cryotherapy reduces the severity of the acute lesion. *Equine Vet J* 36:255–260.

123 van Eps AW: 2010. Therapeutic hypothermia (cryotherapy) to prevent and treat acute laminitis. *Vet Clin North Am Equine Pract* 26:125–133.

124 van Eps AW, Orsini JA: 2016. A comparison of seven methods for continuous therapeutic cooling of the equine digit. *Equine Vet J* 48:120–124.

125 van Eps A, Collins SN, Pollitt CC: 2010. Supporting limb laminitis. *Vet Clin North Am Equine Pract* 26:287–302.

126 Whitfield CT, Schoonover MJ, Holbrook TC, et al.: 2016. Quantitative assessment of two methods of tiludronate administration for the treatment of lameness caused by navicular syndrome in horses. *Am J Vet Res* 77:167–173.

127 Wright IM, Smith MR, Humphrey DJ, et al.: 2003. Endoscopic surgery in the treatment of contaminated and infected synovial cavities. *Equine Vet J* 35:613–619.

128 Wylie CE, Newton JR, Bathe AP, et al.: 2015. Prevalence of supporting limb laminitis in a UK equine practice and referral hospital setting between 2005 and 2013: Implications for future epidemiological studies. *Vet Rec* 176:72. http://doi.org/10.1136/vr.102426.

129 Yorke EH, Judy CE, Saveraid TC, et al.: 2014. Distal border fragments of the equine navicular bone: Association between magnetic resonance imaging characteristics and clinical lameness. *Vet Radiol Ultrasound* 55:35–44.

Revised from "Lameness of the Distal Limb" and "Foot Care and Farriery" in *Adams and Stashak's Lameness in Horses, 7th Edition,* by Gary M. Baxter, Randy B. Eggleston, James K. Belknap, Andrew H. Parks., Katy V. Dern, and Stephen E. O'Grady.

3

Common Conditions of the Forelimb

Pastern

OA of the Proximal Interphalangeal (PIP) Joint

Overview
- The term "high ringbone" is often used synonymously with OA of the PIP and is an important and common cause of lameness in virtually all breeds and ages of horses.
- Older horses are at greater risk and the forelimbs are more frequently affected than the hindlimbs.
- The development of secondary OA from P2 fractures (particularly plantar eminence fractures) or osteochondrosis (OC) occurs more commonly in the hindlimbs than the forelimbs.

Anatomy

- The PIP joint or pastern joint is a diarthrodial joint, which is formed from the distal aspect of the proximal phalanx (P1) and the proximal aspect of the middle phalanx (P2).
- The pastern region is bounded dorsally by the common or long digital extensor tendon together with the dorsal branches of the suspensory ligament (SL; Figure 2.1).
- Palmar/plantar support structures of the pastern region are formed by the distal sesamoidean ligaments (DSLs) (straight, oblique, cruciate, and short), SDFT, DDFT, and the proximal and distal digital annular ligaments within the DFTS.
- The medial and lateral collateral ligaments support the PIP in the sagittal plane and four palmar/plantar ligaments provide further stability (Figure 2.19).
- The PIP joint is a low motion joint, and most horses can still perform following joint arthrodesis.

Imaging
- Radiography is the imaging method of choice to evaluate the PIP joint.
- Ultrasonography is an integral part of characterizing the extent of any soft tissue injury that primarily occurs on the palmar/plantar aspect of the pastern.
- More advanced imaging (scintigraphy, CT, or MRI) can be used to provide additional information necessary for a complete and accurate diagnosis and prognosis.

Etiology
- Chronic overuse or repetitive trauma of the PIP joint and surrounding structures is the most common cause.
- Inherent conformational traits (upright pasterns) and the type of work (Western performance) the horse performs also may contribute to increased concussion to the PIP joint and predispose to pulling/tearing

of the soft tissues surrounding the joint or to incongruences within the joint surfaces.

- Single-event, high-energy trauma that does not cause a fracture or joint luxation also can damage the articular cartilage and subchondral bone, predisposing to subchondral cystic lesions (SCLs) and OA.
- OA may develop secondary to OC, unrecognized palmar/plantar eminence fractures of P2, traumatic blows or lacerations, and septic arthritis.

Clinical Signs

- Abnormalities such as dorsal swelling or diffuse bony enlargement in the pastern region are often obvious due to minimal soft tissue in the area (Figure 3.1).
- Palpable heat and pain with firm digital pressure may be appreciated, depending on the duration.
- Usually there is pain on flexion and rotation of the pastern region.
- Obvious enlargement of the pastern and/or varus deformity of the phalanges may be present in horses with advanced disease.

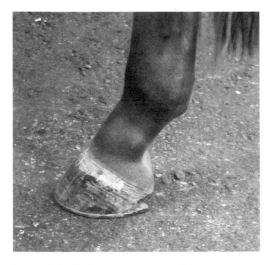

Figure 3.1 Typical enlargement of the pastern that may be visible in horses with OA of the PIP joint. This was a young horse with osteochondrosis of the hindlimb PIP joint.

- Horses with mild disease may have no visual or palpable abnormalities.
- Lameness is often variable depending on the severity and duration of the disease and is usually worsened when the affected limb is on the inside of the circle.
- The lameness should not improve with a very low PD nerve block, but most horses will improve with a basisesamoid or abaxial sesamoid nerve block, or with intra-articular (IA) anesthesia.

Diagnosis

- A tentative diagnosis can often be made based on physical examination findings combined with the responses to local anesthesia and radiography. A tentative diagnosis can often be made based on physical examination findings and responses to local and/or IA anesthesia.
- Radiographic abnormalities may include (Figure 3.2):
  1) Joint space narrowing or collapse
  2) Osteophyte formation
  3) Subchondral bone sclerosis
  4) Periosteal/periarticular bony proliferation
  5) Deformity/collapse of the joint space
  6) Subchondral bone lysis
- Other radiographic features that may be identified include SCLs or OC lesions.

- Radiographs of the contralateral joint should be considered in horses with OC or older horses with advanced OA because these conditions are often bilateral.
- Radiographic abnormalities may be limited in horses with only mild disease or those with acute traumatic injuries. CT or MRI may be performed to determine the exact cause or repeat radiographs in one to two months may reveal evidence of OA.
- Lame horses that do not have radiographic abnormalities may have PIP joint synovitis/capsulitis, subchondral bone bruising, or other unrecognized bone or cartilage damage that can only be recognized with advanced imaging such as CT or MRI (Figure 3.3).

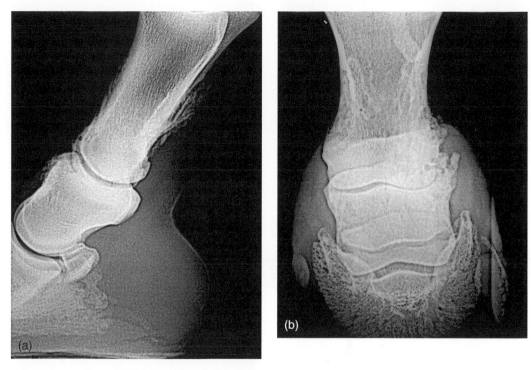

Figure 3.2 Lateral (a) and dorsopalmar (b) radiographs of the pastern region with a marked periosteal reaction, joint space collapse, and subchondral lysis consistent with advanced OA within the joint. This horse was lame at the walk and underwent arthrodesis of the joint.

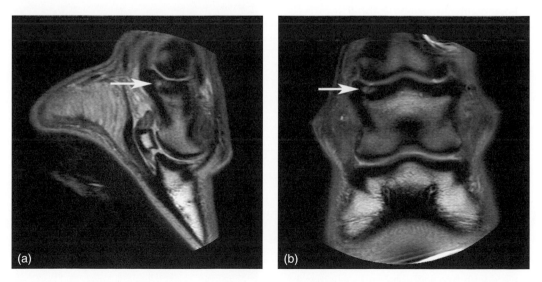

Figure 3.3 Lateral (a) and dorsopalmar (b) proton density (pd) MRI images of a horse with lameness isolated to the pastern region that revealed subchondral bone disease/SCL (arrows) of the palmar aspect of P2.

Treatment

- Treatment is variable and often depends on the severity of the disease, degree of lameness, age and intended use of the horse, and the owner's expectations and financial constraints.
- Horses with severe lameness and advanced radiographic abnormalities (especially asymmetrical joint narrowing) usually are not good candidates for nonsurgical treatments because their effectiveness is often short-lived.
- Horses with a single traumatic injury to the PIP joint may respond well to rest and develop minimal radiographic abnormalities (Figure 3.3).
- Horses with only mild-to-moderate radiographic abnormalities of joint may respond well to conservative treatment, depending on the horse's intended use.
- Conservative management may involve periods of rest, systemic and/or IA anti-inflammatory therapy, trimming and shoeing, and a change in the horse's career.
- In acute cases, rest from exercise is important to prevent further trauma, reduce inflammation, and permit healing to occur. Confinement and rest are rarely effective in horses with chronic OA.
- Oral NSAIDs are often combined with IA medication of the PIP joint in horses with chronic OA to reduce the signs of lameness and improve the effectiveness of both treatments.
- The hoof-pastern axis should be corrected if abnormal because either a broken-forward or broken-back hoof-pastern axis can contribute to problems within the PIP joint.
- Surgical treatment for OA of the PIP joint consists of arthrodesis to eliminate motion within the joint; natural ankylosis may occur but it is often a long, painful process with variable results.
- The current recommended technique is a single dorsal midline 4.5 mm DCP or LCP plate with two additional transarticular 5.5-mm screws (Figure 3.4). This technique is thought to improve the comfort level of horses in the immediate postoperative period and requires casting for only two to three weeks postoperatively.

Prognosis

- Most horses with mild-to-moderate OA can be managed with some combination of non-surgical treatments.
- The prognosis for horses following PIP joint arthrodesis is less predictable in the forelimb than in the hindlimb.
- Approximately 85–95% of horses with hindlimb and 70–85% of horses with forelimb

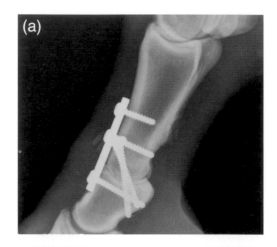

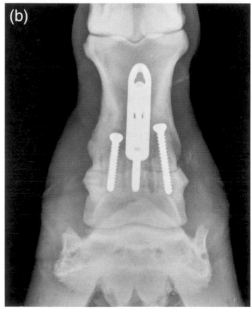

Figure 3.4 Lateral (a) and DP radiographs (b) of the pastern following placement of a three-hole plate with two transarticular 5.5-mm screws for arthrodesis of the PIP joint. A DCP was used in the horse on the top (a) and an LCP was used in the horse on the bottom (b). Image (b) Courtesy of Ashlee Watts.

lameness should return to their intended use, and 85% should return athletic soundness following an arthrodesis.

- Complications that may prevent horses from becoming athletically sound include implant infection, excessive bony proliferation that impinges on the DIP joint, exostosis of the extensor process of the distal phalanx, and soft tissue "irritation" associated with the implants.
- Horses with chronic infectious arthritis treated by PIP joint arthrodesis have a worse prognosis than those treated for non-septic conditions.

Osteochondrosis (OC) of the PIP Joint

Overview

- OC of the PIP joint is identified less commonly than other joints in the horse. However, both osteochondral fragmentation and SCLs can occur.
- Osteochondral fragments tend to occur dorsally (usually from the distal aspect of P1) or palmarly/plantarly (midline from the eminences of P2) (Figure 3.5).
- SCLs usually involve the distal aspect of P1 but occur rarely in the proximal aspect of P2 (Figure 3.6).
- Malformation of the condyles of the distal aspect of P1 without fragmentation can occur and may represent another form of OC that leads to early OA within the joint.

Anatomy (Please refer to previous section on "OA of PIP Joint")

- OC of the PIP joint is assumed to be due to similar factors that cause the condition in other locations.

Imaging

- Radiography is the imaging modality of choice and will detect the majority of OC lesions within the PIP joint.
- Early detection of OC lesions usually requires advanced imaging (CT or MRI) to confirm the abnormality within the joint.

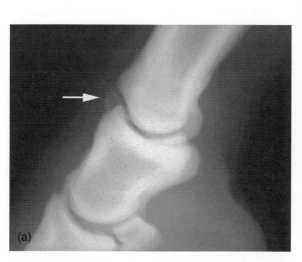
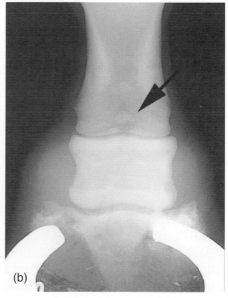

Figure 3.5 (a) Lateral radiograph of a horse with a dorsal OC fragment (arrow) and (b) dorsopalmar radiograph of another horse with fragmentation in the palmar aspect of the PIP joint (arrow). Both fragments were removed with arthroscopy.

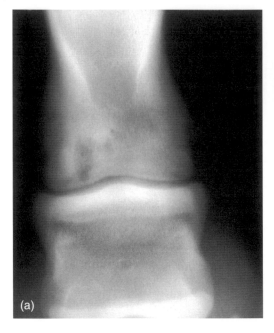 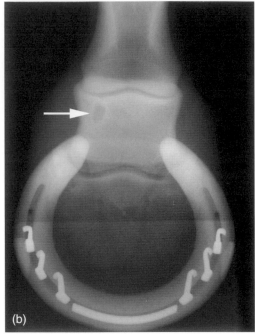

Figure 3.6 Dorsoplantar radiographs of two different young horses demonstrating SCLs of the distal medial condyle of P1 (a) and the proximal aspect of P2 (arrow; b). The SCL in (b) was not considered to be the cause of the lameness in that horse.

Etiology
- OC of the PIP joint is assumed to be due to similar factors that cause the condition in other locations in the horse.
- Traumatic fragmentation and subchondral bone damage leading to SCLs can occur within the PIP joint, and it may be difficult to differentiate between developmental and traumatic causes.

Clinical Signs
- Developmental lesions tend to occur in younger horses and cause less severe clinical signs and traumatic lesions can occur in any age horse and typically have more severe clinical signs.
- Physical examination findings are similar to other problems within the PIP joint and may include no abnormalities, enlargement of the pastern, pain with flexion and manipulation of the pastern region, and positive response to flexion tests.

- Horses with SCLs tend to be more lame than horses with osteochondral fragmentation and occur more commonly in the hindlimb than the forelimbs.

Diagnosis
- The diagnosis of OC is usually confirmed with radiographs. Osteochondral fragmentation usually can be seen on both lateral and dorsopalmar/plantar views (Figure 3.5), whereas SCLs are often only visible on the dorsopalmar/plantar radiographic projection (Figure 3.6).
- Some lesions, particularly osteochondral fragmentation, may be incidental findings.
- Most SCLs that involve the distal condyle of P1 are clinically significant and are often accompanied by radiographic changes consistent with OA.
- Radiography of the opposite PIP joint should be performed because OC lesions can be bilateral.

Treatment

- Arthroscopic removal is the treatment of choice for osteochondral fragments that are causing clinical problems. Both the dorsal and palmar/plantar pouches of the PIP joint are accessible with the arthroscope, but the surgery can be difficult.
- SCLs of distal P1 are often clinically significant and can be managed conservatively or surgically depending on the severity of lameness. Conservative management with NSAIDs and IA medication usually resolves the lameness, but recurrence is common.
- Surgical management may include transcyst screw application, transcortical cyst debridement, corticosteroid injection, or pastern arthrodesis.
- Most horses with SCLs and significant secondary joint OA are best treated surgically with arthrodesis of the joint.

Prognosis

- Horses with OC fragmentation within the PIP joint have a very good prognosis after arthroscopic removal. Some fragments may be incidental findings and horses can perform without removal.
- Horses with SCLs have a worse prognosis than those with fragmentation and the prognosis will depend on the type of treatment and if an arthrodesis was required.

Luxation/Subluxation of the PIP Joint

Overview

- Luxation of the PIP joint is uncommon, can occur in a medial/lateral or palmar/plantar direction, and nearly always involves a single limb.
- Medial/lateral luxation involves the collateral ligaments of the PIP joint and may be open or closed.
- Palmar/plantar subluxation is associated with complete tearing of the straight DSL, branches of the SDFT, or a combination of these injuries (Figure 3.7).

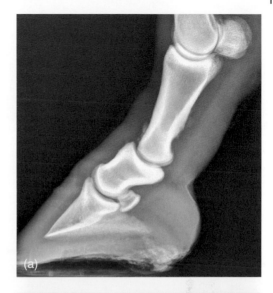
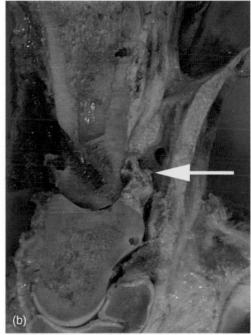

Figure 3.7 Lateral radiographic view (a) and postmortem specimen (b) from a horse that had plantar luxation of the PIP joint. Excessive dropping of the fetlock can be seen in (a) and rupture of the straight DSL can be seen in b (arrow).

- Dorsal subluxations of the PIP joint are most common in young horses secondary to flexural deformities and other developmental orthopedic diseases (Figure 3.8).

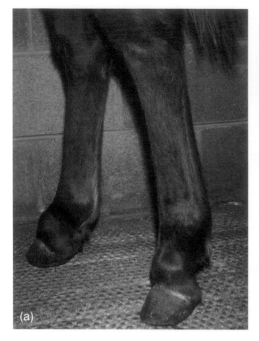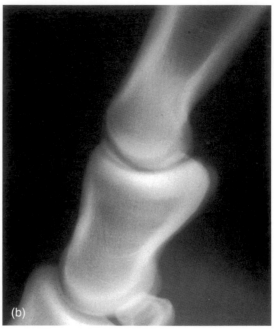

Figure 3.8 Visual (a) and radiographic (b) lateral views of a young horse with bilateral dorsal subluxation of the PIP joints. Dorsal swellings over both rear pastern joints can be seen in (a) and dorsal subluxation of P1 in relation to P2 within the pastern joint is present in (b).

Anatomy

- The medial and lateral collateral ligaments of the PIP joint provide support in the sagittal plane (Figure 2.19).
- The pastern is supported palmarly/plantarly by the distal straight sesamoidean ligament, the SDFT branches that attach to the eminences of P2, and the palmar/plantar ligaments of the pastern (Figure 3.9).
- Dorsally, the PIP joint is supported by the common or long extensor tendon and the extensor branches of the SL.

Imaging

- Radiography is the optimal imaging technique to confirm the diagnosis and identify concurrent abnormalities such as fractures or OA that may be present.
- Stress films may be needed to confirm medial/lateral subluxation because the phalanges can often remain in correct anatomic alignment unless pulled medially or laterally.
- Ultrasonography can be used to evaluate the soft tissue damage to the palmar/plantar support structures but is usually unnecessary to develop a treatment plan.

Etiology

- Lateral/medial luxations are usually caused by severe trauma to the joint capsule and collateral ligament (e.g. distal limb caught in something and the horse struggles and/or falls) or lacerations that transect the collateral ligament.
- Palmar/plantar subluxation generally occurs from acute trauma resulting in overextension of the PIP joint and tearing of the joint capsule, straight DSL, and the branches of the SDFT.
- Palmar/plantar subluxation also can be seen in foals and weanlings that have jumped from heights and in foals with flexor tendon

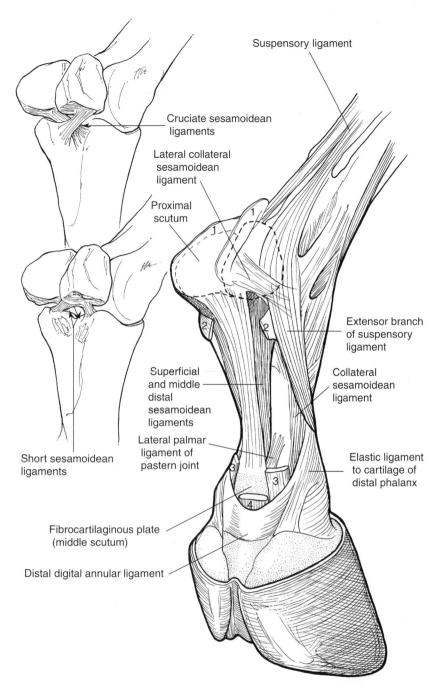

Figure 3.9 Sesamoidean ligaments. Dashed lines indicate positions of the proximal sesamoid bones embedded in the metacarpointersesamoidean ligament. Numbers indicate cut stumps of (1) palmar annular ligament, (2) proximal digital annular ligament, (3) superficial digital flexor, and (4) deep digital flexor tendon.

laxity that overexert themselves during free exercise.

- Dorsal subluxations are thought to be secondary to flexural deformities or limb contracture and may be seen in foals/weanlings that are rapidly growing with an upright conformation (Figure 3.8).
- Dorsal subluxation may also be seen in horses after traumatic disruption of the suspensory apparatus and arthrodesis of the fetlock joint, or progressive, severe suspensory desmitis.

Clinical Signs

- Horses with medial/lateral luxation are often non-weight-bearing or lame at the walk, have swelling of the pastern associated with the ligament injury, and a limb deformity may be present. Instability and pain may be identified with rotation or medial/lateral movement of the phalanges.
- Horses with palmar/plantar subluxation are often very lame in the acute stage but usually remain lame at the walk over time. The dorsal surface of the pastern will appear concave (dished out) and with chronicity, excessive hyperextension of the pastern and sinking of the fetlock may be seen when the horse walks.
- Dorsal subluxation occurs primarily in the hindlimbs in young horses and lameness is usually absent or mild. This type of subluxation is often dynamic in nature; it is seen when the limb is unweighted and usually resolves during full weight-bearing. With chronicity, an obvious swelling over the dorsal aspect of the pastern region similar to high ringbone becomes evident.

Diagnosis

- A tentative diagnosis can usually be made from the history and physical examination of the horse.
- Dorsal and palmar/plantar subluxations/luxations are usually obvious on standing lateral-to-medial views of the pastern (Figures 3.7 and 3.8) and medial/lateral luxations are often obvious with DP stressed views.

Treatment

- The treatment of choice for most horses with medial/lateral and palmar/plantar luxations/subluxations of the PIP joint is arthrodesis of the joint.
- Unlike medial/lateral luxations of the fetlock joint, similar luxations of the PIP joint do not respond well to casting alone and often develop secondary OA and persistent lameness.
- Conservative treatment of palmar/plantar subluxations is usually unsuccessful and with chronicity fibrosis of the PIP joint in an abnormal position occurs, making surgical realignment difficult.
- Horses with intermittent dorsal subluxation with upright conformation and no apparent lameness may be treated conservatively with anti-inflammatory medication and a controlled exercise program. Horses with intermittent dorsal subluxation of the pelvic limb associated with excessive tension of the DDFT have been treated successfully with transection of the medial head of the DDFT.
- Dorsal subluxations also can be treated with arthrodesis if they fail to respond to other methods of treatment. Horses with dorsal luxation that develop secondary OA are best treated with arthrodesis.

Prognosis

- The prognosis appears to be good for survival and fair to good for return to use in horses with luxations/subluxations treated early by arthrodesis.
- The convalescence can be long and up to a year may be required before the horse may return to performance.
- Three cases of bilateral acquired pelvic limb intermittent dorsal subluxation treated by tendonectomy of the medial head of the DDFT responded favorably to the treatment and the subluxation resolved between one to seven days postoperatively.

Fractures of the Middle Phalanx (P2)

Overview

- A variety of fracture types involving P2 have been reported, including osteochondral (chip) fractures, palmar/plantar eminence fractures, axial fractures, and comminuted fractures.
- Osteochondral fractures and axial fractures are rare, whereas eminence and comminuted fractures occur commonly.
- Fractures of P2 occur most commonly in the hindlimbs of middle-aged Western performance horses used for cutting, roping, barrel racing, pole bending, and reining.
- However, these fractures may occur in any horse of any breed during lunging, turnout, after kicks or falls, or from any form of single-event trauma.
- Palmar/plantar eminence fractures can be uniaxial (involving one eminence; Figure 3.10) or biaxial (involving both eminences; Figure 3.11).
- Comminuted fractures are the most common fracture and always involve the PIP

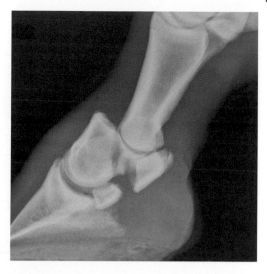

Figure 3.11 Lateral radiograph of the pastern demonstrating biaxial eminence fractures of P2. Internal fixation is recommended for these types of fractures to prevent palmar/plantar luxation of P1.

joint (uniarticular) but often extend distally into the DIP joint (biarticular; Figure 3.12).

Anatomy

- The middle phalanx, P2, or short pastern bone is located between the distal and proximal phalanges and communicates with the DIP joint distally and PIP joint proximally.
- P2 is bounded dorsally by the common or long digital extensor tendon together and palmarly/plantarly by the DSL, the branches of the SDFT, DDFT, and distal digital annular ligaments within the DFTS (Figures 2.1 and 3.9).
- The middle phalanx is stabilized both distally and proximally with collateral ligaments that attach to P3 and P1, respectively.

Imaging

- Radiography is the imaging modality of choice to diagnose suspected fractures of the middle phalanx. With comminuted fractures, radiography typically underestimates the degree of comminution and amount of DIP joint involvement.

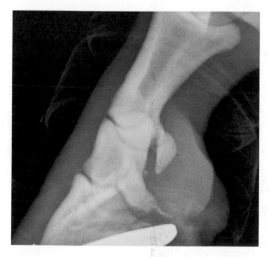

Figure 3.10 Oblique radiograph of the pastern region demonstrating a medial plantar eminence fracture of P2. This horse presented for a hindlimb lameness of two weeks duration.

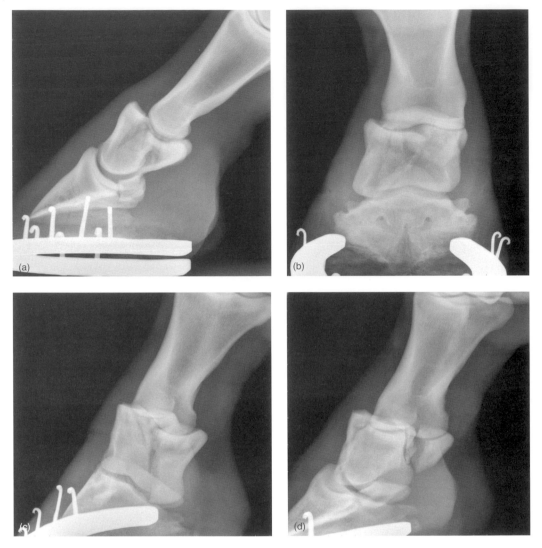

Figure 3.12 Lateral (a), dorsoplantar (b), and two oblique (c and d) radiographic projections of a horse with a comminuted P2 fracture. Multiple fracture lines are commonly seen, and most comminuted fractures involve both the PIP and the DIP joint surfaces.

- Cross-sectional imaging (CT) can be helpful in defining the fracture configuration of comminuted P2 fractures and aids in reconstruction of the DIP joint.

Etiology

- Osteochondral fractures may occur from use, direct trauma to the bone (e.g. penetrating wound), or avulsion of soft tissue attachments (palmar/plantar aspect), or they may be associated with OC.
- Palmar/plantar eminence fractures may occur from compression and rotation that is associated with sudden stops and short turns. They also may occur during PIP joint overextension which results in excessive tension of the SDFT and straight DSL, causing an avulsion of the eminence(s).

- Comminuted fractures are thought to result from a combination of compression and torsion (twisting) forces that occur with sudden stops, starts, and short turns. Most comminuted P2 fractures are thought to occur as a single-event injury, but a history of lameness in the affected limb may precede the fracture in some horses.
- Horses shod with heel calks are believed to be more prone to comminuted P2 fractures because the calks grip the ground, preventing the normal rotation of the foot and phalanges when the horse rapidly changes directions.
- Horses turned out for exercise after long-term confinement also have been reported to be at risk for comminuted P2 fractures.

Clinical Signs

- Lameness associated with P2 fractures that do not disrupt the weight-bearing capabilities of P2 (osteochondral fragments, single eminence and simple axial fractures) can be variable. Some horses may have a history of an acute onset of lameness, whereas others may present for a chronic forelimb or hindlimb lameness that worsens with exercise.
- Swelling of the pastern is not a reliable finding, but fetlock/phalangeal flexion and rotation of the pastern region often elicit a painful response.
- Diagnostic anesthesia with a basisesamoid nerve block or IA anesthesia is often required to localize the lameness to the pastern region. However, diagnostic anesthesia is contraindicated with other types of P2 fractures because of the risk of fracture displacement.
- Horses with comminuted or biaxial P2 eminence fractures often have a history of acute onset of severe lameness. Horses are usually very lame, painful to manipulation of the pastern, and crepitus may be felt but is not a consistent finding. The pastern also may appear to be "unstable" during

manipulation and swelling may be present just above the coronary band with comminuted fractures (due to effusion of the DIP joint).

Diagnosis

- A definitive diagnosis requires a complete radiographic examination – four views are recommended: dorsopalmar (DP), lateromedial (LM), dorsolateral to palmaromedial oblique (DLPMO), and dorsomedial to palmarolateral oblique (DMPLO).
- Osteochondral fractures usually are diagnosed with the routine radiographic views.
- Additional views may be necessary with comminuted fractures – identification of whether the fracture lines extend into the DIP joint and whether there is an intact "strut" of bone is very important information to help decide treatment options.
- The fracture configuration has considerable bearing on the treatment method selected as well as the prognosis for future soundness (Figures 3.10–3.12).
- Computer tomography (CT) is recommended if there is doubt about whether a comminuted P2 fracture can be repaired and the extent of involvement of the DIP joint (Figure 3.13).

Treatment

Osteochondral Fractures

- Fracture fragments (dorsal or palmar/plantar) associated with the PIP joint that contribute to lameness are best removed with arthroscopy.
- Arthrotomy can be used but is less desirable.

Eminence Fractures

- Uniaxial or biaxial eminence fractures of P2 that involve the PIP joint are best treated by arthrodesis of the PIP joint. The use of single or double bone plating is considered

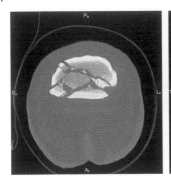
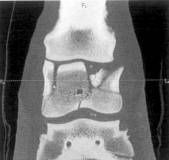
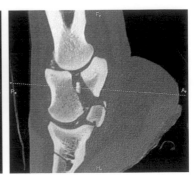

Figure 3.13 CT images of a comminuted P2 fracture that demonstrate the numerous fracture fragments that are present in different orientations. This fracture was repaired with two dorsally applied bone plates and pastern arthrodesis. Courtesy of Ashlee Watts.

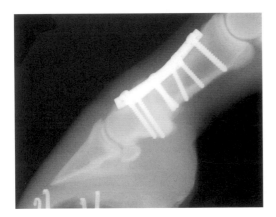

Figure 3.14 Lateral radiograph one year after the biaxial eminence fracture of P2 depicted in Figure 3.11 was repaired with two plates.

mandatory for biaxial eminence fractures (Figure 3.14).

- Single eminence fractures rarely heal back to the parent bone with casting, and secondary OA of the PIP joint leads to chronic lameness. Therefore, casting should be reserved for cases in which pasture or breeding soundness is desired and economic constraints dictate the approach.
- If internal fixation of biaxial P2 fractures is not elected, transfixation pin-casts or another type of external fixator is recommended over casting alone to maintain phalangeal alignment since palmar/plantar subluxation of the PIP joint is common.

Comminuted P2 Fractures

- In general, comminuted P2 fractures should be repaired with some type of internal fixation (bone plating) if at all possible.
- Horses with an intact strut of bone spanning from the PIP to the DIP joint are ideal candidates for internal fixation. Horses that do not have an intact bony strut yet have large-enough bony fragments for screw fixation also often benefit from internal fixation.
- Horses with highly comminuted P2 fractures (so-called "bag of ice") are best treated with transfixation pin-casts or another type of external fixator.
- Casting alone can also be used for some highly comminuted fractures but fracture collapse is not uncommon.

Prognosis

- The prognosis for horses with osteochondral fractures treated by arthrotomy or arthroscopy appears to be very good for return to full serviceability.
- The prognosis for uniaxial or biaxial palmar/plantar eminence fractures treated by arthrodesis also is very good for return to performance and should be considered similar to horses treated for OA of the joint.
- Horses with comminuted fractures that only involve the PIP joint usually have a good prognosis for return to athletic performance, provided they are treated with internal fixation.

- The prognosis for horses with biarticular comminuted P2 fractures is much reduced compared with those with uniarticular fractures because the limiting factor in many cases is related to the health of the DIP joint.
- Internal fixation of comminuted P2 fractures with bone plates increases both survival and return to athletic function. In general, horses with biarticular comminuted P2 fractures should be considered to have a 40–50% chance of returning to performance after internal fixation.

Fractures of the Proximal Phalanx (P1)

Overview

- Fractures of P1 occur frequently and can be broadly categorized into noncomminuted and comminuted fractures.
- Fracture configurations (excluding osteochondral fragmentation) range from small fissures that enter the MCP/MTP joint to highly comminuted biarticular fractures ("bag of ice").
- Stress or fatigue-type fractures that cannot be identified on routine radiographs also may occur in performance horses.
- Noncomminuted P1 fractures have been classified into several types:
  1) Midsagittal or sagittal fractures: Exist primarily in the sagittal plane and begin at the MCP/MTP joint.
     a) Short (extend less than 30 mm in length distally; Figure 3.15a)
     b) Long (extend more than 30 mm in length distally; Figure 3.15b)
     c) Complete (exit the lateral cortex or are biarticular)
  2) Dorsal frontal fractures: Begin at the MCP/MTP joint in the frontal plane and extend to the dorsal cortex or distally

toward the PIP joint; can be incomplete or complete.
  3) Distal joint fractures: Involve the PIP joint.
  4) Palmar/plantar eminence fractures: Involve the MTP/MCP joint (Figure 3.16).
  5) Physeal fractures: Usually Salter-Harris Type 2.
  6) Oblique or transverse diaphyseal fractures.
- Comminuted P1 fractures can range from fairly simple three-piece fractures to the "bag of ice" type injury (Figure 3.17). For treatment purposes, they can be divided into fractures that have an intact cortex (strut) of P1 from the proximal to distal joint surfaces (moderately comminuted) and fractures that do not have an intact bone strut (severely comminuted).
- Less common types of P1 fractures include proximal medial collateral ligament avulsion fractures, dorsal nonarticular fractures, and stress or fatigue fractures.
- Sagittal and other types of noncomminuted P1 fractures are primarily seen in racing Thoroughbreds (forelimbs) and Standardbreds (hindlimbs) but can also occur in other types of performance horses.
- Comminuted P1 fractures also occur commonly in racing Thoroughbreds and Standardbreds but may also occur in other types of performance horses and in any horse at pasture or at exercise from a single traumatic event.

Anatomy

- The proximal phalanx, P1, or long pastern bone is located between the middle phalanx and the MC/MT and communicates with the PIP joint distally and fetlock joint proximally.
- P1 is bounded dorsally by the common or long digital extensor tendon and palmarly/plantarly by the DSLs, SDFT, DDFT, proximal digital annular ligament, and the DFTS (Figures 2.1 and 3.9).

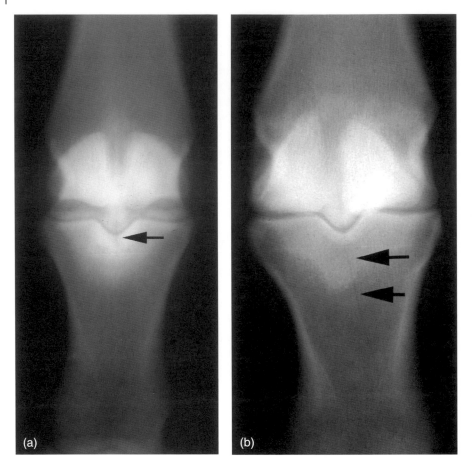

Figure 3.15 Dorsopalmar radiographs of the pastern region revealing short (a) and long (b) incomplete sagittal fractures of P1 (arrows). The fracture in (b) was repaired with two lag screws through stab incisions.

- The proximal phalanx is stabilized both distally and proximally with collateral ligaments that attach to P2 and the MC/MT, respectively.
- P1 articulates with the sesamoid bones on its proximal palmar/plantar aspect and the extensor branch of the suspensory courses from the sesamoid bones over P1 in a palmar/plantar to dorsal direction to join the extensor tendons on its dorsal aspect.

Imaging
- Radiography is the imaging modality of choice to diagnose suspected fractures of P1. A minimum of four views (DP, LM, DLPMO, and DMPLO) is recommended.

- CT can be helpful in defining the fracture configuration of comminuted P1 fractures and aids in preoperative planning for surgery.
- Scintigraphy may be used in horses with suspected stress or fatigue fractures that may not be visible on radiographs.

Etiology
- A combination of longitudinal compression in conjunction with asynchronous lateral-to-medial rotation of P1 or twisting of P1 in relation to the MC/MT may be the cause of some fractures.
- If the alignment between the convex sagittal ridge of the distal end of the MC/MT and the

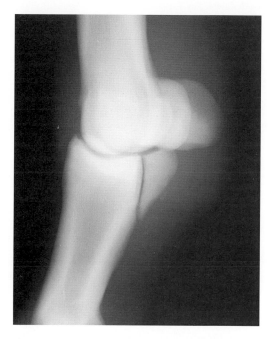

Figure 3.16 Lateral radiograph of the fetlock demonstrating a fracture of the palmar eminence of P1. This fracture was an acute injury and was repaired by lag screw fixation. Smaller, chronic fractures are more common in this location and are often removed if they are problematic.

concave groove in the proximal surface of P1 is not perfect, the convex sagittal ridge may act as a wedge to create a fracture. This may be worsened if the rotary movement is accelerated such as would occur if the foot slips.

- In most cases, a combination of axial weight-bearing and torsional forces usually contributes to P1 fractures.
- Parasagittal P1 fractures in the athletic horse may occur as part of a chronic pathological process characterized as bone maladaptation or fatigue-type fractures. Stress or fatigue-type fractures may precede the development of a radiographic apparent sagittal P1 fracture or may predispose to a comminuted fracture. Stress fractures tend to occur most commonly in the midsagittal groove at the proximal aspect of the bone, the same area where most P1 fractures originate.

Clinical Signs

- The clinical signs associated with P1 fractures are variable and depend on the fracture type and degree of fracture propagation.

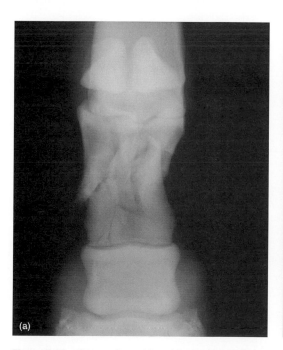

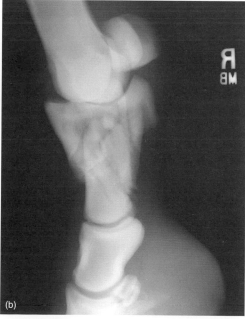

Figure 3.17 Dorsopalmar (a) and lateral (b) radiographs of a horse with a severely comminuted fracture of P1. Internal fixation is typically not possible with these types of fractures and transfixation pin-casts or external fixators are usually used to attempt salvage of these horses.

- Horses with incomplete sagittal fractures may demonstrate moderate pain and lameness initially, but it may be short in duration. However, fetlock effusion is usually present, and a painful response is often elicited with flexion and rotation of the phalanges.
- Horses with complete sagittal fractures are usually quite lame (grade 3–4/5) and fetlock effusion and swelling of the pastern region is usually apparent.
- Horses with comminuted fractures are usually non-weight-bearing and may show signs of physical distress such as sweating. The pastern region is often obviously swollen, and crepitus and instability are palpable.
- Perineural anesthesia is usually unnecessary to make the diagnosis but some horses with short sagittal P1 fractures may present for a routine lameness evaluation. Perineural anesthesia is contraindicated if any type of P1 fracture is suspected because it will increase the risk of fracture propagation.

Diagnosis

- Radiographs are required to characterize the type of P1 fracture and dictate the appropriate treatment. Additional views at varying angles may be necessary to accurately document the fracture configuration, especially in comminuted fractures.
- Midsagittal fractures are often readily apparent on the DP view, but some short, incomplete fractures may be difficult to see radiographically (Figure 3.15).
- The presence or absence of an intact bony strut that spans from the MCP/MTP to the PIP joints is an important radiographic feature (Figure 3.17).
- CT should be used to assess the degree of comminution and aid in preoperative planning for surgery whenever necessary.

Treatment
Noncomminuted P1 Fractures

- The decision on how to treat horses with noncomminuted fractures usually depends on the fracture type, fracture location and length, degree of displacement, and intended use of the horse.
- Most noncomminuted P1 fractures (long sagittal) are best treated with internal fixation using lag screws placed through stab incisions (Figure 3.15).
- Short, incomplete sagittal fractures can be treated with pressure bandaging and stall rest, but most are treated with lag screw fixation because of the risk of fracture propagation and reported improved prognosis.
- Horses with displaced fractures that are not treated with internal fixation have a reduced chance of returning to performance.
- Complete sagittal fractures that extend distally from the MCP/MTP joint to involve the PIP joint or that exit the lateral cortex are best treated by internal fixation and coaptation. These fractures are often displaced and generally can be better reduced with open approaches to P1 followed by lag screw stabilization. A distal limb cast is usually recommended after surgery for two to four weeks, depending on the security of the fixation.
- Bandaging and/or external coaptation has been used alone in cases in which breeding soundness is the objective or if there are economic constraints. These horses may develop considerable exostosis at the fracture site and secondary OA of the MCP/MTP joint.
- Dorsal frontal incomplete or complete nondisplaced P1 fractures can be treated by rest and bandaging or by internal fixation using lag screws, depending on the fracture size. Arthroscopic examination of the fetlock joint should be considered to visualize the dorsal articular margin and debride damaged cartilage if needed.

Comminuted Fractures

- The objective for treatment of most horses with comminuted P1 fractures is usually to preserve the horse for breeding purposes or pasture soundness. Even horses with only moderately comminuted P1 fractures repaired surgically rarely return to racing.

- The goals of surgery are usually to restore the articular congruity of the joint(s) involved and to stabilize the fracture to maintain bone length.
- Methods for treatment include:
  1) External coaptation alone.
  2) External skeletal fixation alone (transfixation pin-casts or Nunamaker skeletal fixator).
  3) Lag screw fixation through stab incisions +/− external skeletal transfixation.
  4) Open reduction with lag screws and external coaptation.
  5) Open reduction with plates and screws and external coaptation.
  6) Reduction combined with transfixation pin-casts.
- Internal fixation is usually recommended in horses with moderately comminuted P1 fractures (those with an intact strut of P1 that extends from the proximal to distal joint surfaces) that permit fracture realignment (Figure 3.18). These horses have a much

greater chance of surviving than do those without an intact strut of bone.

- External skeletal fixation is usually the treatment of choice to repair severely comminuted P1 fractures that lack an intact bony strut (Figure 3.17), and for fractures that are open or have a severely compromised blood supply.
- Internal fixation with either screws alone or plates and screws may be combined with a transfixation pin-cast in some horses. The transfixation pin-cast is used to protect the implants from potential failure in horses that may not have an intact strut of bone.
- Casting alone can be used to treat some horses with comminuted P1 fractures, but it is less than optimal. Case selection is important, and the fracture should be minimally comminuted and be relatively stable to prevent axial collapse of the fracture.

Prognosis
Noncomminuted Fractures

- These horses generally have a very good prognosis for long-term survival and many return to performance, although often at a reduced level.

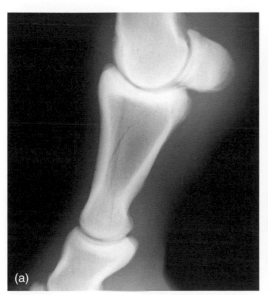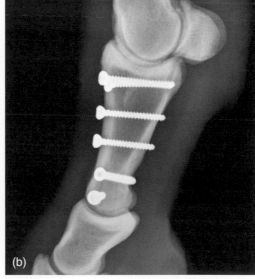

(a) (b)

Figure 3.18 Lateral radiographs of a nondisplaced, moderately comminuted P1 fracture before (a) and after repair (b) with multiple lag screws placed through stab incisions.

- Complete sagittal fractures that extended into the PIP joint have a worse prognosis (46%) than short, incomplete sagittal fractures (71%); long, incomplete sagittal fractures (66%); or complete sagittal fractures that extended to the lateral cortex (71%).
- 89% of the Standardbred racehorses returned to racing although at significantly decreased performance levels and 65–70% of Thoroughbred horses returned to racing following incomplete sagittal fractures.

Comminuted Fractures

- Horses with open or closed severely comminuted fractures that do not permit reconstruction of the fragments remain difficult to treat and have only a fair prognosis for survival, regardless of the treatment approach used.
- Moderately comminuted P1 fractures (those with an intact boney strut) usually can be repaired with internal fixation; a 92% successful outcome has been reported.

Desmitis of the Distal Sesamoidean Ligaments (DSLs)

Overview

- Desmitis of the oblique, straight, and cruciate DSLs occurs in all types of performance horses with injury to the oblique DSL being most common.
- Horses that jump (e.g. event horses, show jumpers, field and show hunters, steeple chasers, and timber racehorses) and race and Quarter horses used for Western performance such as reining, cutting, and barrel racing appear to be particularly prone to these injuries.
- Either branch of the oblique DSL can be injured (medial thought to be most common) and these injuries are thought to more common in the forelimb than the hindlimb.
- Horses with a valgus or varus limb conformation or long, sloping pasterns may be at increased risk for injury.

- Injuries to the DSLs can be the primary injury or can be part of a complex of lesions, all of which contribute to some part of the current lameness.

Anatomy

- The DSLs extend distad from the proximal sesamoid bones (PSBs) and are the functional continuation of the suspensory apparatus to the digit. There are three DSLs: straight (superficial), paired oblique (middle), and paired cruciate (deep) (Figure 3.9).
- All of the ligaments originate from the base of the PSBs and intersesamoidean ligament.
- The straight DSL attaches primarily to the proximopalmar/plantar aspect of P2 and less robustly to the palmar/plantar aspect of P1.
- The paired wedge-shaped oblique DSLs attach to a triangular region on the middle and distal third of P1.
- Deep to the straight and oblique DSLs, the paired cruciate ligaments attach distally to the contralateral eminence of the proximal extremity of P1.
- The DSLs are an important part of the suspensory apparatus that provides resistance to extension of the MCP/MTP joint during the stance phase.

Imaging

- A combination of radiography and ultrasound may reveal findings that may suggest a diagnosis of injury to the DSL.
- MRI is the best diagnostic tool to make a definitive diagnosis (Figure 3.19).

Etiology

- Hyperextension of the fetlock joint can result in supraphysiologic strains in the suspensory apparatus, which may lead to failure of the DSLs.
- The straight DSL would most likely be injured during hyperextension, but injury to this ligament is less common than to the oblique DSL.

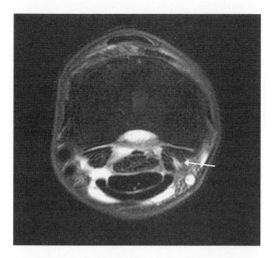

Figure 3.19 Transverse proton density MRI image showing high signal intensity (arrow) in the lateral branch of the oblique DSL in the pastern region.

- Injuries to the oblique DSLs usually occur unilaterally, probably as a result of asymmetric loading caused by abnormal conformation, lateral/medial foot imbalances, a misstep, or poor footing.
- Although injuries to the oblique DSL are more common, concurrent injuries to the straight and oblique DSLs can occur.

Clinical Signs

- With acute injuries (less than three weeks duration), mild swelling of the palmar/plantar surface of the pastern region may be present as a result of (DFTS) effusion. Heat and pain with digital pressure also may be palpable.
- Horses with chronic injuries have a more insidious onset of lameness and often present for a routine lameness evaluation.
- The lameness is usually mild to moderate in severity, positive to fetlock or phalangeal flexion, and worsened when the affected limb is on the inside of the circle.
- Palpation of the DSLs is best performed with the foot held off the ground and the MCP/MTP joint flexed, so the flexor tendons are relaxed. Careful digital palpation dorsal to the flexor tendons midway between the heel

bulbs and the PSBs may reveal firm swellings and/or pain.
- Swelling of a DSL must be differentiated from swelling of the medial or lateral branch of the SDFT, which is also located in the mid-pastern region.
- Perineural anesthesia (basisesamoid block) should improve the lameness in most cases. However, an abaxial sesamoid, low four-point block may be necessary in some cases.

Diagnosis

- Radiographic abnormalities that may suggest a previous or concurrent injury of a DSL include enthesophyte formation on P1 or the sesamoid bones, avulsion fractures/fragments, and dystrophic mineralization within one of the DSLs.
- Bone fragments also have been observed on the nonarticular proximal extremity of P1 and at the base of the sesamoid bones that may involve the oblique, cruciate, or short DSLs.
- Sonographic evidence of acute desmitis is manifested by a diffuse increase in ligament size, fiber disruption, discrete core lesions, and peri-ligamentous fluid surrounding the affected ligament.
- Although ultrasound can be useful to diagnose problems in the DSLs, lack of ultrasound abnormalities does not rule out a problem.
- MRI is usually required to make a definitive diagnosis (Figure 3.19).

Treatment

- Injuries to the DSLs are treated very similarly to other soft tissue problems such as tendinitis.
- In acute cases, confinement, cold therapy, pressure/support wraps, and administration of NSAIDs are recommended. Cold therapy in the form of an ice water slurry applied for 30 minutes twice a day during the acute inflammatory phase is beneficial.
- A six-month rest and rehabilitation program is currently recommended. This usually

involves a short period of stall confinement depending on the severity of the injury (three to six weeks), followed by increasing periods of hand-walking and controlled exercise. Clinical evaluation should be performed at four-to-six-week intervals, and if the horse has improved, controlled exercise can be increased.

- Adjunctive treatments that may be used in addition to the rehabilitation protocol include extracorporeal shockwave, ligament splitting, intrasynovial treatment of the DFTS, and intralesional treatment of the damaged ligament with biologics.
- Nonarticular basal sesamoid fragments that may be associated with DSL avulsion injuries can be removed using a "keyhole" surgical approach through the DFTS.

Prognosis

- The prognosis for horses with DSL injuries to return to performance has historically been guarded because of the high probability of reinjury.
- Approximately 66–90% of horses with DSL injuries or avulsion fractures of the PSBs may return to performance following treatment.
- Recurrence of DSL desmitis is not uncommon, similar to other soft tissue injuries.

SDFT and DDFT Injuries in the Pastern

Overview

- In general, injuries to the SDFT in the pastern region occur most frequently in the forelimb and injuries to the DDFT within the DFTS occur most frequently in the hindlimbs. (Injuries to the DDFT that are associated with navicular syndrome are covered in Chapter 2).
- Injuries involving the SDFT most commonly involve the branches of the SDFT located outside the DFTS, and typically occur in racehorses.

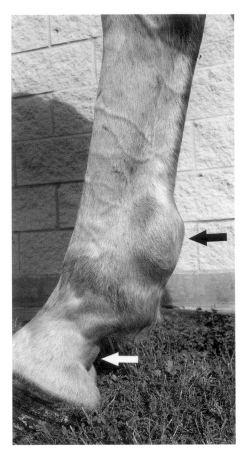

Figure 3.20 This horse was 4/5 lame in the left hindlimb and had severe effusion of the digital flexor tendon sheath and chronic DDFT injury. Arrows demonstrate the largest outpouchings of synovial effusion proximolateral and medial (black) and plantarodistal (white). Lesions of the DDFT within the tendon sheath appear to be more common in the hindlimbs than the forelimbs. Courtesy of Ashlee Watts.

- Injuries to the DDFT within the pastern are nearly always within the DFTS, often cause effusion of the sheath, and may contribute to chronic tenosynovitis of the DFTS (Figure 3.20).

Anatomy

- Both the SDFT and DDFT course along the palmar/plantar aspect of the pastern within the DFTS (Figure 2.1).

- The annular ligament of the fetlock binds the digital flexor tendons and their enclosing sheath in the sesamoid grove. Immediately distal to this, the DDFT perforates through a circular opening in the SDFT called the manica flexoria.
- The SDFT branches at the level of the MCP/MTP joint and the medial and lateral branches insert on the palmar/plantar eminences of P2 outside the DFTS (Figure 3.9).
- The DDFT descends between the two branches of the SDFT and the DFTS enfolds both tendons as far distally as the T-ligament (fibrous partition attaching to the palmar/plantar surface of P2).

Imaging

- Ultrasonography is usually the initial diagnostic method used to diagnose tendon injuries in the pastern even though it may provide false-negative results.
- MRI is thought to be superior to ultrasonography to characterize the location, type, and severity of damage to both the SDFT and DDFT within the pastern.
- When MRI is not available, a contrast tenogram may be useful to define marginal tears of the DDFT as well as tears of the manica flexoria with improved positive and negative predictive values over ultrasound.

Etiology

- Injuries to the SDFT in the forelimbs are usually associated with hyperextension of the MCP joint resulting in non-physiologic stretching and overload of the SDFT.
- Abnormal conformation such as a long pastern or an underrun heel may also predispose to injury of the SDFT branches.
- The cause of DDFT injuries within the DFTS is unknown but hyperextension of the MCP/MTP joint and overstretching of the tendon is also likely.
- Both SDFT and DDFT injuries in the pastern region are thought to occur more frequently as a result from a single traumatic event as

compared with flexor tendon injuries at the level of the MC/MT.

Clinical Signs
SDFT Branch Injuries

- Lameness usually occurs at the onset of injury with focal heat, swelling, and sensitivity noted on palpation. Careful palpation and comparison of the medial to lateral branches is important to detect differences in size, heat, and pain as these injuries can be easily missed.
- The medial SDFT branch appears to be more frequently injured than the lateral branch and avulsion fractures at the insertion of the SDFT branch occur infrequently.
- Some SDFT injuries and damage to the manica flexoria may occur within the DFTS and result in sheath effusion.

DDFT

- Deep digital flexor tendinitis occurs in a variety of sport horses and typically presents as an acute-onset, unilateral, moderate-to-severe forelimb or hindlimb lameness that is persistent.
- Heat, pain, and swelling of the DDFT itself are usually not palpable because the damage is often located within the DFTS.
- Distension of the DFTS often occurs in conjunction with the injury and many horses present with chronic tenosynovitis of the DFTS of undetermined cause (Figure 3.20).
- Lameness is often worse on a soft surface and generally improves with perineural anesthesia above the PSBs or with intrasynovial anesthesia of the DFTS.

Diagnosis

- Ultrasonography is currently the most commonly used method to diagnose branch lesions of the SDFT and abnormalities in the DDFT within the DFTS.
- A DDFT lesion may involve one or both lobes and is typically characterized by enlargement and alteration of the tendon with or without a hypoechoic region.

- False-negative ultrasound results for DDFT injuries are not uncommon because surface and longitudinal lesions are more common than core lesions and more difficult to visualize with ultrasound.
- MRI or contrast tenography is thought to provide more accurate information than ultrasonography in many cases (Figure 3.21).
- Tenoscopy of the DFTS is also a useful diagnostic tool to document lesions of both SDFT and DDFT that may not be visible with ultrasound (Figure 3.21).

Treatment

- Branch lesions of the SDFT are usually treated with a controlled rehabilitation program similar to any SDFT injury; 6–12 months is typically needed.
- If the SDFT lesion is within the DFTS or if DFTS effusion is present, tenoscopy is often helpful to further diagnose the specific problem and to debride the damaged tendon.
- Lesions of the DDFT at the level of the pastern are often within the DFTS and

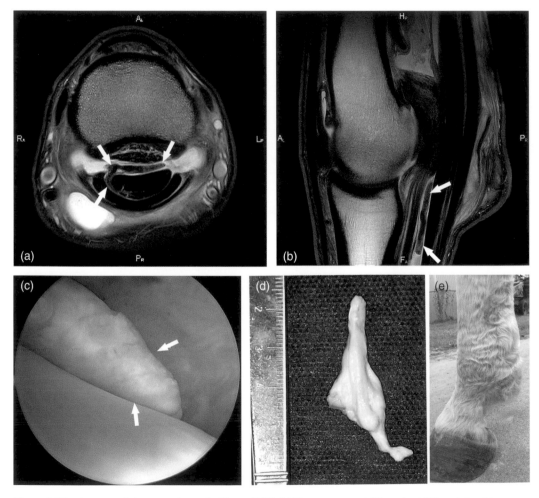

Figure 3.21 Images of the same horse in **Figure 3.20.** (a) Transverse and (b) sagittal PD-weighted images of the extruded fibers from the plantar margin of the DDFT wrapping around the dorsal edge of the DDFT (white arrows) in the proximal pastern. (c) The chronic DDFT extruded fibers at (c) tenoscopy after (d) tenoscopic removal. The plantar annular ligament was also transected. (e) Photograph of the limb eight months later with marked improvement of DFTS effusion and minimal lameness. The DDFT injury was not recognized as a surface split with extruded fibers by ultrasound. Courtesy of Ashlee Watts.

tenoscopy is often beneficial because these lesions are often difficult to diagnose and treat.

- Additional treatment options include medication of the DFTS and intralesional injection of biologics directly into the damaged tendon.

Prognosis

- Soft tissue injures of the SDFT and DDFT in the pastern region can be difficult to diagnose and tend to have a worse prognosis than similar injuries in the MC/MT.
- Injuries to the SDFT and DDFT in the pastern region are prone to recurrence.
- Horses with SDFT branch injuries are thought to have a poorer prognosis to return to racing than horses with SDFT injuries in the metacarpal region, with more frequent recurrence.
- Only 40% of horses with surface lesions of the DDFT within the DFTS returned to previous level of performance following tenoscopic debridement.
- In horses with chronic DFTS tenosynovitis, 68% of treated horses were sound and 54% returned to their preoperative level of performance in one clinical study.

Fetlock

Osteochondral (Chip) Fractures of Proximal P1

Overview

- Dorsal and palmar/plantar chip fractures of P1 are relatively common in racehorses.
- Most fractures of this type involve the dorsal eminences just medial or lateral to midline. The left forelimb and medial aspect of the joint are affected more often.
- Fractures of the lateral or medial palmar/plantar eminences occur less frequently than dorsal fractures and may be traumatic or developmental in origin.

Anatomy

- The distal cannon bone, proximal extremity of P1, the two PSBs, and the fibrocartilaginous metacarpointersesamoidean ligament form the fetlock joint (Figure 2.1).
- The articular surface of MC/MTIII is divided by a sagittal ridge, and this surface fits into an accommodating depression formed by P1, the sesamoid bones, and the metacarpointersesamoidean ligament.
- The CLs of the fetlock joint extend distad from the eminence and depression on each side of the MC/MTIII and attach to P1 and the abaxial surface of the sesamoid bone.
- The fetlock is a high motion joint and accounts for the majority of flexion that occurs within the distal limb.
- Non-physiologic hyperextension of the fetlock joint is prevented by the suspensory apparatus of the fetlock (interosseus muscle, intersesamoidean ligament, and DSLs), the digital flexor tendons, and the CLs of the joint.

Imaging

- Radiography is the imaging modality of choice to document osteochondral fragmentation within the fetlock. A minimum of four views (five views including the flexed lateral) should be obtained.
- Ultrasonography also may be used to diagnose chip fractures of the dorsal aspect of P1 and concurrent proliferative synovitis of the fetlock synovial pad if present.

Etiology

- Excessive concussion and overextension of the joint are thought to contribute to dorsal fractures.
- Overextension compresses the dorsal aspect of P1 against the MCIII/MTIII and the medial aspect of proximal P1 is more prominent and extends slightly more proximal than its lateral counterpart.

- Limb fatigue may contribute to fetlock over-extension as is often noted at the end of races when the back of the fetlock nearly contacts the ground.
- Overextension of the fetlock may also contribute to avulsion fractures of the palmar/plantar aspect of P1, but this is debatable since these fractures may be traumatic or development in origin.

Clinical Signs

- Effusion of the fetlock joint is commonly palpable, and heat may be detected in acute injuries.
- Lameness can be variable but usually increases after exercise, and a workout or a race may cause the horse to be markedly lame.
- Passive flexion of the affected fetlock often elicits pain and a fetlock flexion test usually exacerbates the lameness.
- With chronicity, there may be fibrous enlargement of the dorsal aspect of the fetlock joint.

- Intrasynovial anesthesia is the most specific method to document that the fetlock is the cause of the lameness.

Diagnosis

- A definitive diagnosis is usually made with radiography. Oblique radiographs should be taken to determine whether the chip is on the medial or lateral side of the midline (Figure 3.22).
- For palmar/plantar fragments, oblique radiographs raised ~20° from horizontal can be helpful in limiting the superimposition of the sesamoids on proximal P1 (Figure 3.23).
- Radiography of the contralateral fetlock is recommended because many of these fractures can be bilateral despite lack of clinical signs.

Treatment

- Arthroscopic removal of chip fractures is usually the treatment of choice for both dorsal and palmar/plantar fragments.

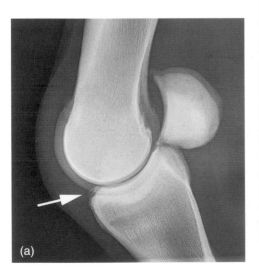
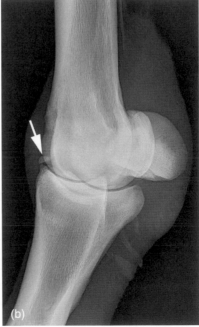

Figure 3.22 (a) Flexed lateral radiograph of the fetlock demonstrating a small fragment off the dorsoproximal aspect of P1 (arrow). (b) DLPMO radiograph of a horse with a rounded fragment off of the dorsomedial aspect of proximal P1 (arrow). Courtesy of Matt Brokken.

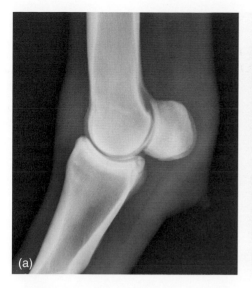 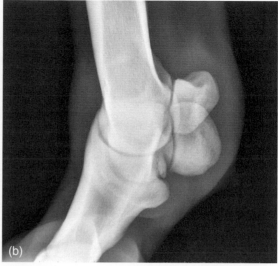

Figure 3.23 Lateral (a) and oblique (b) radiographs demonstrating a typical palmar/plantar osteochondral fragment of the first phalanx.

- Lesions commonly seen in association with P1 chip fracture include proliferative synovitis of the dorsal metacarpal synovial pad and cartilage erosion of the MCIII condyle.
- The benefit of removing palmar/plantar fragments to improve performance has been questioned based on a study that indicated there was no difference in racing speed, career earnings, or lifetime starts between Standardbred racehorses with the fracture and those without.

Prognosis

- The prognosis is usually good to excellent (approximately 70–80%) but it is somewhat dependent on the size and number of chip fractures, their duration, whether or not corticosteroids have been injected, amount of concomitant articular cartilage damage, and degree of OA.
- Factors that lower the prognosis include extreme large size of the fragment, chronicity, and the presence of articular cartilage damage.
- Racehorses that develop dorsal P1 fractures have reduced lifetime earnings compared with racehorses that do not develop these fractures.

Fractures of the Proximal Sesamoid Bones

Overview

- Fractures of the PSBs are common injuries in racing Thoroughbreds, Standardbreds, and Quarter horses.
- Types of sesamoid fractures include apical, abaxial (articular and nonarticular), mid-body, basilar (articular and nonarticular), sagittal, and comminuted.
- The forelimbs are most frequently affected in the Thoroughbred (right forelimb) and Quarter horse, whereas the hindlimbs are more frequently affected in the Standardbred (left hindlimb).
- Apical fractures are by far the most common and are usually articular and involve less than one-third of the bone (Figure 3.24).
- Basilar and abaxial fractures are uncommon and can be articular or nonarticular (Figure 3.25).
- Midbody transverse sesamoid fractures are seen most frequently in Thoroughbreds, older Standardbreds (mean age 6.5 years), and young foals under two months of age.

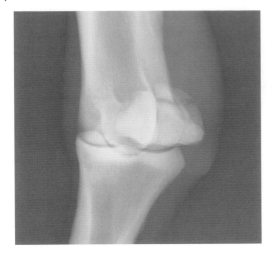

Figure 3.24 Oblique radiograph of a Quarter horse mare with a large apical sesamoid fracture.

- The midbody transverse fracture divides the bone into equal portions and biaxial mid-body fractures cause loss of the suspensory support apparatus.

Anatomy

- The paired PSBs are an integral part of two synovial structures within the fetlock region – fetlock joint and the DFTS (Figure 2.1).
- The dorsal surfaces of the bones together with the intersesamoidean ligament form the palmar/plantar aspect of the fetlock joint.
- Palmarly/plantarly the annular ligament spans the PSBs forming the fetlock canal in which the SDFT and DDFT pass through within the DFTS (Figure 3.9).
- The PSBs are part of the suspensory apparatus of the distal limb that prevents hyperextension of the joint during exercise. The branches of the SL attach to the proximal surfaces of the bones and the DSLs attach distally.

Imaging

- Routine radiography of the fetlock usually confirms the presence of a sesamoid fracture. The flexed LM projection may be helpful in some cases.

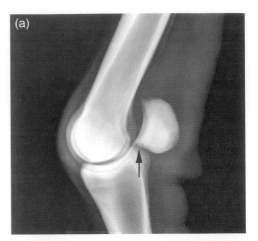

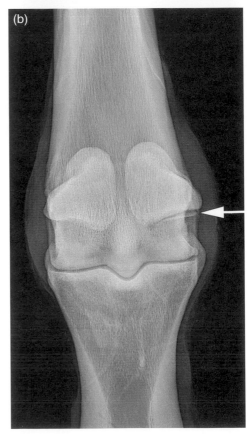

Figure 3.25 Flexed lateral (a) and DP (b) radiographs demonstrating a small articular basilar fracture (arrows) in two different Thoroughbred racehorses. The fracture in (a) extended across the entire base of the medial sesamoid bone. Also note the other degenerative changes present in the fetlock (marked sclerosis of the palmar condyles of the distal third metacarpal bone, remodeling of the fetlock joint space; primarily on the side of the base sesamoid fragment) in (b). Image (b) courtesy of Matt Brokken.

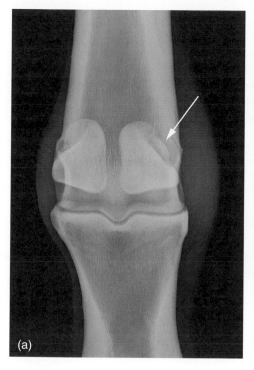
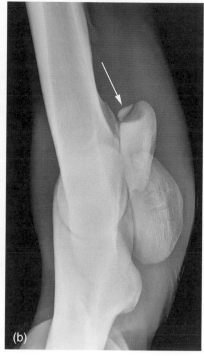

Figure 3.26 (a) DP radiograph of a horse with an abaxial sesamoid fracture (arrow). (b) Skyline projection to highlight the abaxial fragment of the sesamoid (arrow). Courtesy of Matt Brokken.

- The addition of the skyline projection of the abaxial surface of the sesamoid bone is helpful to identify the exact location of fractures on the abaxial surface (Figure 3.26).
- Ultrasonography should be performed on all apical and abaxial fractures to identify the degree of concurrent injury to the SL.

Etiology

- The cause of most PSB fractures is excessive tensile forces related to fetlock hyperextension that maximally loads the sesamoid bones. The bone fails when the sesamoid bone can no longer withstand the distraction forces applied to it by the SL and DSLs.
- Fatigue of the digital flexor muscles that support the fetlock is a critical factor as most fractures occur at the end of races.
- Other factors include poor conditioning, improper trimming and shoeing, training and racing schedules, and poor conformation.

- Foals that have been confined to a box stall for several days and then turned out for free exercise with the dam appear to be at risk for sesamoid fractures.
- Direct trauma to the sesamoid bone such as with interference may also occur and fetlock immobilization for extended periods may result in a pathologic fracture after cast removal.

Clinical Signs

- Horses with different types of sesamoid fractures may have similar clinical signs.
- Lameness is usually very pronounced in acute stages and horses will usually resist the fetlock descending to a normal weight-bearing position.
- Palpable fetlock effusion and heat, pain on direct palpation of the sesamoid bone, and pain with passive flexion of the fetlock are typical findings.
- Horses with chronic fractures will have less severe clinical signs but usually remain lame at a trot and have persistent fetlock effusion.

- Desmitis of the SL and DSLs may occur concurrently with fractured sesamoids.

Diagnosis

- Diagnosis is based on the physical examination findings and confirmed with radiologic examination of the affected fetlock.
- The radiographs should be closely examined for any signs of OA associated with the fetlock and incomplete fractures that may be confused with enlarged vascular channels.
- If an incomplete sesamoid bone fracture is suspected, repeat radiographs should be taken after a period of two to four weeks of stall rest, or nuclear scintigraphy can be performed.

Treatment

- The treatment of PSB fractures is based on the location of the fracture and the intended use of the animal. Treatment options include stall rest, cast application, surgical excision, lag screw fixation, and circumferential wiring and bone grafting.
- Generally, the conservative approach should be used in horses that will not be used for performance and in the majority of foals regardless of the fracture type.
- Stall rest (with or without external coaptation) for three to four months has been successful to obtain fibrous or partial bony union that is relatively weak.
- Surgical removal or repair when possible is the treatment of choice for fractures in horses intended for performance.
- Apical, articular abaxial, and basilar fractures involving less than one-third of the sesamoid bone are best treated by arthroscopic removal of the fragment (Figures 3.24–3.26).
- Midbody transverse fractures and large basilar transverse fractures of the PSBs are best treated with lag screw fixation.
- Biaxial midbody or comminuted sesamoid bones (breakdown injuries) are usually treated by humane euthanasia or arthrodesis of the fetlock.

- Immediate casting or splinting is recommended for midbody and comminuted fractures, or in any fracture if clinical evidence of suspensory disruption is suspected.

Prognosis

- The reported prognosis for apical sesamoid fractures is good to excellent (88% of Standardbreds and 77% of Thoroughbreds return to racing).
- The prognosis for abaxial fractures is good (71% of Thoroughbreds or Quarter horses returned to racing).
- The prognosis for basilar fractures is fair (50–60% of Thoroughbreds return to racing).
- The prognosis for midbody fractures repaired by either lag screw fixation or circumferential wiring is also fair (44–60% return to performance).
- It is presumed that the prognosis is guarded to poor for basilar or midbody fractures that are not treated surgically although comparison reports are not available.
- The prognosis for fractures of the sesamoid bones that result in loss of the suspensory apparatus is poor.
- The prognosis for foals with sesamoid fractures is usually very good unless there is extensive remodeling and distortion of the bone.

Sesamoiditis

Overview

- Sesamoiditis is observed frequently in racing horses and hunters and jumpers between 2 and 5 years of age but can occur in any type of horse.
- Sesamoiditis is characterized by pain associated with the PSBs and insertions of the SL that result in lameness. The pain is thought to result from inflammation at the interface of the SL with the PSBs.
- Concurrent SL branch disease should be suspected in these horses as there is a significant

relationship between the presence of sesamoiditis and the subsequent development of SL injuries.

- Pain, heat, and inflammation can be detected at the insertion of the SL during the active stages of the disease process but marked lameness and limitations on performance can also occur with few detectable signs.
- Radiographs can reveal a range of changes from accelerated early remodeling response in the bones (increased size and number of vascular canals) to marked proliferation of bone along the abaxial margin of the sesamoid and increased bone density of the sesamoid.

Anatomy (Please refer to previous section on "PSB Fractures")

Imaging

- Radiography is usually the cornerstone to diagnose sesamoiditis in horses.
- Ultrasonography should also performed to detect secondary damage to the branches of the SL attaching to the PSBs.
- More advanced imaging techniques such as scintigraphy or MRI can be used in horses suspicious of sesamoiditis with minimal to no radiographic abnormalities.

Etiology

- Any unusual strain to the fetlock region may produce sesamoiditis by increasing stress to the attachment of the SL to the sesamoid bones. Repetitive overextension of the fetlock is thought to damage the interface between the branches of the SL and the DSLs with the PSBs.
- The sesamoid bones undergo intense remodeling in response to training and the progression of radiographic changes correlates to bone response to remodeling and injury.
- Microfracture and bone damage of the PSBs only occurs if the stresses exceed the bones' capability to strengthen.
- The pain is thought to be due to the initiation of the remodeling response to bone stress

and/or may reflect an inflammatory response from tearing of the attachment of the SL.

Clinical Signs

- In the early stage, minimal swelling will be observed, but increased heat may be palpable over the abaxial surface of the sesamoid bones.
- As the disease progresses, a visible enlargement of the soft tissues overlying the palmar surface of the fetlock may be seen due to fibrosis of the SL.
- Firm palpation of the sesamoid bones and flexion of the fetlock usually cause painful responses. Pain may also be elicited by palpation of the branches of the SL.
- The lameness can be variable in severity but is usually most evident during the first part of exercise and when exercised on hard surfaces.
- Perineural and/or intrasynovial anesthesia is usually not necessary to diagnose the condition – horses respond to a low four-point block, but not to an IA fetlock block.

Diagnosis

- The diagnosis is usually confirmed with routine radiography of the fetlock.
- The radiologic changes of true sesamoiditis have been described as bony changes on the abaxial surface or basilar region, increased number and irregularity of the vascular channels, and increased coarseness and mottling of the bone trabeculation (Figure 3.27).
- Careful radiographic interpretations of the mottled trabecular pattern are necessary to differentiate from a fracture; a fracture usually extends to the abaxial surface and the vascular channels do not.
- Nuclear scintigraphy typically indicates increased radiopharmaceutical uptake (IRU) in the region of the sesamoid bones, but the uptake is usually less than what would occur with a fracture.
- Subclinical SL branch change has been reported in Thoroughbred yearlings with

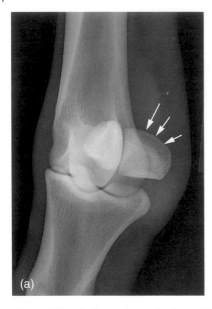 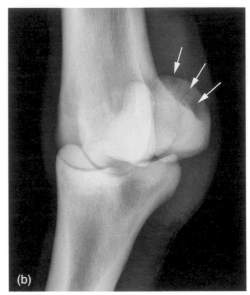

Figure 3.27 Radiographs of the fetlock in two different horses demonstrating mild sesamoiditis (a) and moderate sesamoiditis (b) with increased number of the vascular channels in the lateral proximal sesamoid bone (arrows). Courtesy of Matt Brokken.

evidence of sesamoiditis suggesting that ultrasound examination should be performed in all affected horses.

Treatment

- The initial treatment in acute cases is focused on reducing the inflammation. Both topical and systemic anti-inflammatory medications may be used.
- Rest from performance until soundness at the trot is achieved followed by slow increasing duration and intensity of exercise allows the bone to continue to remodel and strengthen. Exercise must be kept below the level that would reinjure the bones.
- Similar to other SL injuries, convalescence is long (six to eight months) and injury often recurs when horses return to full work.
- In chronic stages, blistering and ESWT have been used but with equivocal success.
- Biologics such as PRP may be injected into the junction between the bone and the SL to reduce inflammation as well as to promote healing.

Prognosis

- The prognosis for return to full athletic performance is usually guarded to unfavorable.
- The prognosis often depends on the amount of periosteal reaction and new bone growth that occurs on the PSBs and the extent of the injury to the SL and the DSLs.
- In yearling racehorses, enlarged vascular canals identified on radiographs have been associated with fewer race starts and reduced earnings compared with horses with normal vascular canals.

Axial Osteitis/Osteomyelitis of the PSBs

Overview

- Osteitis/osteomyelitis of the axial border of the PSBs is specifically associated with the intersesamoidean ligament within the apical to midbody axial margins of the sesamoid.
- The condition has occurred in horses with septic tenosynovitis of the digital sheath, septic

bacterial arthritis of the fetlock, and secondary to an *Aspergillus* fungal fetlock infection.

Anatomy (Please refer to the section on "PSB Fractures")

Imaging

- Routine radiography of the fetlock may be sufficient to make the diagnosis in more advanced cases.
- Ultrasonography along with advanced imaging (CT and/or MRI) of the fetlock is often necessary to determine the surface location of the lytic areas and to assist with the decision for surgery (Figure 3.28).

Etiology

- The cause remains unknown and speculative with vascular, infectious, and traumatic etiologies implicated.
- Clinical signs and radiographic lesions are suggestive of sepsis, although histology revealed infarction and necrosis as well as osteoporosis and chronic inflammation of the intersesamoidean ligament in one study.

Clinical Signs and Diagnosis

- Horses typically present with a consistent lameness that may be severe (often lame at the walk).
- Effusion within the fetlock, DFTS, or both may be present along with diffuse enlargement of the fetlock region. Most horses are painful to distal limb flexion.
- In one report of 12 Friesian horses, all lesions were in the hindlimb, and lameness was acute and severe.
- Radiographs usually reveal bone lysis at the attachment of the intersesamoidean ligament primarily at the midbody and apical regions with varying degrees of joint effusion (Figure 3.28a).
- A single or both sesamoids may be affected, and some lesions appear cystic whereas others appear to erode the axial border more diffusely.

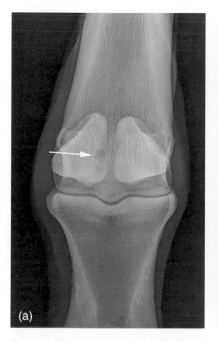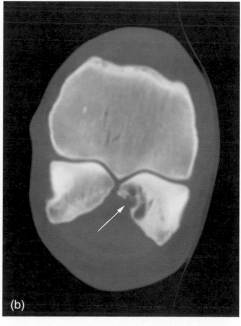

Figure 3.28 DP radiograph (a) and transverse CT image (b) of two different horses demonstrating focal lysis in the axial aspect of the lateral proximal sesamoid (arrows). Courtesy of Matt Brokken.

Treatment and Prognosis

- Small lesions that are internal or only open toward the intersesamoidean ligament may be best treated conservatively without surgery.
- Most lytic lesions have surgical access to the area from the palmar/plantar fetlock joint and/or digital sheath using arthroscopy. Abnormal bone and ligament should be debrided if present, and samples submitted for culture and sensitivity.
- Regional limb perfusion offers the advantage of perfusion of multiple affected sites including the fetlock joint, tendon sheath, and sesamoid bones.
- The prognosis for return to performance is considered guarded to poor, although horses may become pasture sound or return to less strenuous activities.

Traumatic OA of the MCP/MTP Joint

Overview

- Traumatic OA of the fetlock includes a diverse collection of pathologic and clinical states that develop after single or repetitive episodes of trauma to a joint.
- Predisposing conditions may include synovitis, capsulitis, ligamentous sprain/strains, IA fractures, cartilage injury/damage, and subchondral bone injuries.

Anatomy (Please refer to the anatomy section under "Osteochondral Fractures of P1")

Imaging

- Radiography remains the initial imaging technique often used despite its limitations in evaluating articular cartilage damage and subchondral bone disease.
- Radiography can help diagnose an underlying cause in many cases, such as osteochondral fragments (either as part of OC or as an IA fracture), SCLs, subchondral bone erosion, osteophytosis, or joint space narrowing.
- Both CT and MRI are considered to be superior to digital radiography to detect subchondral bone pathology and cartilage disease in the fetlock joint.

Etiology

- Many types of acute or chronic (repetitive) traumatic joint injuries can progress to OA within the fetlock.
- Soft tissue injury to the joint commonly occurs in horses in full work and often represents overuse of the joint or a single event injury.
- Many types of bone and articular injuries may occur from overextension of the fetlock joint at speed and subchondral bone disease is known to occur in racing Thoroughbreds and predispose to OA.
- Abnormal limb conformation may also predispose horses to joint soreness and eventually OA of the fetlock.

Clinical Signs

- In mild cases, joint inflammation may occur without lameness and is noted as joint soreness on flexion and joint effusion in a young, recently worked or maximally performing horse.
- Cases that involve capsulitis of the fetlock, particularly the dorsal fetlock, often have palpable heat and a more severe response to fetlock flexion.
- In moderate cases, joint soreness and effusion persist and lameness often worsens with exercise.
- In severe cases of injury or advanced joint degeneration, lameness can be severe, and obvious joint enlargement and decreased range of motion can ensue.
- Subchondral bone damage and/or articular cartilage damage should be suspected in horses with signs of chronic synovitis with severe lameness.

- Digital nerve blocks do not block fetlock OA, but a low four-point block may improve the lameness. IA anesthesia of the fetlock is the preferred approach.

Diagnosis

- The history and clinical findings often provide a tentative diagnosis of a fetlock problem and routine radiography can often confirm the presence of OA as well as determine the underlying cause.
- Radiographic abnormalities can range from negative to obvious signs of OA which often include osteophytosis, joint space narrowing, and subchondral bone sclerosis and or lysis (Figure 3.29).
- Advanced imaging (CT or MRI) can usually provide a more accurate identification of the pathology and determination of whether a horse is a candidate for arthroscopic surgery or medical therapy (Figure 3.30).

Treatment

- Management of fetlock OA should address any primary problem and potentially include the following: rest, physical therapy, bandages, shoeing changes, and systemic and IA joint medications.
- Arthroscopic surgery is recommended in horses that have concurrent predisposing conditions such as OC or osteochondral damage/fragmentation.
- Performance horses that are lame from fetlock joint soreness should be rested until lameness resolves, frequently a minimum of 30 days. Return to work should be gradual and can be supplemented with systemic joint medications and shoeing alterations to promote break-over of the foot and an easy landing (rim pads, remove caulks and toe grabs, etc.).
- Many jumping horses and racehorses are treated with icing and wrapping of the fetlocks after workouts as a routine.

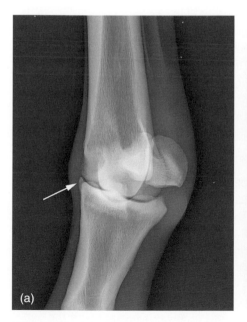
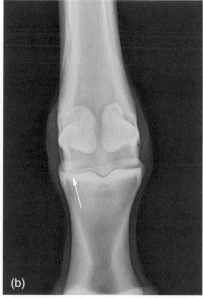

Figure 3.29 DLPMO radiograph of the fetlock (a) of a horse with a large periarticular osteophyte on the dorsomedial aspect of proximal P1 (arrow). DP (b) and oblique (c) radiograph of another horse with severe narrowing of the medial aspect of the fetlock joint (arrow) due to marked cartilage loss. Note that there are minimal other radiographic signs of OA in this horse other than subchondral bone sclerosis in proximal P1. Courtesy of Matt Brokken.

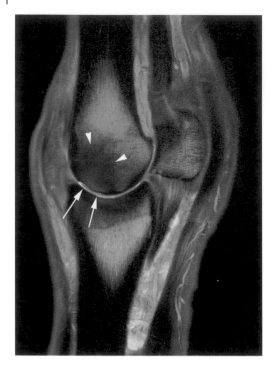

Figure 3.30 Sagittal proton density MR image depicting marked cartilage damage of the distal third metacarpal bone (arrows) along with marked sclerosis of the adjacent subchondral and medullary bone (arrowhead). Courtesy of Michael Schramme.

- Joint medications (IA and/or systemic) can be effective for horses with OA of the fetlock. Biologic therapies, such as autologous conditioned serum and stem cells, have also been promoted for IA treatment of OA.
- Horses that respond to an IA block but do not respond to treatment are often candidates for either further imaging (CT or MRI) an exploratory arthroscopy.
- Confining horses with chronic OA often worsens their stiffness and discomfort. Regular exercise and turn-out often provide the greatest longevity with this condition.

Prognosis
- Early recognition and management of traumatic arthritis of the fetlock are key to keeping the joint in good health and continuing training in racehorses.

- Once degenerative changes in the joint are visible on radiographs, the prognosis is still fair with management if the horse is sound enough to perform.
- Once horses are no longer sound with medical management, an extended period of rest may permit some horses to return to training, usually at a reduced expectation.
- Many top equine athletes can continue to perform at some level of activity with fetlock OA.

Palmar/Plantar Osteochondral Disease

Overview

- Palmar osteochondral disease (POD) is considered to be repetitive high-impact injury of the palmar metacarpus that nearly exclusively occurs in Thoroughbred racehorses.
- The subchondral bone damage of the condyle is thought to cause lameness and loss of training days.
- The pathology is reportedly worse in the medial condyle of the forelimbs and lateral condyle in the hindlimbs.
- Horses with POD often develop performance-limiting lameness but severe cases can result in career-ending lameness and significant OA.

Anatomy

- The MC/MTIII condyles together with the PSBs and P1 make up the fetlock joint.
- The somewhat cylindrical articular surface of the MC/MT condyles is divided by a sagittal ridge and this surface fits into an accommodating depression formed by P1 (Figure 3.31a).
- The palmar/plantar aspect of these condyles is thought to receive greater than twice the amount of stress compared with the dorsal surface of the bone at racing speeds.
- These excessive forces make this area vulnerable to bone necrosis and cartilage injuries (Figure 3.31b).

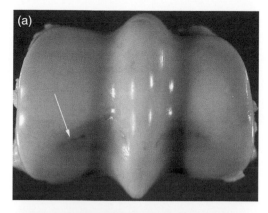

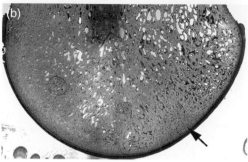

Figure 3.31 (a) The distal aspect of the third metacarpal condyles demonstrating subchondral bone bruising in this Thoroughbred racehorse (arrow). (b) A histologic section through the palmar metacarpal condyle in a racehorse demonstrating changes in the subchondral bone associated with exercise. Courtesy of Chris Kawcak.

Imaging

- Radiography may not reveal abnormalities except in the later stages of the disease.
- Scintigraphy often reveals increase uptake in the condyle but there has been no correlation with the degree of uptake and prognosis for return to racing.
- MRI is currently the imaging modality of choice to evaluate horse with POD.

Etiology

- Repetitive overloading to the palmar/plantar aspect of the MC/MTIII condyles at training and racing speeds contributes to focal areas of fatigue to the subchondral bone at the articulation of the condyles with the PSBs.

- With continued stress, microtrauma occurs due to the decreased compliance of the sclerotic bone, resulting in edema and hemorrhage in these regions usually accompanied with microfracture.
- Subchondral bone resorption and eventual collapse of the overlying articular surface adjacent to the subchondral bone lesions with eventual articular cartilage degeneration is often the end result.
- Postmortem lesions can range grossly from discoloration of the subchondral bone with minimal to no cartilage erosion to severe subchondral bone discoloration and associated cartilage damage (Figure 3.31).

Clinical Signs

- The primary clinical sign of POD is performance-limiting lameness localized to the fetlock region in racehorses.
- Joint effusion is an uncommon finding and only about 60% of horses will be positive to flexion of the fetlock joint.
- Perineural anesthesia (low 4-point block) is usually more useful than IA anesthesia due to the pathology originating within the subchondral bone.

Diagnosis

- Diagnosis of POD can be difficult with radiographs alone in the early stages of the disease. Common radiographic features of POD are focal radiopacities and/or radiolucencies in the palmar/plantar condyles along with flattening of the condyle and osteophytosis (Figure 3.32).
- Scintigraphy usually reveals abnormalities within the condyles and can help with locate the site of the lameness.
- MRI has improved the understanding of the relationship between pathology and prognosis in cases of POD and is the preferred imaging technique.
- The primary clinical sign of POD is performance-limiting lameness localized to the fetlock region in racehorses.

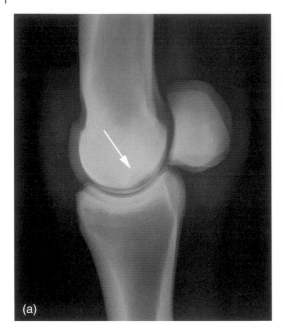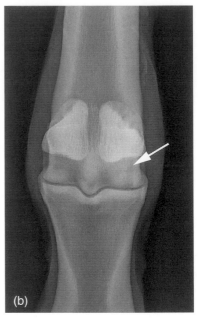

Figure 3.32 Flexed lateral (a) and dorsopalmar (b) radiographs of two different fetlock joints demonstrating radiolucent defects and severe sclerosis of the palmar condyles of the distal third metacarpal bone (arrows). Courtesy of Matt Brokken.

Treatment and Prognosis

- Treatment options are limited and range from rest, which allows for bone remodeling in the early stages of the POD, to systemic and IA anti-inflammatory therapies.
- A period of 60- to 120-day small paddock turn-out has been reported to permit 95% of horses diagnosed with POD to return to racing.
- With advanced disease, pain control is difficult and typically unrewarding in the majority of cases.
- The prognosis is usually good if POD is diagnosed and treated early but advanced disease will likely be career ending.

Fetlock Subchondral Cystic Lesions (SCLs)

Overview

- SCLs occur most commonly on the weight-bearing surface of the metacarpal condyle and less commonly on the weight-bearing surface of proximal P1.
- Cystic lesions of the distal metacarpus/tarsus that open into the fetlock joint can occur in young horses and are possibly considered part of the OC syndrome.

Anatomy (Please refer to section on "Osteochondral Fractures of P1")

Imaging (Please refer to section on "OA of Fetlock Joint")

Etiology

- MCIII SCLs that occur in younger horses are thought to be developmental in origin.
- Some SCLs are thought to be associated with subchondral bone trauma and are more common in adult horses but can occur at any age (Figure 3.33a).
- SCLs of proximal P1 are more often traumatically induced and can occur in horses of any age (Figure 3.33b).

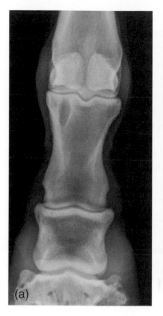
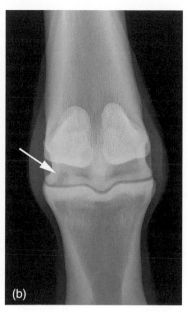

Figure 3.33 (a) DP radiograph of a horse with a subchondral cystic lesion in the medial aspect of the distal third metacarpal bone (arrow). (b) Dorsopalmar fetlock radiograph with a SCL of proximal P1. Image (a) Courtesy of Matt Brokken.

Clinical Signs

- Lameness is usually moderate with pain on fetlock flexion and fetlock effusion in approximately 50% of the cases.
- Some horses with P1 SCLs may present with an acute onset of lameness, joint heat and effusion, and severe pain to fetlock flexion.
- The degree of lameness can vary considerably depending on the location and age of the SCL.

Diagnosis

- Radiography usually confirms the diagnosis of an SCL. Some lesions may not be apparent early in the disease process, and follow-up radiographs should be considered.
- SCLs are characterized by defined lucent defects in MCIII or P1 and can be articular or nonarticular (Figure 3.33).
- Nuclear scintigraphy should be able to identify a focal area of increased uptake in the bone as the SCL is developing but may not be detectable with chronic lesions.
- Advanced imaging (CT or MRI) is often helpful to document the extent of the SCL

and any secondary articular pathology that may be present in horses with trauma-induced lesions.

Treatment

- Surgical debridement of MCIII SCLs by an arthroscopic approach is the preferable treatment if the diagnosis is made before significant signs of OA have developed.
- Medical therapy with IA PSGAGs or biologics, systemic joint medications, and periods of inactivity may be helpful depending on the location and characteristics of the SCLs.
- For SCLs that do not respond to conservative treatment or debridement or are not accessible with arthroscopy (nonarticular), osteostixis by an extra-articular approach can be performed. The SCL is decompressed and debrided using this approach.

Prognosis

- The prognosis for return to performance appears to be good for developmental lesions of MCIII (80% of horses treated surgically returned to their intended use in one report).

- The prognosis for SCLs of proximal P1 is less favorable than lesions of MCIII, particularly if they are traumatically induced.
- Horses with trauma-induced SCLs typically have a more guarded prognosis for performance than those with developmental lesions regardless of their location.

Traumatic Rupture of the Suspensory Apparatus

Overview

- Traumatic rupture of the suspensory apparatus with or without fractures of both PSBs is a common cause of acute breakdown in the racing Thoroughbreds.

- Proximal luxations of the sesamoid bone without fracture also can occur with traumatic rupture of the DSLs (Figure 3.34a).
- Transverse or comminuted fractures of both PSBs allow the apical portions to be drawn proximally by the pull of the SL while the basilar fragments remain attached to the DSLs (Figure 3.34b).
- Besides the severe trauma sustained by the supporting soft tissues and bone, the adjacent vasculature may be damaged sufficiently to result in ischemic necrosis of the hoof.

Anatomy

- The suspensory apparatus of the distal limb supports the fetlock during weight-bearing and prevents hyperextension of the joint during exercise.

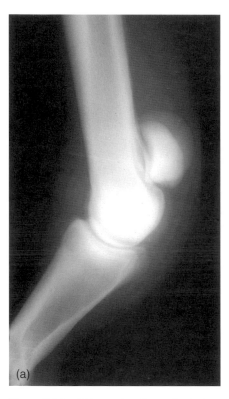
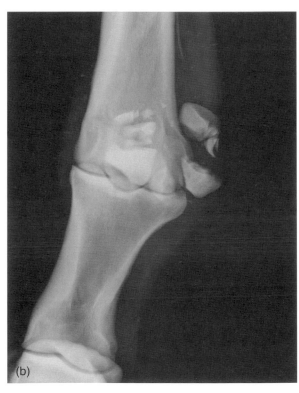

Figure 3.34 (a) Lateral radiograph of a horse with disruption of the distal suspensory apparatus that has permitted the sesamoid bones to luxate proximally, and (b) oblique radiograph of the MCP joint illustrating a suspensory ligament breakdown injury where comminuted fractures of both proximal sesamoid bones have occurred. Image (b) courtesy of Robert Hunt.

- The suspensory apparatus of the distal limb is composed primarily of the body and branches of the SL, the PSBs, and the DSLs. The branches of the SL attach to the proximal surfaces of the PSBs while the DSLs attached to the distal surfaces of the PSBs.
- The function of the suspensory apparatus of the distal limb can be lost by either complete tearing of the DSLs, biaxial fractures of the PSBs, or disruption of the SL in the MT/MT region.

Imaging

- Radiography can be used to document failure of the DSLs or biaxial PSB fractures.
- Ultrasound is used to document damage to the SL in the MC/MT region.

Etiology

- Extreme overextension of the fetlock is the likely cause for disruption of the suspensory apparatus.
- Pre-existing pathology of the PSBs or SL may contribute to the breakdown – lesions identified in the SL branches or DSLs were more likely to occur in horses that died from suspensory apparatus failure or metacarpal condylar fractures than in horses that died from nonmusculoskeletal causes.
- Factors that increase the strain on the flexor surface of the limb, such as toe grabs, are thought to increase the risk of suspensory apparatus failure.
- Injuries to the suspensory apparatus may be more likely to occur in males, older horses, and horses in training without any starts.

Clinical Signs

- The horse is usually completely non-weight-bearing, and the fetlock will usually sink to the ground when the limb is weighted.
- The fetlock region is usually very swollen, and palpation may reveal the proximal displacement of either the intact sesamoid bone or the apical fractured fragment.

- Immediate stabilization of the limb is critical to prevent rupture of the neurovascular bundles. The vascular supply is best evaluated after the horse has been treated for shock and the limb stabilized.

Diagnosis

- Radiographic examination usually reveals either the proximal displacement of the intact sesamoid bone or proximal displacement of the apical portions of the fractured sesamoid bones (Figure 3.34).
- Associated swelling of the soft tissues is usually quite evident, and pre-existing degenerative lesions within the sesamoid bones and fetlock joint also may be present.

Treatment

- Treatment options include humane euthanasia, casting and splinting, or surgical arthrodesis of the fetlock.
- Management of the horse on the racetrack is critical for success in treatment. Immediate immobilization of the affected limb is required to decrease the chances of further injury to the soft tissue and vascular supply.
- Casting and splinting to promote fetlock ankylosis is not currently recommended because it is problematic and rarely successful.
- Arthrodesis should be considered for horses that are intended for breeding or when there is sentimental value, because a normal gait will not be achieved.
- Arthrodesis with implants can achieve a pain-free stable fusion of the fetlock joint if the soft tissues are intact and risk of infection is minimal.

Prognosis

- The prognosis appears to be good for pasture and breeding soundness with preselection of cases. In one study, 32 of 54 horses with arthrodesis of the fetlock survived and were eventually allowed unrestricted activity.
- The prognosis is better for horses in which fetlock arthrodesis was elected as the primary treatment rather than as a last resort.

- The prognosis is also better for horses in which fetlock fusion was elected for OA rather than rupture of the suspensory apparatus.
- Contralateral limb laminitis is one of the major complications of surgical arthrodesis of the fetlock.

Palmar/Plantar Annular Ligament (PAL) Constriction and DFTS Tenosynovitis

Overview

- DFTS tenosynovitis is often characterized by effusion within the sheath, with or without clinical signs of lameness.
- DFTS effusion associated with lameness can be due to several disease conditions of the SDFT, DDFT, PAL, and the sheath itself, such as previous infection.
- Primary or secondary desmitis of the PAL often accompanies DFTS tenosynovitis and PAL constriction can be a cause of lameness in all breeds and uses of horses.
- Both PAL constriction and DFTS tenosynovitis appear to be more common in the hindlimb than the forelimb.

Anatomy

- The DFTS is located on the palmar/plantar aspect of the fetlock and pastern and extends from just proximal to the fetlock joint distally to the T-ligament on the palmar/plantar aspect of P2 (Figure 2.1).
- The PAL spans the palmar/plantar aspects of PSBs forming the fetlock canal in which the SDFT and DDFT pass through within the DFTS (Figure 3.9).
- The PAL is a tough, fibrous, thickened, relatively inelastic part of the DFTS strategically located to support the tendons as they course around the palmar/plantar aspect of the fetlock joint.
- Narrowing of the fetlock canal within the DFTS can occur from either desmitis and

thickening of the PAL, tendinitis and enlargement of the SDFT, DDFT, or manica flexoria, or thickening of the DFTS itself.

Imaging

- Ultrasonography can usually document most abnormalities within the PAL, SDFT, DDFT, and DFTS.
- More subtle lesions involving the DDFT, SDFT and manica flexoria are often best document with MRI or contrast tenography.

Etiology

- DFTS tenosynovitis associated with lameness or marked swelling of the sheath is usually secondary to trauma to the flexor tendons, PSBs, intersesamoidean ligament, PAL, or the DFTS itself.
- Constriction of the fetlock PAL usually occurs as a result of trauma and/or infection and can be primary (desmitis and thickening) or secondary (from damage to the flexor tendons within the DFTS).
- Tendinous defects within the sheath can involve the DDFT (longitudinal tears), the SDFT, and the manica flexoria of the SDFT.
- Wounds such as wire cuts or nail punctures may cause generalized thickening in the region contributing to tenosynovitis and constriction of the PAL.
- Synovial masses within the DFTS may also produce a constriction of the PAL and signs of tenosynovitis.
- With chronic tenosynovitis, permanent swelling and fibrosis of the tendons, the annular ligament, and the lining of the sheath can lead to stenosis of the fetlock canal.

Clinical Signs

- Effusion of the DFTS is usually visible and palpable palmar/plantar to the SL and proximal or distal to the PSBs (Figures 3.20 and 3.35).
- The most notable feature of PAL constriction is swelling of the palmar/plantar soft tissues around the fetlock together with a

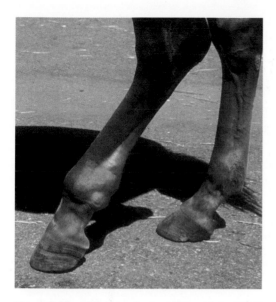

Figure 3.35 This horse had swelling of the DFTS and evidence of constriction of the fetlock annular ligament of the left hindlimb and was lame at the walk.

visible proximal border of the annular ligament ("notching"; Figure 3.20).

- Lameness is usually persistent, worsens with exercise, and is characterized by a decreased extension (dorsiflexion) of the fetlock during weight-bearing.
- Pain can often be elicited with deep palpation of tendons within the DFTS and with fetlock flexion.
- Intrasynovial anesthesia of the DFTS is usually the most reliable method to document painful conditions within the sheath.

Diagnosis
- Ultrasonography is usually the most important diagnostic tool to identify abnormalities within the DFTS. Lesions identified at ultrasound vary and can include core tendon lesions or longitudinal tearing of the DDFT and SDFT, fibrosis and thickening of the tendons, synovial proliferation, adhesions or masses, and thickening of the PAL.
- Radiographs of the fetlock region should always be performed to evaluate possible osseous involvement, particularly of the

sesamoids that may be contributing to PAL desmitis or tenosynovitis. This is especially true in horses with a history of wounds.
- MRI or contrast tenography should be considered in cases where ultrasound findings are equivocal since many lesions can be missed with ultrasound.

Treatment
- Medical management of DFTS tenosynovitis and PAL constriction may include controlled exercise, cold hydrotherapy, bandaging, NSAIDs, and intrasynovial medication of the sheath.
- Tenoscopy of the DFTS is currently the preferred treatment method to address synovial masses and tendon lesions, and to perform PAL transection if indicated (Figure 3.36).
- If tenoscopy is not an option and PAL constriction is present, the PAL can be transected percutaneously either above or in the middle of the PAL over the abaxial surface of the PSB.

Prognosis
- The prognosis for soundness in horses with DFTS tenosynovitis is considered to be good, with 68% returning to soundness and 54% returning to levels of previous work.
- Horses with PAL desmopathy alone that was not accompanied by abnormalities in the

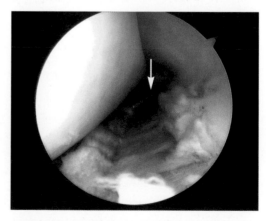

Figure 3.36 Tenoscopic view within the DFTS following transection of the annular ligament with a curved radiofrequency probe (arrow).

tendons usually have a good prognosis following surgical transection.

- Horses with concurrent SDFT or DDFT lesions with or without PAL constriction usually have a reduced prognosis.

Metacarpus/Metatarsus

Bucked Shin Complex and Stress Fractures of Dorsal MCIII

Overview

- Periostitis and stress fracture of the dorsal surface of MCIII constitute a spectrum of diseases that are commonly observed in young (two to three years of age) fast gaited horses.
- It is most common in young racing Thoroughbreds but can also occur in young Quarter horses and racing Standardbreds.
- Dorsal metacarpal bone failure or stress fractures occur on the dorsolateral cortex of MCIII in older horses (three to five years of age) that have had a history of bucked shins.

Anatomy

- MCIII is a long cylindrical-shaped bone located between the fetlock and carpal joints that undergoes constant remodeling and modeling during exercise (Figure 3.37).
- The cortex under the rounded dorsal surfaces of MCIII is thicker than the cortex under the concave palmar surface and nearly devoid of soft tissue coverage.
- Under stress such as occurs with training and racing, MCIII changes shape by adding periosteal new bone formation to the dorsal cortex. The thickening of the dorsal cortex is likely a natural response to the demands on the bone to withstand stress without developing microfractures or dorsal cortical fractures.

Imaging

- Radiography can assist with the diagnosis of dorsal cortical stress fractures is less helpful in horses with acute dorsal metacarpal disease and bucked shins.
- Scintigraphy can be beneficial in horses without radiographic abnormalities and racehorses may have scintigrams performed to determine whether training should continue or to identify focal uptake indicative of impending fracture.
- Standing robotic cone-beam computed tomography (CT) or other types of standing CT might be useful in defining difficult-to-see fractures.

Etiology

- The MCIII in young horses (two-year-olds) is less stiff, and therefore greater strains (bone movement) are measured on the dorsal cortex during high-speed exercise as compared with older horses. This high-strain environment may lead to cyclic fatigue of the bone, microdamage, and subsequent bone pain (bucked shins, sore shins).
- The majority (more than 80%) of two-year-old racing Thoroughbreds and many racing Quarter horses demonstrate dorsal cortical pain.
- It is estimated that approximately 12% develop acute failure or dorsal cortical fracture, usually within six months to one year of showing dorsal cortical pain.
- Training horses at longer distances at slower speeds is thought to predispose to bucked shins and the incidence of bucked shins has decreased now that Thoroughbred horses are trained at shorter distances at higher speeds.
- The incidence of fatigue failure of MCIII is greater in Thoroughbreds than Standardbreds, presumably due to different stresses on the bone during training and racing.

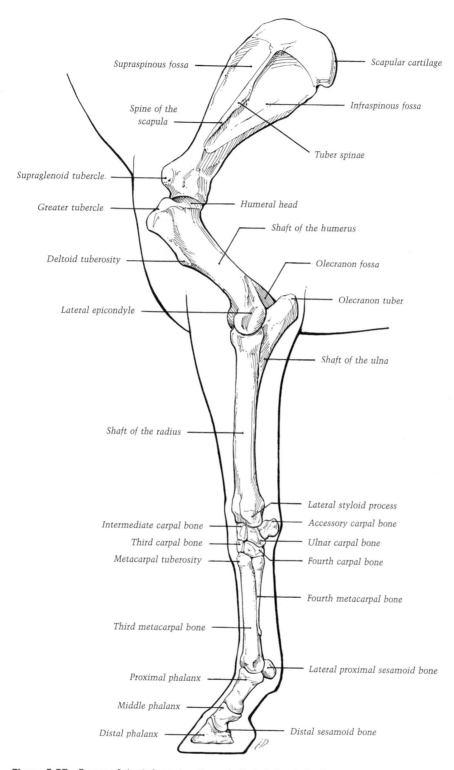

Figure 3.37 Bones of the left equine thoracic limb (lateral view).

Clinical Signs

- Early dorsal metacarpal disease (two to three-year-olds) usually has an acute onset and is most obvious after intense exercise. Horses often have a short, choppy gait without overt lameness.
- A visible convex swelling overlying the surface of the affected portion of the cannon bone is common.
- The dorsal cortex of MCIII is usually painful to pressure or concussion.
- With subacute or chronic dorsal metacarpal disease (two to four-year-olds), lameness may be mild, but a painful enlargement on the dorsomedial cortex of MCIII is usually present. The pain response is typically more profound after strenuous exercise, and the left limb is usually more severely affected.
- In horses with dorsal cortical fractures (three to five-year-olds), the lameness becomes prominent after strenuous exercise, and a discrete painful area can be palpated on the dorsolateral surface of the left MCIII at the junction of the middle and distal third (Figure 3.38).

Diagnosis

- A tentative diagnosis of bucked shins or dorsal cortical stress fracture can be made from the clinical findings and the age relationship.
- Little information is derived from local direct infiltration anesthesia of the painful area because it provides only partial relief in the lameness.
- Radiographs (four standard views) can usually confirm the diagnosis in cases of chronic bucked shins and dorsal cortical stress fractures.
- The DPLMO and the LM will best identify the dorsal medial bone proliferation and the DPMLO and LM will best identify the dorsal lateral cortical fractures.
- Cortical fractures usually enter the cortex distally and progress proximad at a 35–45° angle. They usually appear as a straight or slightly concave fracture line (tongue frac-

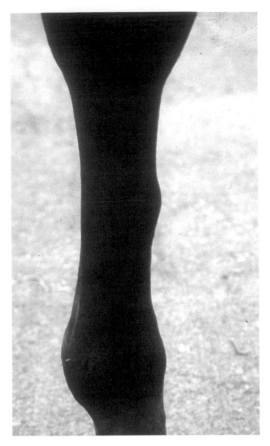

Figure 3.38 A racing Quarter horse with the classical metacarpal profile of a dorsal cortical stress fracture. Courtesy of Kyla Ortved.

ture [Figure 3.39]) but occasionally exit through the dorsal cortex (saucer fracture).
- Repeated radiographs at 7- to 10-day intervals may be necessary to identify a fracture that is suspected but not observed on initial radiographic examination.
- Nuclear scintigraphy can provide information about the stage of disease in horses showing dorsal cortical pain without radiographic abnormalities or in those with undiagnosed forelimb pain.

Treatment

- The goal of treatment with acute disease is to gradually increase the stress to the dorsal surface of MCIII at such a rate that this surface can model (form new bone) according

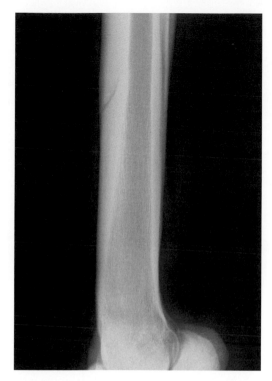

Figure 3.39 Lateromedial radiograph showing a dorsal cortical fracture of MCIII. Courtesy of Robert Hunt.

to compressive demands without producing structural damage.

- Most horses with dorsal metacarpal disease are removed from training and put on a convalescent exercise program to provide time for the early acute changes to subside. Many horses with acute bucked shins can continue to train after 5–10 days of rest and anti-inflammatories.
- Hand walking, ponying, cold water hosing, or icing and bandaging should continue until the MCIII is free of palpable pain. Initially, daily galloping distance is reduced to 50%. An overall modification of the training program with less galloping miles and more short-distance breezing may be necessary. If speed is increased, distance should be decreased.
- Subacute and chronic dorsal metacarpal disease can be the most difficult to treat. Many of these horses may not be suitable for the modified training regimen described above and pain will immediately return with any

sustained galloping. These horses may have marked periosteal new bone formation and may require more prolonged rest.

- Some dorsal cortical fractures in young horses may resolve with an altered exercise program but may require four to six months for the fracture to heal.
- Surgical treatment of dorsal cortical MCIII fractures include placement of a Unicortical lag or positional screw, and dorsal cortical drilling. The screw may or may not need to be removed but most surgeons recommend removal.
- Adjunctive treatments that have been recommended (with or without surgical treatment) include electrical stimulation, shock wave therapy, injection of osteogenic substances (sodium oleate), chemical vesication (blistering), and cryotherapy (point freezing).

Prognosis

- The prognosis is good to excellent (80–98%) for return to racing with surgical treatment of dorsal cortical fractures.
- Horses with acute periostitis given adequate time to convalesce also have a very good prognosis.
- Adjustment of training regimens (regular short-distance breezing and less to long-distance galloping) may assist with prevention of this problem, and training on grass, wood fiber, or softer surfaces without toe grabs is recommended.

MCIII/MTIII Condylar Fractures

Overview

- Fractures of the condyles of MCIII/MTIII occur most frequently in racing Thoroughbreds, less frequently in Standardbreds, and occasionally in Quarter horses and Polo ponies; they comprise a subset of catastrophic breakdowns on racetracks.
- Fractures occur at speed and males are overrepresented.

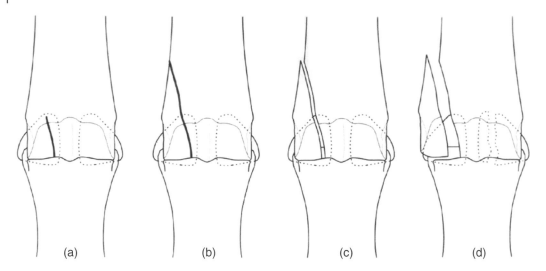

Figure 3.40 Condylar fractures. (a) Incomplete, (b) complete nondisplaced, (c) complete separated, (d) complete displaced.

- The distribution of fractures is approximately one-third incomplete-nondisplaced, one-third complete-nondisplaced, and one-third complete-displaced (Figure 3.40).
- In Thoroughbreds, fractures of the lateral condyles of the either forelimb are most common, and these fractures tend not to spiral proximally.
- Condylar fractures of the hindlimb are more common in Standardbreds and are more likely to be medial and to not exit the cortex. These fractures can propagate proximally or progress to a complete "Y" fracture, even with stall confinement.
- Articular comminution can occur, usually at the palmar/plantar articular margin, in about 15% of fractures.
- Concurrent axial sesamoid fractures are associated with displaced lateral condylar fractures that disrupt the collateral ligament and avulse the intersesamoidean ligament complex.

Anatomy (Please refer to previous section on "POD")

Imaging
- Radiography is usually adequate to diagnosis most condylar fractures.

- In addition to the standard radiographic projections (DP, LM, DLPMO, and DMPLO), a flexed DP view should be obtained to highlight the palmar/plantar surface of the condyles and evaluate the fracture line for comminution.
- Long cassettes are recommended so that the fetlock joint as well as the proximal cannon bone can be included in the study (Figure 3.41).
- Standing robotic cone-beam CT and nuclear scintigraphy can also be used to locate bone damage prior to fracture or to identify a fracture that is difficult to detect radiographically.

Etiology
- The etiology is trauma from high compressive loads, asynchronous longitudinal rotation of the cannon bone, and exercise on uneven surfaces.
- The risk of fatal condylar fractures in Thoroughbred racehorses is seven times and 17 times more likely if horses are shod with low or regular toe grabs, respectively. The toe grab presumably places more stress on the suspensory apparatus and plants the foot

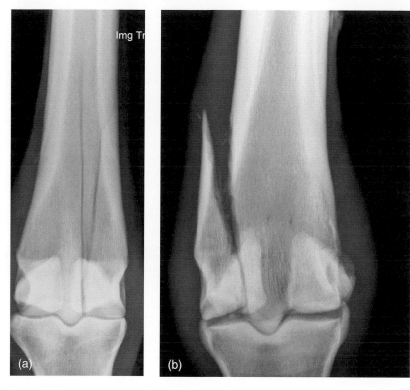

Figure 3.41 Radiographs of a spiraling medial condylar fracture in a racing Standardbred (a) and a displaced lateral condylar fracture in a racing Thoroughbred (b). Courtesy of Alicia Bertone.

more securely altering the compressive and rotatory forces on the distal MCIII.

- The palmar MCIII condyle is the site of maximum loading in racing and the bone responds by increasing density (sclerosis). Bone fatigue failure occurs, and due to the normal columnar arrangement of the bone trabeculae, acute failure of the bone propagates in the configuration seen in condylar fractures.

Clinical Signs
- The clinical signs may vary from a mild lameness that is exacerbated by exercise with little heat or swelling with nondisplaced, incomplete fractures, to severe lameness with heat, pain, and swelling in the acute displaced fracture.
- Incomplete nondisplaced fractures often have very subtle physical examination findings with minimal lameness.

- Nearly all horses have fetlock effusion because all fractures originate at the articular surface, and most horses will be positive to fetlock flexion and rotation.
- Radiographs should be taken immediately if a fracture is suspected based on history, clinical signs, and joint effusion.
- Perineural and intrasynovial anesthesia should be considered only after it is confirmed that a fracture is not present.

Diagnosis
- Radiographs usually confirm the diagnosis. The exception may be very short, incomplete, nondisplaced fractures that may be difficult to detect.
- Displaced fractures are obvious on the radiographs as longitudinal lines propagating up MCIII/MTIII and exiting the lateral cortex (Figure 3.41).

- Lesions that have been associated with condylar fractures include proximal fractures of P1, fractures of the PSBs, OA of the fetlock, evidence of POD, SL desmitis, and longitudinal fractures of MTIII.
- CT can be performed on fractures that spiral up MCIII/MTIII to further define the fracture propagation, especially if surgery is being contemplated.

Treatment

- The recommended treatment of most condylar fractures is internal fixation with transcortical lag screws either standing or with the horse anesthetized.
- Arthroscopic evaluation of the articular alignment can be helpful in displaced fractures, particularly if other bone fragments need to be removed, such as P1 eminence fractures or comminution of the palmar fracture line.
- Incomplete, nondisplaced fractures can be treated conservatively with successful return to racing, and surgery is not always required.
- Lag screw fixation offers the advantage of preventing fracture displacement, shorter convalescence, a reduced incidence of refracture at the same site, and decreased risk of OA within the fetlock.
- Horses with condylar fractures that spiral proximally (typically the medial MTIII) can be repaired with lag screws in the standing, sedated horse or with plates and screws or screws alone with the horse under general anesthesia. CT is recommended to aid with fracture planning and minimally invasive approaches are recommended.

Prognosis

- General prognosis for athletic performance and returning to racing is excellent for nondisplaced incomplete fractures, whether treated conservatively or following internal fixation.
- Prognosis for athletic performance and returning to racing is fair for complete displaced and nondisplaced fractures following internal fixation.
- In cases of complete displaced fractures when there was a delay in diagnosis and treatment and/or improper immobilization, a guarded to poor prognosis can be expected.
- The prognosis for return to racing is considered poor for comminuted fractures or subchondral erosive lesions in the palmar/plantar surface of the distal MCIII/MTIII.
- The prognosis to return to racing in Thoroughbreds is significantly reduced with complete fractures, forelimb fractures, or evidence of sesamoid fracture, or if the horse is female (presumed retired for breeding).

Complete Fractures of the MCIII/ MTIII (Cannon Bone)

Overview

- Fractures of the cannon bone can occur in any age or breed of horse but are most common in younger animals.
- Younger horses sustain simpler fractures than adults, possibly because of more elastic, less brittle bone. The fracture can occur anywhere along the bone length and can enter either the proximal or distal joint.
- Because of the minimal soft tissue around the cannon bone, the fractures are commonly open or become open after injury occurs, and more than half of referred MCIII/MTIII fractures are open.
- Stress fractures of MCIII/MTIII in racehorses can progress to acute and complete failure of the bone.

Anatomy

- The equine MC/MT region consists of the large MC/MTIII bone, the second (medial) and fourth (lateral) small MC/MT bones (splint bones), and the structures associated with them (Figure 3.37). The shaft of each small splint bone is united by an interosseous ligament to the large MC/MT bone.

- MC/MTIII is a long cylindrical-shaped bone located between the fetlock and the carpus or tarsus that is prone to injury because of its lack of soft tissue coverage (Figure 3.37).
- The common (MCIII) or long (MTIII) are the primary extensor tendons that course along the dorsal aspect of the cannon bone and the SL, inferior check ligament (ICL) in the forelimb, DDFT and SDFT are located palmar/plantar to the bone.
- The MC/MT is particularly susceptible to fracture because of its distal location and because little soft tissue covers the bone to help absorb impact energy in blunt trauma.

Imaging

- Radiography is the best diagnostic method to diagnose complete MC/MT fractures.
- Repeat radiographs may be necessary to aid diagnosis of nondisplaced fractures from blunt trauma.

Etiology

- External trauma in any form is the usual cause of cannon bone fractures. This often include kicks; halter breaking accidents; injuries associated with ground holes, fences, or cattle guards; slipping accidents and falls.
- When foals are affected, the dam has often stepped on the limb.
- Propagation of stress fractures or propagation of forces through screw or transfixation pin holes can result in similar complete cannon bone failure.

Clinical Signs and Diagnosis

- Complete yet nondisplaced fractures of the cannon bone secondary to direct trauma can occur and may be difficult to diagnose initially (Figure 3.42). The lameness may be nonspecific and other signs suggestive of a fracture are often variable.

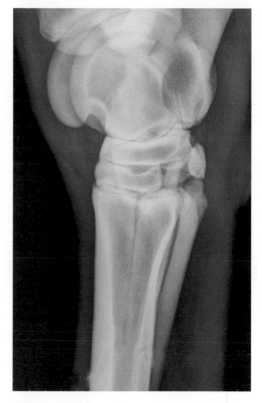

Figure 3.42 This oblique radiograph of the tarsus revealed an incomplete proximal metatarsal fracture. The fracture occurred from an accident at a jump and was initially thought to be a proximal suspensory injury. Courtesy of Ty Wallis.

- Heat, swelling of the soft tissues overlying the fracture, and pain on deep digital palpation are usually present in most types of fractures.
- With complete fractures, the diagnosis is usually obvious. Horses are often non-weight-bearing, and the limb has an abnormal angulation. These fractures should be immediately supported and then radiographed to identify the type (simple vs. comminuted) and location of the fracture.
- A tentative diagnosis can often be made based on physical examination of the limb and can usually be confirmed with radiography.
- Approximately 50% of complete cannon bone fractures open.

Treatment

- The selection of treatment of cannon bone fractures depends on the type of fracture (open vs. closed, simple vs. comminuted), the location of the fracture (articular vs. nonarticular, proximal vs. distal), the animal's age, its intended use, the presence of wounds, vascular compromise, and the economics.
- The preferred treatment for most cannon bone fractures is internal fixation with one or two DCP or LCP plates combined with individual lag screws where appropriate (Figure 3.43).

- LCPs are ideal for minimally invasive plate fixation extending the length of the bone.
- Severely comminuted fractures may heal with transfixation pins and external fixators or casts. These methods are more successful in foals with rapid healing and low body weight.

Prognosis

- In general, transverse, slightly oblique, and mildly comminuted (one butterfly fragment) fractures in the midcannon bone region in foals under seven months of age have a good

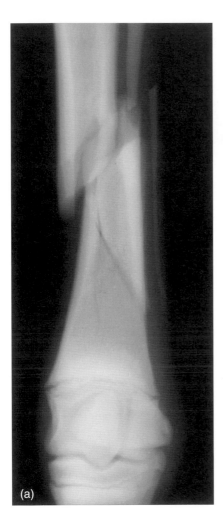
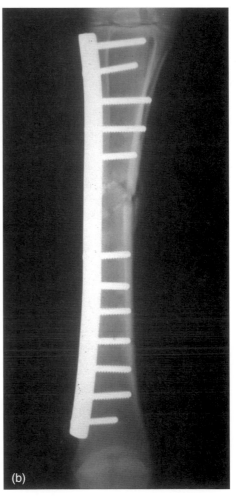

Figure 3.43   (a) Open comminuted mid-diaphyseal fracture of MTIII in a seven-month-old weanling that was successfully repaired with two broad dynamic compression plates. (b) A transverse MTIII fracture that was repaired with a single broad plate.

to excellent prognosis with internal fixation (Figure 3.43).

- Older horses with similar fractures have a more guarded prognosis due to their size and the risk of complications.
- Older horses with open, comminuted, or articular fractures have a guarded-to-poor prognosis for recovery.

Metacarpal/Metatarsal Exostosis (Splints)

Overview

- Exostoses of the second and fourth MC/MT bones, or "splints," are a condition most commonly diagnosed in young, immature horses but can be seen in older horses.
- Splints are most commonly seen in the proximal half of the bones and MC II is most commonly affected (Figure 3.44).
- The terminology used to identify the condition is variable. A true splint refers to a sprain or tear of the interosseous ligament that can be observed 6–7 cm below the carpus on the medial aspect of the cannon bone. A blind splint refers to an inflammatory process of the interosseous ligament that is difficult to detect on physical examination.
- The condition is most common in young skeletally immature horses (two-year-old) undergoing heavy training but can affect horses of any age.

Anatomy

- The shafts of the second (medial) and fourth (lateral) small MC/MT bones (splint bones) are united by an interosseous ligament to the large MC/MT bone.
- The "heads" of the splint bones articulate with the carpometacarpal joint (MC II + IV) or tarsometatarsal joint (MTII + IV) and are exposed to loads during weight-bearing (Figure 3.37).

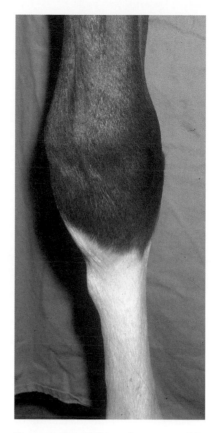

Figure 3.44 Visible enlargement of the medial splint area just distal to the carpus, typical of horses with "splints." Courtesy of Alicia Bertone.

- The head of MCII is entirely articular and is thought to absorb more weight-bearing and torsional forces than the other splint bones.
- The interosseus ligament consists of dense fibrous tissue that can tear with the strains applied during independent motion of the splint bones and the cannon bone.
- The splint bones are covered with periosteum that can respond very actively to external trauma resulting in proliferative periostitis of the bones.
- The palmar/plantar surfaces of the splint bones form the MC/MT groove, which contains the SL.
- The splint bones gradually taper as they extend distally along the MC/MTIII and terminate at the "button" of the splint just proximal to the fetlock joint capsule (Figure 3.37).

Imaging

- Radiography should be used to confirm the presence of a splint.
- Ultrasonography is helpful to demonstrate concomitant injury to the SL and possible ligament impingement.
- In some cases, scintigraphy may be needed to confirm a blind splint or other types of splint bone disease if radiographs are normal.

Etiology

- The condition is associated with tearing of the interosseous ligament between the splint bones and MC/MTIII, external trauma such as kicks or interference, or subsequent to healing of splint bone fractures.
- Conformation abnormalities such as offset carpi, improper hoof care, mineral imbalances, and overnutrition may exacerbate the condition.
- Excessive loading of MCII with or without conformational abnormalities such as "bench knees" can contribute to tearing of the interosseous ligament.
- Direct trauma is thought to cause subperiosteal hemorrhage and periosteal bone proliferation or instability between the splint bones and MC/MTIII.
- Initially, a desmitis and periostitis occurs, with subsequent fibrous tissue enlargement and ossification (proliferative exostosis) of the splint bone.

Clinical Signs

- Acute splints are characterized by palpable heat, pain, and swelling in the proximal, medial cannon bone area. With time, the inflammation subsides, and the resultant exostosis is much smaller and firmer than the initial swelling.
- Horses have variable lameness but generally worsen with work and seem to be worse on hard ground.

- Palpation of the exostosis usually elicits a very painful response when the splint is active whereas horses with chronic exostosis of the splint bones usually have minimal evidence of palpable pain or lameness.
- Palpation of the axial aspect of the splint bone is useful to determine if new bone formation may be causing impingement of the SL.

Diagnosis

- A tentative diagnosis can usually be made based on physical examination findings.
- Diagnostic anesthesia is usually unnecessary but may be required to prove that the splint is the true cause of lameness.
- Radiographs are necessary to confirm the diagnosis as fractures of the splint bone can be confused with splints. A periosteal reaction associated with the splint bone is usually present (Figure 3.45).
- Ultrasonography should be used to document SL injuries if necessary.

Treatment

- Treatment for splints includes anti-inflammatories and rest for the acute phase, and occasionally surgery in the more chronic stages.
- NSAIDs combined with hypothermia, pressure support wraps, topical Surpass®, and rest appear to be most beneficial to decrease the heat, pain, and swelling in acute cases.
- Intralesional corticosteroid in the acute stage may reduce inflammation and prevent excessive bone growth.
- Other treatments depending on potential contributing factors include ESWT, acupuncture, massage, splint or shin boots (guards), and corrective farriery.
- Surgical removal of the exostosis with or without the splint bone may be necessary if the exostosis is causing lameness or for cosmetic reasons (Figure 3.44).

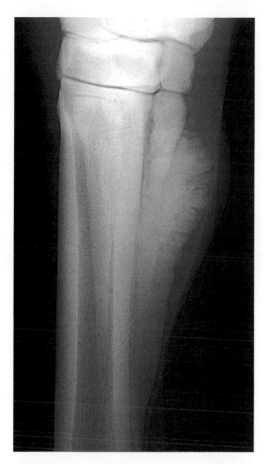

Figure 3.45 This large exostosis of the medial splint contributed to lameness and was removed surgically. Just the exostosis was removed, and the underlying splint bone was left intact.

- It is recommended to retain the splint bone lever arm if possible and reflect the periosteum to prevent excessive new bone formation.

Prognosis
- Prognosis is good to excellent for soundness except for those cases in which the exostosis is large and encroaches on the SL or the carpal joint.
- Chronic recurring lameness can occur in horses that are not rested long enough, which can be five to six months.

- Surgery to remove the excess bone callus can successfully alleviate lameness and recurrence does not occur in most cases.

Fractures of the Small MC/MT (Splint) Bones

Introduction

- Fractures of the splint bones can occur anywhere along their length but are most common in the distal one-third.
- Fractures of the middle and proximal aspects are usually due to external trauma and are often open and complicated by comminution, osteomyelitis, and bone sequestration. The lateral splint bones are at greatest risk.
- Fractures of the distal splint bone are usually due to internal forces associated with exercise and can be associated with SL desmitis, sesamoiditis, and fetlock OA. These fractures tend to occur in older horses (five to seven years of age) and the forelimbs (MCIV) are more frequently involved than the hindlimbs.

Anatomy (Please refer to previous section on "Splint Exostoses")

Imaging (Please refer to previous section on "Splint Exostoses")
Etiology
- Distal fractures are usually due to internal trauma from increased axial compression forces on the splint bones during exercise, pressure from the SL, or increased tension on the bones from fascial attachments. Although the exact association is unknown, a higher incidence of SL desmitis is noted in the forelimb in association with distal splint bone fractures.
- Distal splint fractures can also occur from external trauma such as interference, kicks, and direct blows from hitting another object.

- Fractures of the middle and proximal aspects of splint bones are usually due to external trauma such as kicks or interference and may be associated with a wound.
- Proximal fractures of MCII in racehorses may be due to excessive torsional forces that may occur in the starting gate.

Clinical Signs

- With distal fractures, swelling of the distal cannon bone region and pain on palpation over the fracture may or may not be present. Lameness can be variable and perineural anesthesia may be indicated to isolate the site of the lameness.
- Swelling and lameness are usually prominent features of proximal splint fractures.
- Horses with closed middle and proximal fractures usually present with variable severity of lameness and swelling in the cannon bone area. Focal pain, heat, and swelling can usually be palpated over the fracture site. A firm exostosis may be palpable, depending on the duration of the injury.
- Horses with open middle and proximal fractures usually present with a wound or draining tract and severe swelling in the cannon bone area. Bone fragments may be palpable within the wound and purulent drainage is often seen with sequestration and osteomyelitis.
- Palpation of the entire splint bone and the SL including its branches should be performed to gain full appreciation of all structures that may be involved.

Diagnosis

- A fractured splint bone is confirmed with radiography in most cases. Oblique views should be taken to isolate the affected splint bone from superimposition with MCIII/MTIII or the opposite splint bone (Figure 3.46).
- Most fractures are obvious on radiographs, but some nondisplaced fractures can be difficult to identify, and others may resemble a splint exostosis in the chronic stages.
- Other radiographic abnormalities that may be visible include periosteal proliferation, sequestration, and osteomyelitis.

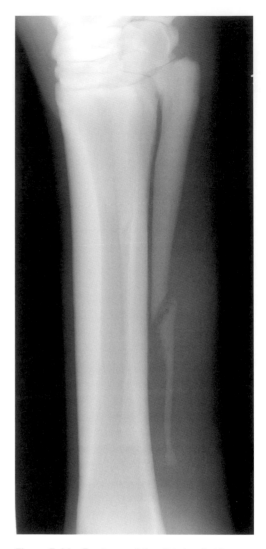

Figure 3.46 Fractures of the distal splint bones such as this rarely heal and are usually removed.

- Proximal fractures may extend toward or into the carpometacarpal or tarsometatarsal joint (Figure 3.47).
- Ultrasonography should be performed in any horses with suspected SL involvement.

Treatment

Distal Fractures

- Distal fractures of the splint bones are traditionally treated by surgical removal, but this may be unnecessary if the fracture does not cause swelling or lameness.

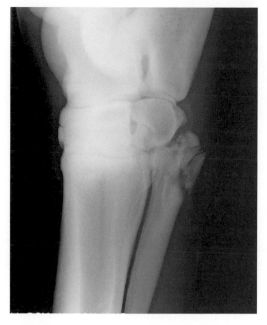

Figure 3.47 Proximal fractures of the fourth metatarsal bone are often comminuted and open and are due to traumatic injuries. This fracture also entered the TMT joint.

- Some closed distal splint fractures can heal spontaneously and not cause lameness, but open fractures are often best removed.
- 70% of horses with distal splint fractures have SL desmitis, which is often the cause of continued lameness.

Middle Fractures
- Closed middle fractures can heal without treatment in two to four months but may develop significant callus at the fracture site that may contribute to lameness.
- Open middle fractures of the splint bone often lead to draining tracts and sequestra (Figure 3.48). Removal of the fracture with or without the remaining distal splint bone is usually the recommended treatment. Up to 80% of the splint bone can be removed without complications.

Proximal Fractures
- Closed nonarticular and nondisplaced proximal comminuted fractures of the splint bones usually heal without surgical treat-

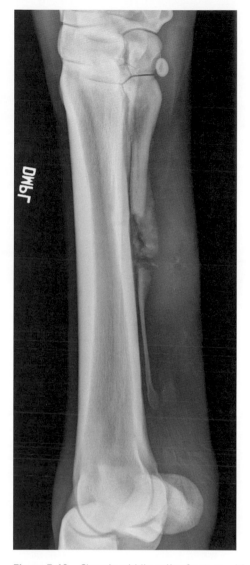

Figure 3.48 Chronic middle splint fracture with secondary drainage and periosteal reaction that is typically best treated with surgical debridement and removal of the distal fragment. Courtesy of Kyla Ortved.

ment. However, avulsion of the proximal fragments is much more likely to occur in fractures of MCII and MCIV than MTII and MTIV.
- Closed articular fractures of MCII and MCIV are usually best treated with internal fixation using a small bone plate to prevent displacement of the proximal fragment (Figure 3.49).

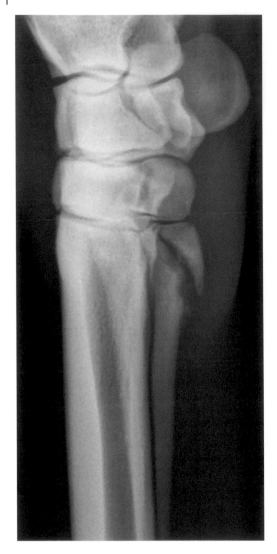

Figure 3.49 A dorsomedial-palmarolateral oblique radiograph of the carpus showing an oblique articular fracture of the second metacarpal bone that should be repaired with a small bone plate. Courtesy of Kyla Ortved.

- Open proximal fractures of the splint bones are the most difficult to treat. Many will heal with conservative treatment if no infection develops. Wound lavage and debridement and local and systemic antimicrobials should be performed to prevent complications.
- If more than 80% of the splint bone must be removed and it appears unstable and active

infection is not present, a small bone plate can be secured to the proximal portion of the splint and the cannon bone using 3.5-mm screws.
- Infected, proximal MTIV fractures can be treated with complete removal of the bone but only if other treatments have failed (Figure 3.47).

Prognosis
- The prognosis for most horses with open or closed distal splint bone fractures is usually very good and is often more dependent on concurrent musculoskeletal problems such as SL desmitis than the fracture itself.
- The prognosis for comminuted closed splint bone fractures is good to excellent with or without surgery, particularly if the horse is used for something other than racing.
- The prognosis for horses with open or closed middle splint bone fractures is also good to excellent with or without surgery if approximately one-third of the proximal splint bone remains.
- The prognosis for horses with open comminuted fractures of the proximal splint bones is more guarded with about 60% returning to performance without lameness.

Suspensory Ligament (SL) Desmitis

Overview
- Injuries to the SL are usually based on location: proximal (proximal suspensory desmitis), middle (body lesions), and distal (branch lesions).
- Proximal suspensory desmitis (PSD), or inflammation of the origin of the SL, is the most common cause of soft tissue injury to the limbs, comprising approximately 30% of all tendon/ligament injuries.

- PSD occurs most commonly in sport horses, such as event horses, jumpers, dressage horses, racehorses, and Western performance horses. The hindlimbs are more frequently affected than the forelimbs and typically have a worse prognosis.
- Injury to the body of the SL is less common than PSD and occurs most frequently in racehorses, especially Standardbred racehorses. Degenerative suspensory ligament desmitis (DSLD) also usually affects the body of the SL.
- Injury to the SL branches occurs most commonly in Standardbred racehorses or jumping horses.

Anatomy

- The SL originates on the proximal palmar/plantar surface of MCIII/MTIII, divides into two branches in the distal fourth of the cannon bone, and inserts on the proximal medial and lateral sesamoid bones (Figure 3.50).
- The SL branches cross the abaxial surface of PSB and an extensor branch continues on to join the tendon of the common or long digital extensor muscle on the dorsal surface of P1.
- The SL lies within the metacarpal/metatarsal groove on the palmar/plantar aspect of MC/MTIII between the axial surfaces of the second and fourth splint bones (Figure 3.37).
- Proximally, the body of the SL separates and attaches into two palmar depressions just distal to the carpometacarpal or tarsometatarsal joints (Figure 3.50).
- There are variable amounts of striated muscle fibers within the mainly collagenous ligament that are organized into two longitudinal bundles within the proximal part and body of the SL (hence the term interosseus medius "muscle").
- The percentage of muscle in the SL differs between Standardbreds and Thoroughbreds and the strength of the suspensory apparatus increases with training.

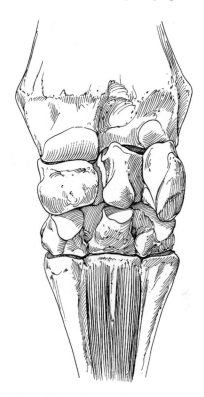

Figure 3.50 The attachments of the suspensory ligament at the proximal palmar surface of the third metacarpal bone. Courtesy of TS Stashak.

Imaging

- Ultrasonography is by far the most commonly used modality to help diagnose SL disease as it is accessible and relatively simple to perform. However, lesions in the proximal SL are often subtle and difficult to detect.
- Advanced imaging such as MRI or contrast CT is often beneficial to diagnose abnormalities within the proximal aspect of the SL.
- Radiography should be performed to rule out other potential problems within the limb but is usually not that beneficial in diagnosing SL disease.

Etiology

- Overloading of the SL may cause trauma to any portion of the ligament. Hyperextension of the carpus/tarsus in conjunction with

- severe overextension of the fetlock joint has been proposed to cause proximal lesions.
- Working horses in deep, soft arenas or in eventing where there is excessive rotational movement of the limbs may increase the risk of injuries.
- Lesions in the body or branches of the SL also occur in sport horses worked in soft ground and in racehorses that race and train on turf.
- Lesions within the branches are also associated with fetlock lameness and suggest that high rotary motion of the fetlock may predispose to suspensory branch injury as may occur in racehorses and horses with dropped fetlock conformation.
- The presence of upright hindlimb (straight hock) conformation is overrepresented in horses with hindlimb SL injury and may predispose to injury and recurrence.

Clinical Signs

- Most horses with PSD present with a history of intermittent lameness that is exacerbated with exercise. Heat and swelling may be palpable in the proximal cannon bone region in acute cases but can be difficult to detect especially in chronic cases.
- Firm digital pressure overlying the proximal SL usually elicits a nonfatiguable painful response (Figures 1.22–1.24).
- Horses with hindlimb PSD can exhibit moderate-to-severe hindlimb lameness.
- Lower limb flexion exacerbates the lameness in 50% of horses with forelimb suspensory problems and hock flexion exacerbates the lameness in 85% of horses with hindlimb suspensory problems.
- Horses with injury to the body or branches of the SL usually have visible and palpable swelling and pain at the site of injury and are usually painful to fetlock flexion.
- A lateral palmar nerve block in the forelimb and the deep branch of the lateral plantar nerve (DBLPN) in the hindlimb are the most specific nerve blocks to help document PSD in each limb.

- Perineural anesthesia is usually not necessary for lesions within the branches and body of the SL.

Diagnosis

- Ultrasonography of the body and branches of the SL is the imaging technique of choice to diagnose lesions in these locations. Radiographs should be included to identify any concomitant bone abnormalities such as distal splint bone fractures.
- Definitive diagnosis of PSD is more difficult, and combinations of ultrasound, radiography, scintigraphy, MRI, and contrast CT may be needed to document damage within the origin of the SL (Figure 3.51).
- Radiographic abnormalities of proximal MCIII/MTIII such as bone sclerosis, fractures, and enthesiophyte formation appear to be more common with hindlimb PSD than forelimb PSD (Figure 3.51).
- Ultrasound can be difficult in the proximal MC/MTIII region. Abnormalities with PSD include enlargement of the ligament (linear width and circumference), poor definition of margins, central or peripheral areas of hypoechogenicity, diffuse reduction in echogenicity, hyperechogenic foci, and irregularity of the plantar cortex of MC/MTIII (enthesiophyte formation or avulsion fracture).
- MRI should be considered in horses with lameness localized to the proximal SL with diagnostic analgesia but without ultrasonographic abnormalities.
- MRI is currently the most accurate and definitive imaging modality to identify abnormalities within the proximal SL (Figure 3.52).

Treatment

- Immediate first aid treatment in acute cases of SL injury should include NSAIDs, hydrotherapy or icing, and bandaging to reduce swelling and support the fetlock.
- Treatment for horses with body or branch lesions includes a convalescence program of confinement and slow return to controlled exercise.

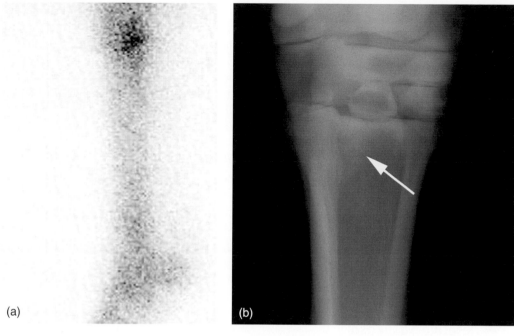

(a)

(b)

Figure 3.51 (a) Nuclear scintigraphy can identify bone injury at the origin of the suspensory ligament. Radiographic lesions such as sclerosis (arrow) can be subtle (b) and usually only identified on the craniocaudal view due to the overlap with the splint bones on the lateral view. Courtesy of Alicia Bertone.

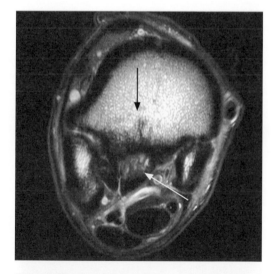

Figure 3.52 Transverse proton density image of the proximal metatarsal region of the left hindlimb of a horse with marked proximal suspensory desmitis and enthesopathy of the proximal plantar metatarsal cortex. There is a large central area of abnormal signal hyperintensity in the suspensory ligament (white arrow). There are irregular areas of low signal in the medullary cavity of MTIII reflecting the presence of osteosclerosis (black arrow). The plantar metatarsal cortex is thickened and has an irregular endosteal margin. Courtesy of Michael Schramme.

- Intralesional therapies with stem cells, PRP, or other biologics have shown some efficacy and can be used to improve healing if indicated.
- Total healing time is often eight months and return to full competitive performance may not be possible for one year. Recurrence of injury is always a concern, especially in horses that are inadequately rested and for abnormalities in the hindlimbs.
- Treatment of PSD can be difficult, especially in the hindlimb. Reported nonsurgical treatments include rest and rehabilitation, ESWT, local infiltration with sarapin, and intralesional therapy with biologics. Surgical treatments have included fasciotomy alone, ultrasound-guided desmotomy and fasciotomy, fasciotomy and osteostixis of MCIII/MTIII, and fasciotomy and neurectomy of the DBLPN in the hindlimb.

Prognosis
- The prognosis for acute forelimb PSD is good (greater than 80%) for return to full work in

sport horses with forelimb PSD following three to six months of rest and controlled exercise.

- The prognosis is less favorable for horses with PSD of the hindlimbs with only 14–69% of horses returning to full athletic function without detectable lameness.
- Neurectomy of the DBLPN has been reported to result in an 80% return to performance for hindlimb PSD.
- Concurrent bone abnormalities are thought to negatively impact the overall prognosis of treatment in horses with PSD.
- Recurrence of PSD is highest in dressage (37%) and show jumping horses (46%) and the prognosis is guarded for return to performance if PSD recurs after one year.

Degenerative Suspensory Ligament Desmitis (DSLD)

Overview

- DSLD is a debilitating disorder thought to be limited to the suspensory ligaments of Peruvian Pasos, Peruvian Paso crosses, Arabians, American Saddlebreds, Quarter horses, Thoroughbreds, and some European breeds.
- It primarily affects the body and proximal aspects of the SL and is often bilateral.

Anatomy (Please refer to previous section on "SL Desmitis")

Imaging (Please refer to previous section on "SL Desmitis")

Etiology

- The etiology of DSLD is unknown, but the disease tends to run in families, suggesting hereditary influences.
- Excessive accumulation of proteoglycans within the SL and other tissues in affected horses has been found and the authors suggested that DSLD is actually a systemic disorder of proteoglycan accumulation and

propose the term equine systemic proteoglycan accumulation (ESPA) as a more appropriate name for the condition.

- It has also been proposed that DSLD in non-Peruvian Paso breeds is due to progressive exercise-induced degeneration of the SL and not associated with a proteoglycan disorder.

Clinical Signs

- Both forelimbs or hindlimbs can be involved, and the condition often leads to persistent incurable lameness requiring euthanasia.
- Many horses have excessive fetlock extension (dropping) on presentation and horses with hindlimb involvement often have the combination of straight hocks and fetlock hyperextension (Figure 3.53).
- Affected horses often have generalized thickening of the cannon bone region and palpable enlargement and pain of the SL.

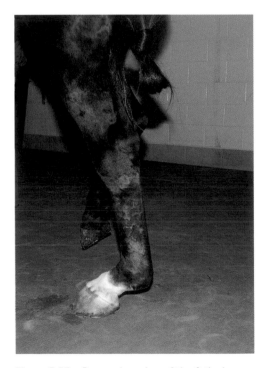

Figure 3.53 Severe dropping of the fetlock together with a straight hock conformation is typical of horses with DSLD.

Diagnosis

- The diagnosis is usually based on patient signalment and history, clinical examination, and ultrasonographic abnormalities within the affected SLs.
- Radiographs may be normal but calcification within the ligament or enthesiophyte formation on the palmar/plantar aspect MC/MTIII may support the diagnosis.

Treatment

- There is no known treatment for this condition. Treatment is empirical and supportive but often not effective in altering progression of the disease.
- Use of support bandages and heel extension shoes, such as an egg bar, are recommended but usually not helpful.
- Horses often remain lame or worsen over time as the disease is almost always progressive.

Prognosis

The prognosis is poor for recovery and most horses are euthanized.

Superficial Digital Flexor (SDF) Tendinitis (Bowed Tendon)

Overview

- Tendinitis of the superficial digital flexor tendon (SDFT) is a common soft tissue injury in horses working at high speeds including Thoroughbred and Standardbred racehorses.
- SDFT injury is almost exclusively a forelimb problem, most commonly occurs in the mid-to-proximal aspect of the cannon bone and often appears as a convex "bow" to the visual profile of the metacarpus on the side view, hence the term "bowed tendon" (Figure 3.54).

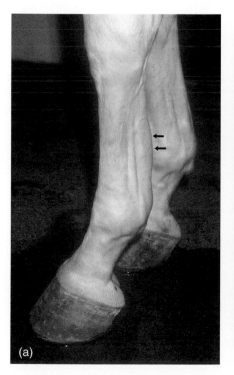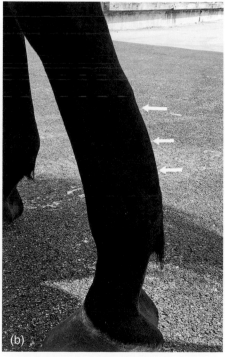

Figure 3.54 Classic appearance of mild (a) and more severe (b) SDF tendinitis of the left forelimb. Note the convex palmar surface to the middle region of the metacarpus (arrows). Image (b) Courtesy of Kyla Ortved.

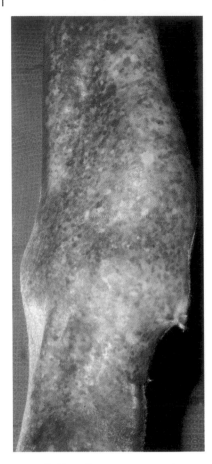

Figure 3.55 A "low bow" of the SDFT, as shown in this image, can be associated with concurrent digital tendon sheath tenosynovitis.

- Less common locations include the distal MC/MT ("low bows"), the branches of the SDFT in the pastern region, and the caudal aspect of the carpus.
- Lesions in the distal cannon bone are often referred to as "low bows" and can be associated with DFTS tenosynovitis or constriction of the PAL (Figure 3.55).
- Damage to the SDFT at or above the level of the carpus is a syndrome that more commonly affects older (>15 years) nonrace-horses and can be subtle and easily missed on lameness evaluation.

Anatomy

- The SDFT is deep to the skin and subcutaneous fascia throughout the length of the metacarpus.

- Dorsally, it is intimately related to the fascial covering of the DDFT, which lies against the palmar surface of the SL.
- The carpal synovial sheath encloses both digital flexor tendons proximally and extends distad as far as the middle of the metacarpus. At this level, the DDFT is joined by its accessory ligament ("inferior" check ligament), the distal continuation of the palmar carpal ligament.
- The SDFT musculotendinous unit originates on the caudal humerus and extends to a bivalved attachment on the palmar/plantar eminences of P2.
- Excessive hyperextension of the fetlock associated with exercise places the SDFT under very high tensile loads, contributing to strain injuries within the tendon.

Imaging

- A complete ultrasound examination remains the primary imaging tool to diagnose SDF tendinitis in most horses.
- Color Doppler ultrasound and elastography are newer techniques to evaluate soft tissue injuries that may be used to complement routine ultrasound in the future.
- MRI has demonstrated an advantage over ultrasound for distinguishing fibrosis from normal tendon in chronic tendinitis.

Etiology

- As the forelimb contacts the ground at the gallop, the fetlock is hyperextended, and the flexor tendons are placed under very high tensile loads.
- The high demands placed on the SDFT put it at risk of overstrain injury.
- Overstrain injury can occur as a single overloading but is more commonly due to repetitive trauma leading to microdamage of the collagen structure that contributes to final failure of fibrils.
- Increasing age and exercise demands can lead to subclinical tendonitis due to accumulation of microtrauma without adequate repair making older horses more susceptible to injury.

Clinical Signs

- The clinical signs are variable and usually parallel the severity and acuteness of the SDFT damage.
- Early focal swelling, heat, and tenderness may occur before a detectable lameness. Intervention at this early phase can prevent structural damage to the tendon.
- Classic signs of acute tendinitis include diffuse enlargement of the cannon bone region, palpable tendon thickening, heat, and pain, and moderate lameness.
- Severe tendon injuries are recognized clinically as horses that do not want to put the hoof flat on the ground, thereby putting tension on the flexor surface of the limb.
- Chronic tendinitis is manifested by fibrosis and firm swelling on the flexor surface of the cannon bone (Figure 3.54b). Signs of inflammation or lameness may or may not be present.

Diagnosis

- Ultrasonography enables initial and reasonably accurate determination of the extent and location of the lesions.
- A complete ultrasound examination extends from proximal aspect of MC/MTIII distally to the heel bulbs and determines the CSA of the SDFT and the lesions at multiple locations from proximal to distal. Comparison to the contralateral side should nearly always be done and longitudinal scans permit the validation of structural lesions and the assessment of fiber alignment.
- Ultrasound abnormalities may include tendon enlargement and focal or diffuse loss of the normal echogenicity (hypoechoic areas) due to hemorrhage, edema, cellular infiltration, or fibrillar disruption (Figure 3.56).
- Repeat ultrasound after the initial signs of inflammation have resolved (two to three weeks) is recommended to more accurately determine the extent of fiber disruption.
- MRI can usually provide further information on SDFT injuries but is usually unnecessary for a diagnosis except in horses with chronic tendonitis.

Treatment

- Immediate medical treatment of SDF tendinitis is recommended to reduce or eliminate the acute swelling and inflammation as rapidly as possible to prevent fiber damage or early fibrous tissue formation. Routine physical therapy such as icing, cryotherapy, pressure wraps, and topical hyperosmotic

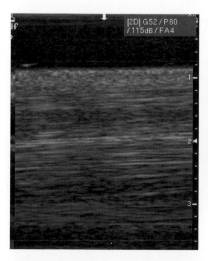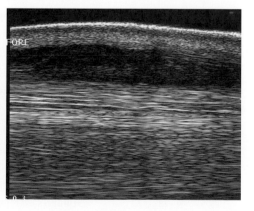

Figure 3.56 Ultrasound longitudinal sections through the midportion of a normal SDFT (left) and SDFT with acute tendonitis. Note the hypoechoic area (black) in the middle of the SDFT that usually corresponds to edema or hemorrhage in acute cases. Courtesy of Alicia Bertone.

sweats or diclofenac liposomal cream, along with systemic NSAIDs, is instituted along with rest until the ultrasound can be performed.

- In acute, severe injury such as rupture, a soft cast, resin cast, or Kimzey Leg Saver splint (Kimzey Welding Works, Woodland, CA) may be indicated.
- The duration of inactivity and the rehabilitation program depends on the severity of the lesion on ultrasound. If ultrasound examination is normal, then hand walking followed by a return to exercise in 30 days may be effective. Severe injuries may require a year or more of rest and rehabilitation.

- Injectable autologous biologic therapies such as bone marrow, BMAC, MSCs, acellular collagen, platelet-rich plasma (PRP), and concentrated plasma are commonly used to treat SDF tendonitis. Use of ultrasound guidance for injection facilitates the injection into the lesion.
- Potential surgical treatments include tendon splitting and proximal accessory ligament transection on the affected limb and frequently on both forelimbs. These treatments seem to have fallen out of favor in recent years.
- Proper rehabilitation and convalescent exercise program remain paramount to success with any of the above treatments (Table 3.1).

Table 3.1 A standard exercise program recommended following tendon injury. This protocol can be modified based upon ultrasound recheck examinations.

Exercise level	Week	Duration and nature of exercise
0	0–2	Box rest
1	3	10 minutes walking daily
1	4	15 minutes walking daily
1	5	20 minutes walking daily
1	6	25 minutes walking daily
1	7	30 minutes walking daily
1	8	35 minutes walking daily
1	9	40 minutes walking daily
1	10–12	45 minutes walking daily
Week 12: repeat ultrasound examination		
2	13–16	40 minutes walking and 5 minutes trotting daily
2	17–20	35 minutes walking and 10 minutes trotting daily
2	21–24	30 minutes walking and 15 minutes trotting daily
Week 24: repeat ultrasound examination		
3	25–28	25 minutes walking and 20 minutes trotting daily
3	29–32	20 minutes walking and 25 minutes trotting daily
Week 32: repeat ultrasound examination		
4	33–40	45 minutes exercise daily, gradually increasing in amount
4	41–48	45 minutes exercise daily with fast work three times a week
Week 48: repeat ultrasound examination		
5	48+	Return to full competition/race training

(Davis CS, Smith RKW: 2006. Equine Surgery. *In:* Auer JA, Stick JA (eds) *Equine Surgery*, Philadelphia, Saunders, 1110.)

Prognosis

- The incidence of reinjury is often used as an outcome measure for successful management of SDF tendinitis. Published reports of reinjury in horses treated conservatively with rest alone are 48 and 56%.
- Stem cell therapy reports significantly reduced a reinjury rate of 18% and surgical transection of the accessory ligament of the SDFT reports a reduced reinjury rate of 25% but increased the risk of SL desmitis 5.5-fold.
- In general, the prognosis for return to racing is often dictated by the severity of the initial tendon injury regardless of the treatments used.
- It is currently thought that optimal conditioning of a young horse may result in improved performance and reduced tendon injury later in life.

Carpus

Common Digital Extensor (CDE) Tendon Rupture

Overview

- Rupture of the CDE tendon is a bilateral or unilateral condition seen in foals shortly after birth.
- It has been reported to occur concurrently with other congenital conditions such as decreased endochondral ossification at other sites, decreased pectoral muscle mass, and prognathic conformation to the jaw.
- It is overrepresented in Arabian horses, Quarter horses, and Arab-Quarter horse crosses.

Anatomy

- On the dorsal carpus, the tendon sheaths of the extensor carpi radialis (ECR), extensor carpi obliquus (abductor digiti I longus), and the CDE muscles are enclosed in fibrous pas-

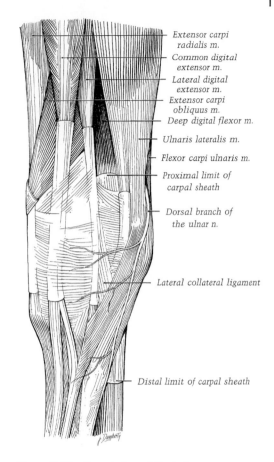

Extensor carpi radialis m.
Common digital extensor m.
Lateral digital extensor m.
Extensor carpi obliquus m.
Deep digital flexor m.
Ulnaris lateralis m.
Flexor carpi ulnaris m.
Proximal limit of carpal sheath
Dorsal branch of the ulnar n.
Lateral collateral ligament
Distal limit of carpal sheath

Figure 3.57 Dorsal view of the left carpus.

sages through the deep fascia and then through the extensor retinaculum.
- The tendon sheaths of the CDE and extensor carpi obliquus tendons extend from the carpometacarpal articulation proximad to 6–8 cm above the carpus (Figure 3.57).
- The tendon sheath of the ECR muscle terminates at the middle of the carpus, and then the tendon becomes adherent to the retinaculum as it extends to its insertion on the metacarpal tuberosity (Figure 3.57).

Imaging

- Ultrasonography is usually the imaging modality of choice to document the location and severity of the tendon injury.

- Radiography of the carpus and distal antebrachium should also be performed to check for other contributing problems.

Etiology

- It is speculated to be a heritable situation, especially if other congenital defects are present.
- Rupture of the CDE tendon is often found together with other flexural deformities of the limb and it is often uncertain which comes first.
- Chronic changes to the CDE tendon also have been reported to occur *in utero*.

Clinical Signs

- Clinical signs include swelling on the dorsolateral aspect of the carpus, mainly in the form of effusion in the CDE tendon sheath (Figure 3.58).
- Forward buckling of the carpi and/or knuckling of the fetlock may exist concurrently, and affected foals can be easily confused with those with simple flexural deformities.

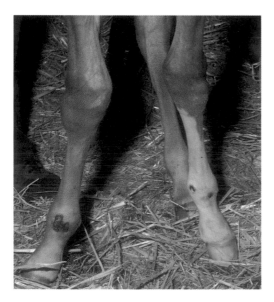

Figure 3.58 Bilateral symmetrical fluid swellings of the lateral aspects of both carpi in neonatal foals are characteristic of rupture of the common digital extensor tendons.

- Heat and palpable pain are usually not present, but the separation of the tendons can sometimes be palpated.

Diagnosis

- The diagnosis is usually based on physical findings alone.
- Radiographs and ultrasound of the carpi can be performed to check for other musculoskeletal problems and to document the amount of tendon separation.

Treatment and Prognosis

- Treatment commonly includes confinement with or without bandaging and splinting to address the concurrent flexural deformities if present.
- Bandaging is recommended to protect the dorsal aspect of the fetlock that may occur due to hyperflexion of the carpus.
- Primary repair of the tendons has been advocated by some but is usually unnecessary because the tendon ends are unlikely to heal, and rather adhere to the sheath.
- The prognosis is often very good for uncomplicated forms of rupture of the CDE tendon but is reduced if severe flexural deformities are present concurrently.

Extensor Carpi Radialis (ECR) Tendon Damage

Overview

- Rupture or tearing of the tendon of the ECR muscle can occur in both foals and adults.
- A tendon sheath encircles the ECR tendon from about 8 cm above the distal end of the radius to the middle carpal joint (3.57).
- Swellings of the ECR tendon sheath can be confused with effusion of the carpal joints, carpal hygroma, and effusion of the CDE tendon sheath.

Anatomy (Please refer to previous section on "CDE Tendon Rupture")

Imaging (Please refer to previous section on "CDE Tendon Rupture")

Etiology

- Inflammation of the ECR tendon sheath can occur from rupture or tearing of the ECR tendon, direct trauma to the sheath/tendon, or from infection secondary to wounds.
- Tenosynovitis of the ECR sheath in adults has been reported to occur mostly in jumpers and in horses that have exostoses on the distal radius. This is typically traumatic in origin from hitting the dorsal aspect of the carpus.
- Infection of the ECR tendon sheath leading to septic tenosynovitis is usually secondary to puncture-type wounds.

Clinical Signs and Diagnosis

- Swelling and effusion of the sheath over the carpus is palpable in most cases (Figure 3.59).
- With acute injuries, pain is usually present with flexion of the carpus and subsides with chronicity.
- With infection, there is usually palpable heat, pain and swelling, moderate-to-severe lameness, and severe pain with carpal flexion.
- Overflexion of the carpus as the foal or horse walks occurs with complete rupture.
- There may or may not be ECR muscle atrophy and a palpable defect is often detected within the swelling of the ECR tendon sheath if the tendon has ruptured.
- Ultrasonography is the imaging modality of choice to assess the ECR tendon and sheath. Radiographic abnormalities are rarely present.

Treatment

- Nonseptic tenosynovitis usually responds to rest, topical and intrasynovial medication, and bandaging.

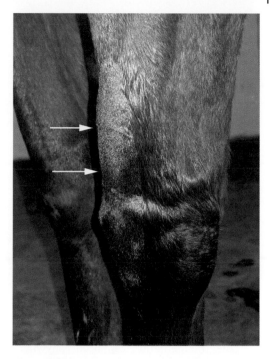

Figure 3.59 An adult horse with synovial effusion of the ECR tendon sheath proximal to the carpal joints (arrows). Courtesy of Ty Wallis.

- Surgical repair in adults with complete rupture in the acute stages has been advocated, with casting for two to four weeks after surgery.
- Tenoscopy and debridement of the ruptured ends also has been advocated but is rarely performed.
- Resection of the infected ECR together with the tendon sheath has been recommended in horses with chronic infection that is not responding to treatment.

Prognosis

- The prognosis for complete rupture of the ECR tendon in adults is guarded for athletic use but horses with partial tears can do reasonably well.
- Resection of the ECR due to infection does not preclude an athletic career, but only a few cases have been reported.

Intra-Articular (IA) Carpal Fractures

Overview

- There are three types of fractures that can occur within the carpal joints of the horse:
  1) Osteochondral fragmentation: one articular surface
  2) Slab fractures: two articular surfaces
  3) Comminuted fractures: multiple pieces
- Osteochondral fragmentation typically occurs at consistent locations in racchorses (distal radiocarpal, proximal intermediate, distal lateral radius, and proximal third carpal bone), which reflects the chronic nature of the disease.
- Standardbreds appear to be prone to problems in the middle carpal joint, especially on the third carpal bone.
- Acute fragmentation can occur anywhere within the carpus including the palmar aspects of both the middle carpal and radiocarpal joints.
- Slab fractures commonly occur on the third carpal bone of Thoroughbreds and Standardbreds but can involve the intermediate and radial carpal bones as well.
- Comminuted fractures primarily involve the third carpal bone, but they can also involve the radial carpal, intermediate carpal, and fourth carpal bones. These horses may be axially unstable and have concurrent ligamentous damage, contributing to a poor outcome.

Anatomy

- The carpus is composed of two rows of small carpal bones that form three articulations (carpometacarpal, middle carpal, and radiocarpal joints). The carpometacarpal joint provides minimal flexion and is formed by the heads of the splint bones, MCIII, and distal row of small carpal bones (first, second, third and fourth carpal bones; Figure 3.37).

- The middle carpal joint is located between the two rows of carpal bones – second, third, and fourth carpal bones distally and the radial carpal, intermediate carpal and ulnar carpal proximally (Figure 3.60).
- The radiocarpal joint is the most proximal articulation in the carpus and is formed by the distal radius proximally and the radial carpal, intermediate carpal, ulnar carpal, and accessory carpal bones distally.
- The medial collateral carpal ligament extends from the medial styloid process of the radius and widens distally to attach to the proximal ends of MCII and MCIII. Bundles of fibers also attach to the radial, second, and third carpal bones (Figure 3.60a).
- The lateral collateral carpal ligament extends distad from its attachment on the styloid process of the radius to primarily MCIV. Palmar to the lateral collateral ligament, four ligaments support the accessory carpal bone; the accessorioulnar, accessoriocarpoulnar, accessorioquartal, and accessoriometacarpal ligaments (Figure 3.60b).
- Tendons of two muscles, the extensor carpi ulnaris muscle (formerly ulnaris lateralis m.) and the flexor carpi ulnaris muscle, attach to the proximal border of the accessory carpal bone.

Imaging

- Radiography is initial imaging tool to document potential IA fractures in the carpus. A minimum of six views is necessary to characterize the carpal joints.
- Scintigraphy can be useful in racehorses to document sclerosis and lysis that may occur from intense remodeling of the carpal bones.
- Both CT and MRI can be helpful to characterize subtle lesions within the carpus and may be necessary to fully recognize the amount of bone damage.

Etiology

- It is hypothesized that fatigue of the soft tissues, increased speed, poor racing surface,

(a)

Accessory carpal bone

Intermediate carpal bone

Medial collateral ligament

Radial carpal bone

Third carpal bone

Second metacarpal bone

Third metacarpal bone

Figure 3.60 Carpal ligaments, medial view (a) and lateral view (b).

(b)

Accessorioulnar ligament

Lateral collateral ligament

Accessoriocarpo-ulnar ligament

Dorsal intercarpal ligaments

Accessorioquartal ligament

Dorsal carpometacarpal ligament

Accessoriometacarpal ligament

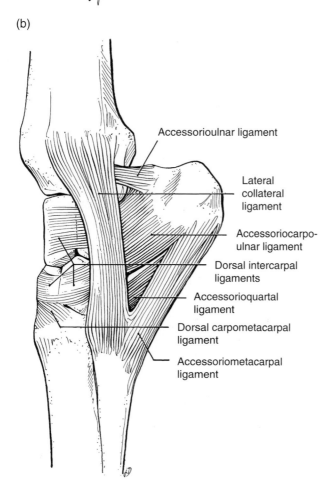

poor trimming, and uncoordinated movement may contribute to hyperextension of the carpus and/or incongruent articulation among the carpal bones, predisposing to fractures.

- Subtle geometric abnormalities within the carpal joints may also predispose these horses to fracture at speed.
- Increased axial loading that occurs with speed also leads to increased dorsal compression between opposing carpal bones. Chronic high loads as well instantaneous maximum loading likely contributes to the bone disease.
- Bone microdamage and intense bone modeling and remodeling at the sites of osteochondral fragmentation are seen with histology. Chronic repetitive stress leads to a chronic pathologic process that ultimately leads to bone failure.

Clinical Signs

- Varying degrees of synovial effusion, soft tissue swelling, pain with carpal flexion, and lameness are usually present in horses with IA carpal fractures.
- A common characteristic of their movement is abduction of the forelimbs, which some have hypothesized is an attempt to minimize carpal flexion.
- Palpation of the dorsal aspect of the carpal bones may demonstrate focal pain of specific bones, especially in horses with subchondral bone disease.
- The severity of clinical signs often indicates the severity of articular damage. Horses with fragmentation alone may have minimal lameness but palpable synovial effusion, while horses with comminuted fractures are often severely lame and have significant soft tissue swelling.
- Horses with fractures of the palmar aspect of the joints are often significantly responsive to flexion, which is reflective of the concurrent soft tissue damage.

- IA anesthesia may or may not be necessary to document the carpus as the site of the lameness and performing radiography prior to performing IA anesthesia may be advisable if there are obvious signs of osteochondral fracture.

Diagnosis

- Radiography is used to document IA fragmentation and both carpi should be radiographed in racehorses, because more than 50% will have fragmentation in both carpi (Figure 3.61).
- The third carpal skyline view is very important for detecting sclerosis, lysis, and fracture and has been shown to give a good impression of third carpal bone density.
- Images should be evaluated for osteochondral damage, the presence of OA such as osteophytes, enthesophytes, and joint space narrowing, and subchondral bone lysis.
- Fragmentation is often best seen on a flexed lateral view (Figure 3.62), while slab fractures of the carpus are often most easily seen on the standing LM projection. Damage to the third carpal bone may only be seen the skyline projection (Figure 3.63).
- Nuclear scintigraphy may be beneficial, especially in racehorses, to identify early remodeling of the carpal bones and help identify subchondral bone disease.
- Arthroscopy can be used as both a diagnostic and treatment tool for osteochondral fragmentation in some horses.

Treatment

- Arthroscopic surgery is usually the best method to fully characterize the disease process, treat the primary problem, and give an accurate prognosis for return to athletic use. The severity of articular cartilage and bone damage is correlated with the outcome.
- Arthroscopy or advanced imaging (MRI or CT) is usually recommended for horses that

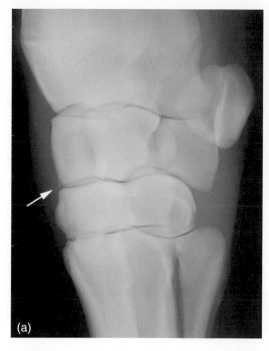
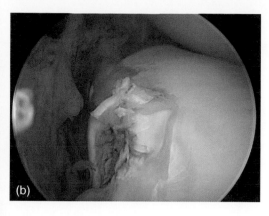

Figure 3.61 (a) A radiographic image showing a subtle fragment on the distal aspect of the radial carpal bone (arrow). (b) The corresponding surgical image is shown as well. This demonstrates how radiographs typically underestimate the severity of articular cartilage damage within the joint. Courtesy of Chris Kawcak.

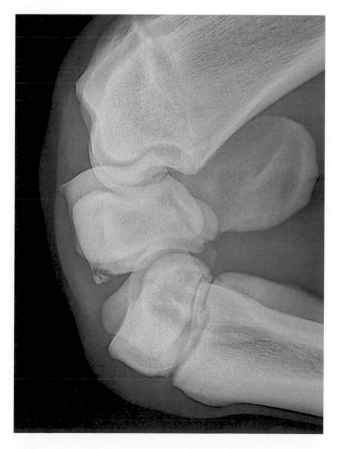

Figure 3.62 Radiograph demonstrating osteochondral chip fragments off the proximal intermediate and distal radial carpal bones (a common combination in the racing Quarter horse). Courtesy of CW McIlwraith.

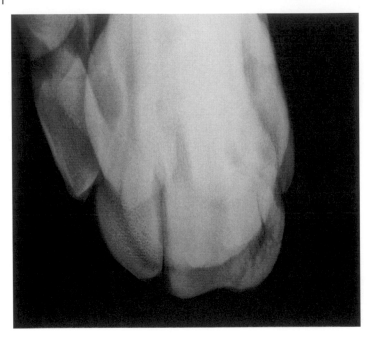

Figure 3.63 30° degree flexed dorsoproximal dorsodistal oblique radiograph showing a slab fracture of the third carpal bone with frontal and sagittal components. Courtesy of Robert Hunt.

block to one or both of the carpal joints but lack radiographic abnormalities.

- Slab fractures usually require internal fixation with lag screw fixation to have the best chance of achieving athletic soundness. The degree of joint surface damage, which is common with slab fractures, often dictates the prognosis of return to athletic use.
- Thin slab fractures of the third carpal bone (less than 5 mm) can be removed because they will not support lag screw repair.
- Sagittal slab fractures can be treated conservatively but most experienced surgeons believe that internal fixation is needed for the best prognosis.
- Comminuted fractures usually require internal fixation or arthrodesis of the carpus to restore axial stability to the limb. Conservative therapy with casting and/or splints may be used but often results in more prolonged lameness and complications (limb deviation and chronic lameness).

- In addition to rehabilitation, some form of IA therapy is recommended to reduce inflammation and speed healing, especially if there was articular cartilage damage.

Prognosis

- For Thoroughbreds and Quarter horses, the chance of racing at the same or increased level following arthroscopic surgery for osteochondral fragmentation is approximately 68%; for Standardbreds it is reported to be 74%.
- For slab fractures of the third carpal bone, approximately 65–77% of horses race after treatment but at a reduced level.
- In general, many horses that return to racing after surgery do so at a reduced level.
- Horses with comminuted fractures of the carpus usually do not return to racing, and salvage for breeding or light riding is the goal.

Accessory Carpal Bone Fractures

Overview

- Fracture of the accessory carpal bone can occur in any breed and primarily occurs in the frontal plane through the lateral groove of the bone (Figure 3.64).
- It is thought that most of these fractures heal by fibrocartilaginous nonunion due to the constant pull from the flexor muscles that attach to its proximal aspect.

Anatomy (Please refer to previous sections on "IA Carpal Fractures Carpal Sheath Tenosynovitis")

Imaging (Please refer to previous sections on "IA Carpal Fractures and Carpal Sheath Tenosynovitis")

Etiology

- Most accessory carpal bone fractures are thought to result from external trauma although it is rare to see primary skin damage over these sites.

- It is also hypothesized that they may be due to extreme internal forces such as asynchronous contraction of the flexor carpi ulnaris and ulnaris lateralis muscles or horses landing partially flexed, leading to a bowstring effect of the flexor carpi ulnaris lateralis and flexor tendons.

Clinical Signs and Diagnosis

- Horses typically have acute lameness with or without dorsal carpal or carpal canal swelling, are very painful with flexion, and may stand with their carpus flexed.
- There is often palpable pain over the accessory carpal bone, crepitus is sometimes felt, and sometimes with flexion, lateral to medial instability can be palpated.
- One frequent clinical sign is a decrease in digital pulses with flexion.
- Radiographs can usually document the fracture and it is important to image distally to the mid MCIII because fracture fragments can displace in multiple planes and even displace within the carpal canal distally.

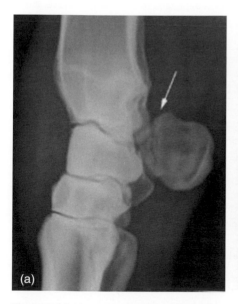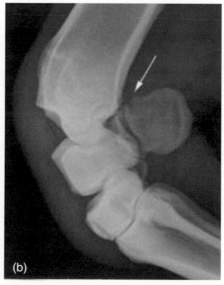

Figure 3.64 Lateromedial (a) and flexed lateromedial (b) radiographs of a fracture of the accessory carpal bone (arrows). Courtesy of Chris Kawcak.

- A complete ultrasound examination of the carpal canal should be performed as fracture fragments can cause damage to the soft tissues of the carpal canal.

Treatment and Prognosis

- Damage to the accessory carpal bone can be treated conservatively with three to six months of stall rest, small fragments can be removed via arthroscopy, or lag screw fixation of larger fractures can be performed.
- Small fragments involving the proximal dorsal aspect of the accessory carpal bone may involve the palmar aspect of the radiocarpal joint and can be removed arthroscopically.
- If possible, fragments that involve the carpal canal may also need to be removed and any soft tissue damage debrided using tenoscopy.
- Periodic radiographs should follow treatment since distraction and further lysis of the fracture due to the fibrocartilaginous nonunion may be seen over time.
- Prognosis for return to soundness is generally good but is usually reduced with carpal canal involvement.
- Horses typically have acute lameness with or without dorsal carpal or carpal canal swelling, are very painful with flexion and may stand with their carpus flexed.

OA of the Carpus/ Carpometacarpal OA

Overview

- OA is common in the carpus and can occur from joint trauma leading to secondary OA or as an insidious, progressive onset of disease regardless of the previous history.
- OA of the carpometacarpal joint is a separate syndrome that predominantly involves older Quarter horses and Arabian horses.

- OA of the carpus is often a progressive condition that may become unmanageable to the point that even pasture soundness is questionable.

Anatomy (Please refer to previous section on "IA Carpal Fractures")

Imaging (Please refer to previous section on "IA Carpal Fractures")

Etiology

- Carpal OA usually occurs in young athletes, such as racehorses, secondary to stress-related bone damage that causes physical damage to the joint.
- Carpal OA also may develop in older horses without a history of trauma. These horses often demonstrate an insidious, progressive onset of disease.
- The etiology of carpometacarpal OA is unknown, but there is a suggestion that an anatomic abnormality may exist between the second and third carpal bones.

Clinical Signs

- Carpal OA most commonly involves the middle carpal joint, and horses have varying degrees of carpal effusion, joint capsule thickening, pain on flexion, and lameness.
- Many horses have an obvious visual swelling on the medial aspect of the carpus and in severe cases the limb deviates axially (varus deformity of the carpus; Figure 3.65).
- The severity of lameness is often reflective of the severity of the OA and horses with advanced disease will have reduced range of motion and pain with carpal flexion.

Diagnosis

- Early radiographic signs of carpal OA may include mild osteophytes, enthesophytes, and osteochondral fragmentation (Figure 3.66).
- More severe abnormalities may include subchondral bone sclerosis and/or lysis, severe osteophytosis, and joint space narrowing.

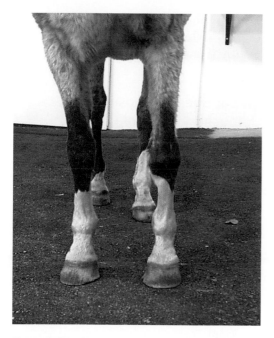

Figure 3.65 Aged mare with varus deviation of the left forelimb and swelling of the left carpus secondary to chronic OA of the carpus.

- Carpometacarpal OA is seen radiographically as osteoproliferation and joint space narrowing medially between the second carpal and second MC bone (Figure 3.67).

Treatment

- Horses with early signs of OA can be treated with controlled exercise and NSAIDs.
- Stall confinement is rarely helpful in these horses, and this supports the fact that strengthening of periarticular soft tissues is of benefit in other species.
- Paddock turn-out seems to help these horses, although their activity should be monitored to avoid excessive exercise.
- Horses with OA and osteochondral fragmentation may benefit from arthroscopy, but the goal is usually to help relieve pain and slow the progression of the disease.
- IA medication with a variety of products (corticosteroids, PSGAGs, IRAP, and other

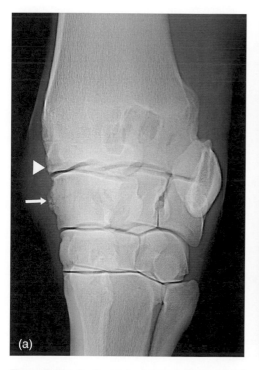

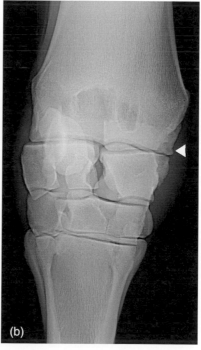

Figure 3.66 Radiographs demonstrating mild signs of osteoarthritis, including enthesiophyte (arrow) (a) and osteophyte (arrowhead) (b) formation. Courtesy of Chris Kawcak.

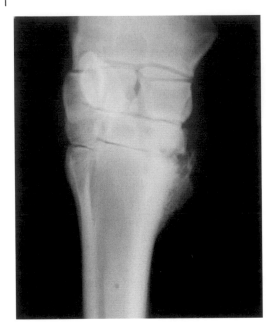

Figure 3.67 A radiograph demonstrating collapse of the medial aspect of the joint space and osteoproliferation typical of OA of the carpometacarpal joint.

biologics) can be used to primarily control the pain associated with the disease.

- A shoe with a lateral extension or a full shoe may help alleviate pain and lameness in horses with varus deformities of the carpus (Figure 3.65).
- In severe cases of OA, partial or pancarpal arthrodesis is often advocated to reduce the pain and prevent laminitis in the opposite limb.
- Carpometacarpal OA may be treated with IA drilling of the joint similarly to horses with tarsal OA or with partial carpal arthrodesis using internal fixation.

Prognosis
- The prognosis for athletic performance in horses with carpal OA is usually guarded to poor, depending on the severity.
- Most horses can be managed with a combination of systemic and IA treatments and controlled exercise, but the disease is most likely to progress.

- Horses with a varus deformity, medial joint space collapse, and significant lameness often do poorly.

Carpal Sheath Tenosynovitis/ Osteochondroma of Radius

Overview
- Effusion of the carpal sheath usually indicates a clinical problem within the sheath, and several different conditions can contribute to the effusion.
- Either the sheath itself or the structures contained within the sheath may contribute to an inflammatory response leading to effusion and lameness.

Anatomy
- The carpal canal (Figure 3.68) contains the SDFT and DDFT enclosed in the carpal synovial sheath and the medial palmar nerve and artery, and the lateral palmar nerve, artery, and vein.
- Medial to the carpal canal, the tendon of the flexor carpi radialis, enclosed in its tendon sheath, descends to its attachment on the proximal part of the second metacarpal bone.
- The carpal synovial sheath enclosing the digital flexor tendons extends from a level 8–10 cm proximal to the radiocarpal joint distad to near the middle of the metacarpus.
- An intertendinous membrane attaches to the palmaromedial surface of the DDFT and the dorsomedial surface of the SDFT, dividing the carpal synovial sheath into lateral and medial compartments.
- The accessory ligament of the SDFT is located at the most proximal aspect of the carpal sheath and can be accessed through the sheath (Figure 3.68).

Imaging
- The carpal sheath is best imaged with both radiography and ultrasonography.

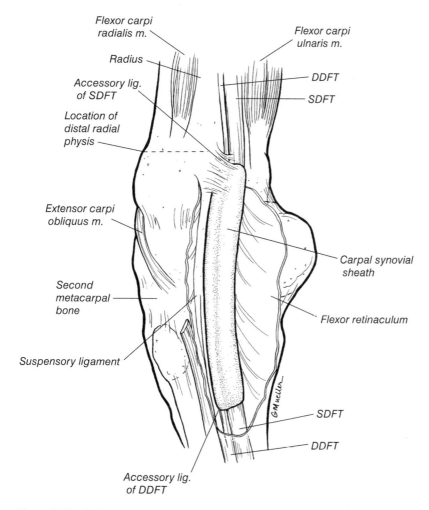

Figure 3.68 Palmaromedial view of carpus with flexor retinaculum cut and reflected. SDFT = superficial digital flexor tendon; DDFT = deep digital flexor tendon.

- Tenoscopy of the carpal sheath can serve as both a diagnostic tool as well as be therapeutic depending on the cause of the tenosynovitis.

Etiology

- Causes of carpal tenosynovitis include osteochondromas at the distal end of the radius, physeal remnants or exostoses of the distal radial physis, damage to the flexor tendons within the sheath, or desmitis of the superior check ligament of the SDFT, or as a sequela to an accessory carpal bone fracture.

- All of these predisposing conditions cause an inflammatory response within the sheath that is manifested as effusion.
- Healing of accessory carpal bone fractures may contribute to later development of carpal sheath tenosynovitis and possibly retinacular constriction.

Clinical Signs

- Affected horses often present with a history of intermittent lameness that increases with exercise.
- An obvious swelling of t.he carpal sheath cranial to the ulnaris lateralis laterally or on

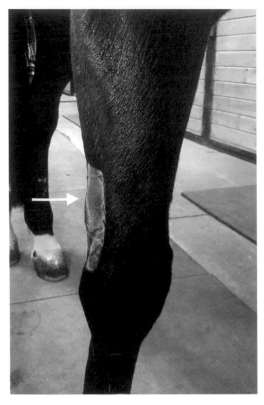

Figure 3.69 Carpal canal swelling visible (arrow) and palpable on the lateral aspect of the limb. Courtesy of Chris Kawcak.

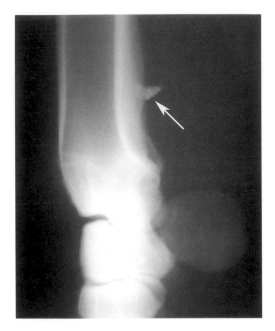

Figure 3.70 Lateral radiograph of the carpus demonstrating an osteochondroma on the caudal aspect of the distal radius (arrow).

the medial aspect of the carpus is often present (Figure 3.69).

- An osteochondroma may be palpable on the caudodistal aspect of the radius with the limb held flexed at the carpus.
- There is usually reduced range of motion to the carpus and a carpal flexion test worsens the lameness.
- In many cases, intrasynovial anesthesia of the carpal sheath is necessary to document the site of lameness.

Diagnosis

- Radiography is usually used to document the potential cause of the tenosynovitis (osteochondroma, physeal remnant, or accessory carpal bone fracture). Osteochondromas usually appear as conically shaped bony protuberances located on

the caudomedial aspect of the distal radius adjacent to the physis (Figure 3.70).

- Fractures of the accessory carpal bone are usually obvious but distal migration of small fragments contributes to carpal sheath tenosynovitis (Figure 3.71).
- Ultrasonography should be performed to determine the presence of tendon lesions, damage to the superior check ligament of the SDFT, or thickening of the retinaculum flexorum that may occur in chronic cases.
- Diagnostic tenoscopy of the carpal sheath may be required to document the cause of the tenosynovitis if other imaging modalities are nondiagnostic.

Treatment

- Surgical excision of the osteochondromas and physeal remnants via tenoscopy is the treatment of choice for these conditions.
- Tenoscopy is also recommended to facilitate debridement of lesions of the DDFT, SDFT, or superior check ligament that are visible on ultrasound.

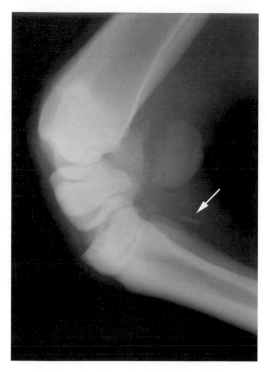

Figure 3.71 Flexed lateral radiograph of the carpus of a horse with a chronic accessory carpal bone fracture. A fragment from the accessory carpal bone (arrow) has migrated distally within the sheath, contributing to carpal sheath tenosynovitis.

- Intrasynovial medication of the sheath often reduces the effusion and lameness, but the signs will often recur if the primary problem is not addressed.
- In more chronic cases, tenoscopic examination of the carpal canal can be performed to aid in characterization of the damage and perform tenoscopic release of the carpal flexor retinaculum if necessary.

Prognosis
- The prognosis for surgical excision of solitary osteochondromas and physeal remnants is good for return to performance.
- Horses with osteochondroma or physeal remnants together with significant damage to the DDFT have a reduced prognosis.
- Prognosis for horses with accessory carpal bone fractures is usually reduced if significant carpal canal involvement occurs.

- Horses with damage to the superior check ligament and/or SDFT have a fair to good prognosis to return to performance.

Antebrachium, Elbow, and Humerus

Fractures of the Radius

Overview

- Fractures of the radius can occur in horses of any age and can occur in a variety of configurations with comminuted fractures being most common (Figure 3.72).
- Approximately 25% of radial fractures can be open and these usually involve the medial

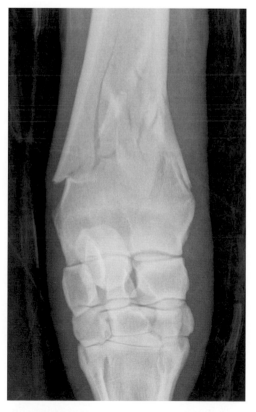

Figure 3.72 A cranial-caudal view of a distal diaphyseal comminuted fracture of the radius. Courtesy of Martin Waselau.

surface of the antebrachium where there is minimal soft tissue covering.

- Incomplete or fissure fractures are relatively common fractures of the radius, the majority of which occur along the longitudinal plane.
- Stress fractures of the radius can occur in racehorses but are uncommon compared with other locations.
- Only about 50% of radial fractures are considered repairable and young horses are more successfully treated than adults.

Anatomy

- The antebrachium includes the radius and ulna and the muscles, vessels, nerves, and skin surrounding these bones.
- The radius is a large bone that is slightly convex cranially with musculature protecting the bone except for the medial aspect. The cranial surface is the tension side of the bone and the caudal surface is the compression side (Figure 3.37).
- The antebrachial extensor muscles are located primarily on the cranial and craniolateral aspects of the radius and the flexor muscles are located more on the caudal and caudomedial aspects.

Imaging

- Radiography is the initial imaging modality to use to document a suspected radial fracture.
- Scintigraphy may be required to document stress fractures in racehorses or other types of nondisplaced fractures (i.e. kick injuries).
- CT may be useful for surgical planning of complex fractures destined to be repaired.

Etiology

- Radial fractures are usually a result of high-impact blunt trauma such as a kick from another horse.
- Kick injuries to the medial aspect of the radius often cause a fissure fracture (incomplete

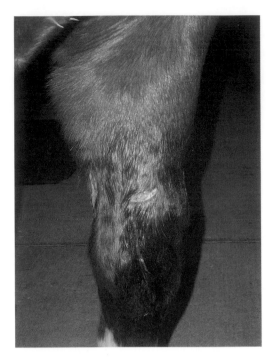

Figure 3.73 Wound on the medial aspect of the antebrachium from a kick injury. This horse had a concurrent distal radial fracture. Radiographs of the radius should always be taken in horses with these injuries.

fracture) that can run longitudinally along the diaphysis (Figure 3.73).
- Age affects fracture configuration since comminuted or butterfly fragment fractures are usually noted in older horses (older than two years), whereas simple oblique and transverse fractures occur in younger horses (Figure 3.74).

Clinical Signs

- Horses with complete fractures usually present with non-weight-bearing lameness, varying degrees of swelling in the antebrachium, and instability associated with the fracture site.
- Crepitation may be felt, and pain elicited when the distal limb is manipulated.
- Wounds or penetration of the skin from the fracture on the distal medial side of the antebrachium is common (Figure 3.73).

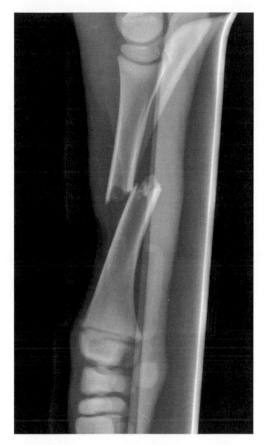

Figure 3.74 A transverse complete midshaft fracture of the radius of a foal. Courtesy of Martin Waselau.

- Horses with incomplete nondisplaced fractures are usually very lame but are willing to bear some weight on the limb.
- Horses with stress fractures can be difficult to identify on examination but often have a history of acute lameness that subsides with rest and reoccurs with exercise.

Diagnosis
- Radiography can usually identify the fracture and several views are often needed to completely evaluate the configuration and extent of the fracture.
- Comminuted and displaced fractures are easily identified whereas acute nondisplaced fractures may not be visible at all.

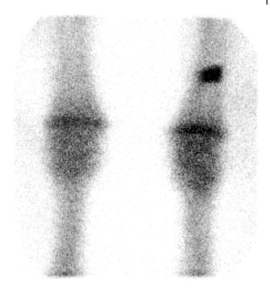

Figure 3.75 A nuclear scintigraphic examination of increased uptake of radioactive isotope in the distal radius, indicating a stress fracture of the metaphysis. Courtesy of Dan Burba.

- Nuclear scintigraphy is often necessary to identify incomplete and stress fractures (Figure 3.75), Alternatively, radiography can be repeated in a few days to a week to hopefully identify the fracture.

Treatment
- Fractures that are nondisplaced or incomplete with minimal displacement can be treated with stall confinement. It may be necessary to prevent the horse from laying down initially to prevent catastrophic breakdown of the fracture.
- Immobilization of displaced radial fractures is very important if surgery is anticipated (please refer to Chapter 7 on musculoskeletal emergencies).
- Internal fixation of complete displaced fractures of the radius is the preferred method of treatment. A single plate may be used in young foals, but two plates are recommended in most horses.
- Transfixation-pin-casts may be considered for open, contaminated fractures in which the chances of successful plate fixation are poor.

- Cast application alone has been used to successfully treat some closed distal radial fractures when there are economic constraints.

Prognosis

- Horses with nondisplaced complete and incomplete fractures and those with stress fractures appear to have a good prognosis with conservative treatment.
- The prognosis for displaced radial fractures treated with internal fixation is best for horses under two years of age (64% discharged from hospital).
- Displaced closed simple fractures including proximal physeal fractures in foals have a favorable prognosis.
- Most adult horses with complete fractures have an unfavorable prognosis for survival no matter what treatment is selected.

Fractures of the ULNA

Overview

- The ulna is a common site of fracture in young horses (79% of ulnar fractures were in horses under two years of age).
- Ulnar fractures are classified as Types I through VI (Figure 3.76). Type I and II fractures involve the apophysis in very young foals and Types III through VI involve the diaphysis of the olecranon.
- Fractures in adults often involve the articular surface and are displaced due to contracture of the triceps apparatus and fractures located distal to the level of the elbow joint typically have less distraction.

Anatomy

- The cubital (elbow) joint is formed by the radius distally, the ulna caudally, and the humerus proximally. The elbow joint contains two articulations – the radiohumeral articulation that is weight-bearing and the humeroulnar articulation that is primarily non-weight-bearing (Figure 3.37).
- The elbow joint is relatively large joint with pouches extending caudally and proximally along the ulna and distal humerus.
- The muscles adjacent to the elbow include two principal flexors, the biceps brachii and the brachialis and three principal extensors, the tensor fascia antebrachia, the triceps brachii, and the anconeus (Figure 3.77).
- All three principal extensors insert on the olecranon tuberosity of the ulna, which serves to transmit the extensor function of the triceps apparatus to the distal limb.
- Medial and lateral collateral ligaments often closely associated with the musculature serve to stabilize the elbow joint (humeroradial articulation).
- The ulna is a non-weight-bearing long bone and therefore, more amenable to internal fixation than most other equine long bones (Figure 3.37).

Imaging

- Radiography is the imaging modality of choice to document ulnar fractures.
- Ultrasonography may be used to evaluate the numerous soft tissue attachments surrounding the elbow joint.

Etiology

- Direct impact or trauma is the most common cause of most ulnar fractures.
- Kick injuries appear to be a common cause in adults and may be associated with wounds on the lateral aspect of the elbow.
- Type I and II fractures can occur from excessive tensile load of the triceps apparatus primarily in foals.

Clinical Signs

- Fractures of the ulna usually result in an acute non-weight-bearing lameness with a classic dropped elbow appearance (the carpus is flexed, and the horse will not bear weight on the limb; Figure 3.78).

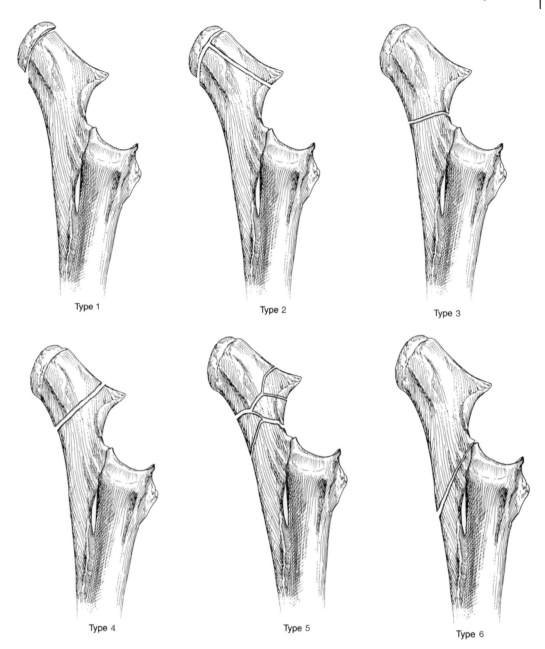

Type 1   Type 2   Type 3

Type 4   Type 5   Type 6

Figure 3.76 Classification of equine ulnar fractures.

- Nondisplaced fractures may initially show the dropped elbow appearance but will show progressive weight-bearing of the limb.
- Varying degrees of soft tissue swelling, crepitation, and skin wounds can be apparent especially in displaced fractures.

- Limb manipulation is resisted, and efforts to get the horse to load the leg, even with a splint in place, are unsuccessful until the triceps apparatus has been restored.

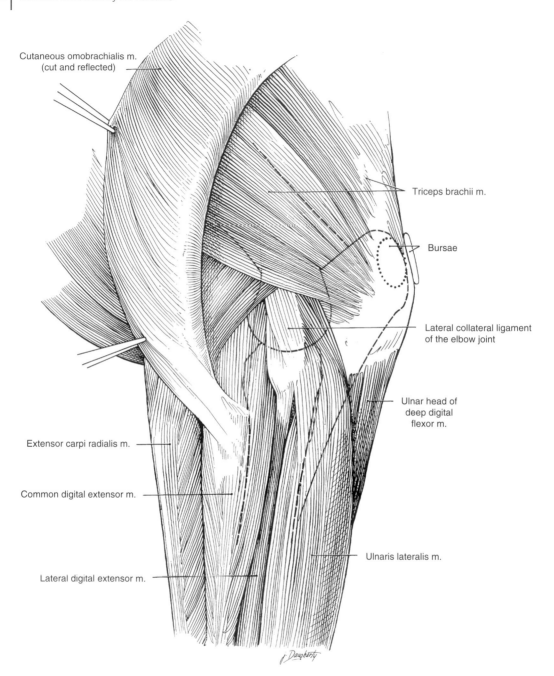

Cutaneous omobrachialis m.
(cut and reflected)

Triceps brachii m.

Bursae

Lateral collateral ligament
of the elbow joint

Ulnar head of
deep digital
flexor m.

Extensor carpi radialis m.

Common digital extensor m.

Ulnaris lateralis m.

Lateral digital extensor m.

Figure 3.77 Lateral view of the left elbow. Dashed lines represent the locations of bony elements. Note that the ulnaris lateralis is now called extensor carpi ulnaris.

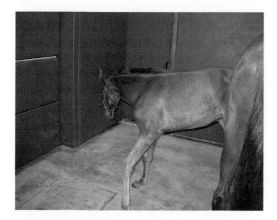

Figure 3.78 Typical dropped elbow appearance and the inability to extend the limb that can be seen in horses with fractures of the humerus or olecranon. Courtesy of Robert Hunt.

Diagnosis

- A tentative diagnosis can be made based on the classic appearance of the limb and palpation findings. Differential diagnoses may include humeral fractures, radial nerve paresis, or joint sepsis if a wound is present.

- Lateral and craniocaudal radiographs of the elbow usually provide a definitive diagnosis (Figure 3.79). It may be necessary to take a flexed-lateral view to provide distraction of the fragment to identify a Type I fracture in foals.

Treatment

- Horses with nondisplaced nonarticular ulna fractures or comminuted fractures may be treated conservatively with stall rest alone or combined with external coaptation (bandage plus caudal splint from the ground to the elbow; Figure 3.80).
- Horses with articular fractures with minimal displacement may be treated conservatively, but better results are obtained with internal fixation.
- In young horses (under six months) internal fixation may be performed using a combination of screws, pins and tension band wires, or plating.
- In older horses, application of a plate (LCP or DCP) along the caudal aspect of the ulna is

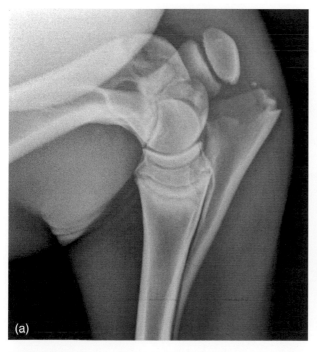
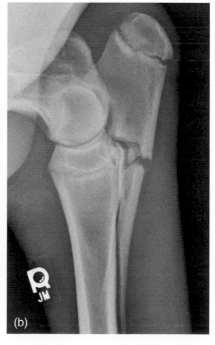

Figure 3.79 (a) Type III ulnar fracture. Courtesy of Lorrie Gaschen. (b) Type VI ulnar fracture. Courtesy of Martin Waselau.

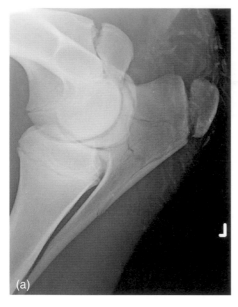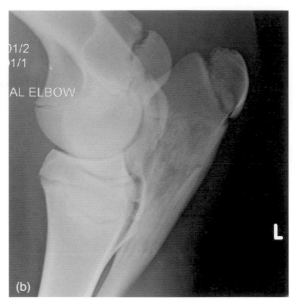

Figure 3.80 Comminuted ulna fracture in a young foal (a) that healed flowing conservative treatment (b).

recommended. The plate counteracts the tension forces of the triceps brachii muscle and is biomechanically stronger than pins and wires.

Prognosis

- The prognosis for conservative management of nondisplaced fractures, nonarticular fracture Types I and IV of the ulna are considered to be good.
- Nondisplaced articular fractures, especially Type VI fractures, also respond well to conservative treatment. One retrospective study reported 70% of affected horses becoming sound.
- The prognosis for internal fixation of displaced Type III, IV, V, and VI fractures is also considered good to very good, depending on the technique used and the intended use of the horse.

Subchondral Cystic Lesions (SCLs) of the Elbow

Overview

- SCLs of the elbow joint have been observed in a wide variety of horse breeds of all ages and usually occur on the weight-bearing surfaces of the joint.
- SCLs typically communicate with the joint, and are most commonly found on the medial side, involving either the proximal medial radius or distal medial condyle of the humerus (Figure 3.81).

Anatomy (Please refer to previous section on "Ulnar Fractures")

Imaging (Please refer to previous section on "Ulnar Fractures")

Etiology

- The two proposed causes for SCLs, regardless of location, are either development associated with OC or trauma secondary to damage to the cartilage and subchondral bone plate.

Clinical Signs

- Horses often present with a history of an acute onset of lameness that may wax and wane with use.
- On physical examination, there are usually no localizing signs other than lameness. Palpation of the caudal aspect of the elbow joint capsule may reveal fluid distension and thickening.

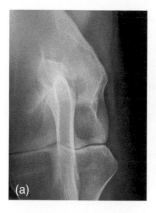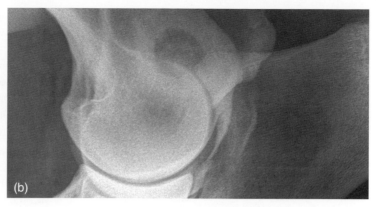

Figure 3.81 Subchondral cystic lesion located on the axial aspect of the lateral epicondyle of the humerus demonstrated on craniocaudal (a) and lateral (b) radiographic views. This cyst was observable arthroscopically. Courtesy of Alanna Zantingh.

- Flexion and extension of the elbow region often elicits a painful response and usually exacerbates the lameness. Intrasynovial anesthesia often eliminates the lameness.

Diagnosis

- Radiographs are required to make the diagnosis. The craniocaudal view often identifies the SCL on the proximal medial aspect of the radius or humerus.
- Nuclear scintigraphy may be necessary to localize the lameness and help identify the site of the SCL in cases of early traumatic lesions.

Treatment

- SCLs may be treated conservatively with rest and IA medications or surgically using an extra-articular or arthroscopic approach. Surgical extra-articular nucleation of the cyst is thought to provide a better long-term success with less evidence of OA than conservative therapy.
- Debridement or osteostixis with or without steroid injections either via arthroscopic guidance or in an extra-articular manner is recommended by some.
- Injection of the SCL with corticosteroids either via arthroscopic guidance or in an extra-articular manner can also be performed.

- If horses that are treated conservatively do not appear to be resolving or the lameness does not improve, surgical intervention may be advised.

Prognosis

- The prognosis appears good for conservative treatment of SCLs as long as there is no radiographic evidence of OA.
- The prognosis for horses treated surgically is difficult to predict but is thought to improve the outcome of horses that do not respond to conservative treatment.

Bursitis of the Elbow (Olecranon Bursitis)

Overview

- "Shoe boil" or "capped elbows" are two common names for this condition.
- It may occur on one or both elbows and is characterized by a movable swelling over the point of the olecranon tuberosity.
- Bursal enlargement usually results in a painless swelling that does not typically interfere with function unless it becomes greatly enlarged.
- With chronicity, thickening of the bursal wall by fibrous tissue develops and fibrous

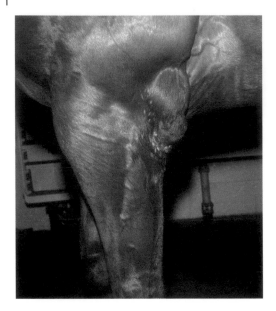

Figure 3.82 A chronic, infected, acquired capped elbow of the left forelimb.

bands and septa may develop within the bursal cavity and subcutaneous tissue.
- An infected bursa is usually painful, causes lameness, and may break open and drain (Figure 3.82).

Anatomy

- All three principal extensor muscles of the elbow insert on the olecranon tuberosity and a subcutaneous bursa may cover its caudal aspect.
- A subtendinous bursa lies deep to the tendon of insertion of the long head of the massive triceps brachii muscle (Figure 3.77).
- In most cases, inflammation of the subcutaneous bursa leads to visible swelling that is associated with olecranon bursitis.

Imaging

- Ultrasonography is usually the initial imaging modality that can determine the content and extent of the swelling.
- Radiography including contrast radiography can help to determine any underlying bone

involvement as well as the precise location and extent of the fluid distention.

Etiology

- Acquired bursitis is commonly caused by repetitive trauma from the shoe of the affected limb hitting the point of the elbow during motion, or more commonly when the horse is lying down.
- The trauma results in a transudative fluid accumulating in the subcutaneous tissue, which becomes encapsulated by fibrous tissue. A synovial-like membrane develops, producing fluid that is similar to joint fluid.
- American Saddlebreds and Standardbreds may hit their elbows during exercise repeatedly.
- The bursae may become infected by a puncture wound or following intra-bursal treatment.

Clinical Signs

- The condition is characterized by a prominent, often freely movable, fluid-filled swelling over the point of the elbow.
- With chronicity, the swelling may be comprised primarily of fibrous tissue and may be fixed in position (Figure 3.82).
- Lameness usually is not present, unless the bursa is greatly enlarged or infected.
- Infected bursae are typically warm and painful to firm palpation with or without purulent drainage.

Diagnosis

- The diagnosis can usually be made on physical exam findings alone.
- If infection is suspected, radiographs should be taken to rule out trauma or infection involving the olecranon process.
- Ultrasound can be helpful to determine the content of the swelling (fluid vs. scar tissue), where the fluid extends, and whether deeper structures are involved.

Treatment

- In the acute stage, the condition may resolve by preventing further trauma to the region with the use of a shoe boil roll or boot.

- The fluid can be removed aseptically, and corticosteroids injected into the bursa, although this treatment does not appear to be very successful.
- Intralesional injection of dilute iodine or iodine-based radiographic contrast material or packing the incised bursa with iodine-soaked gauze also has been recommended, with variable success.
- Surgical intervention, either by placing drains or en bloc resection, appears to have the greatest success.

Prognosis

- The prognosis for conservative treatment to achieve an acceptable cosmetic outcome is guarded.
- En bloc resection is regarded as a superior way to manage olecranon bursitis with good results.

Fractures of the Humerus

Overview

- Fractures of the humerus can occur in horses of any age, breed, or sex, but most often affect foals under one year of age, racing or race training Thoroughbreds, and horses that are used for jumping or steeplechase events.
- Most humeral fractures are complete, closed, and displaced, involve the middle third of the diaphysis, and have considerable overriding of the fracture fragments (Figure 3.83a).
- It is uncommon for proximal complete humeral fractures to become displaced because of the stability provided by the surrounding muscles (supraspinatus, infraspinatus, subscapularis, and deltoid), biceps

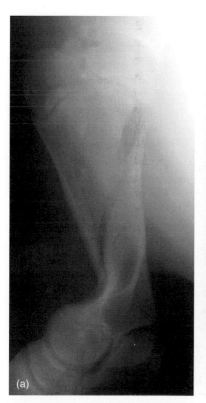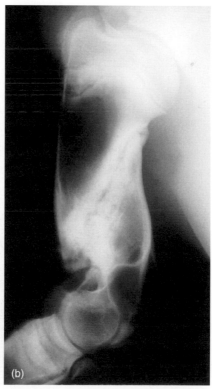

Figure 3.83 (a) Oblique lateral view of a spiral nonarticular fracture of the midhumerus. (b) Lateral view of a healing spiral nonarticular fracture of the midhumerus treated conservatively for five months.

tendinous insertions, and periarticular capsular attachments of the shoulder.

- Incomplete stress fractures occur in two typical locations in racehorses: the proximal caudal lateral cortex and the distal cranial medial cortex.

Anatomy

- The "arm" is the region of the limb between the elbow and the shoulder and includes the humerus and its surrounding musculature.
- The humerus has a short, thick configuration that is surrounded by heavy musculature making it less likely to fracture (Figure 3.37).
- The cutaneous omobrachialis muscle covers the entire humeral region arising lateral to the scapula and extending as far distally as the elbow (Figure 3.77).
- The radial nerve courses in the musculospiral groove of the humerus and may be traumatized to varying degrees as a result of the fracture or during surgical repair.

Imaging

- Radiography is used to confirm humeral fractures in most cases. Oblique views may be required as craniocaudal views can be difficult to obtain in standing horses.
- Scintigraphy is required to document incomplete or stress fractures of the humerus.
- Ultrasonography is primarily used to document problems within the bicipital bursa or the proximal aspect of the humerus.

Etiology

- Humeral fractures frequently occur in foals and weanlings secondary to falls or other impact injuries.
- In racing breeds, they occur subsequent to falling during a race or catastrophic failure of the bone as a result of accumulated stress and microfracture.
- Deltoid tuberosity fractures and proximal humeral fractures may occur from kick injuries or running into objects.

- The configuration of the fracture is usually predictable – when a force is applied in a craniocaudal direction, the humerus fractures transversely and when a force is applied in a lateral to medial direction, the humerus fractures obliquely.
- Horses sustaining stress fractures are at an increased risk to develop a complete fracture if they are not managed properly.

Clinical Signs

- Horses with nondisplaced or minimally displaced fractures may present with a history of a severe lameness that quickly improved. Swelling and pain on deep palpation are usually present at the site of injury.
- Horses with complete displaced fractures usually present with an acute onset of severe non-weight-bearing lameness. Moderate-to-severe swelling of the muscles overlying the humerus is often seen, the elbow is usually dropped, and there is an increased range of motion when the limb is manipulated.
- Horses with stress fractures often present as a nondescriptive lameness with no palpable findings. The lameness usually improves quickly, and manipulation of the elbow and shoulder often exacerbates the lameness.

Diagnosis

- Radiography is used to confirm the fracture and define the configuration in most cases except with stress fractures. Usually lateral-medial and slightly oblique lateral-medial views can be taken in the standing, sedated horse, but foals can often be restrained in lateral recumbency.
- Craniocaudal views of the entire humerus are more difficult to obtain and may require general anesthesia, depending on the size of the animal.
- Nuclear scintigraphy is usually needed to document stress fractures within the humerus (Figure 3.84).

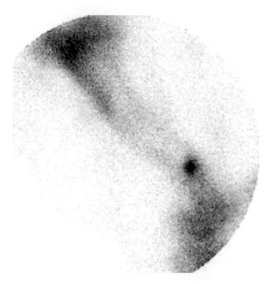

Figure 3.84 Nuclear scintigraphic examination of the humerus with increased isotope uptake indicative of a distal metaphyseal stress fracture. Courtesy of Dan Burba.

Treatment

- Currently, three options are considered when managing a horse with a humeral fracture: nonsurgical management with prolonged stall rest (three to six months), surgical stabilization, and euthanasia. The majority of older horses with complete, displaced diaphyseal fractures are euthanized.
- Nonsurgical management is recommended to treat stress fractures and most minimally displaced fractures, regardless of the location. Some complete, displaced mid-diaphyseal fractures can be treated conservatively because the heavy musculature helps to stabilize the fracture while it heals. A better outcome is usually obtained in foals, compared with adults (Figure 3.83).
- Surgical management using intramedullary pinning, bone plating, and interlocking intramedullary nailing or any combination have been used successfully to treat young horses and ponies with humeral fractures.
- In general, the smaller the horse, the greater the chance for success regardless of the type of for internal fixation that was used.

- Small open fractures of the deltoid tuberosity or greater tubercle are often best removed surgically, especially if concurrent infection is present.

Prognosis

- The prognosis for stress fractures, nondisplaced complete or incomplete fractures, or minimally displaced complete nonarticular fractures managed conservatively appears very good.
- The prognosis for complete displaced nonarticular fractures is guarded but appears better for horses managed conservatively. Diaphyseal fractures that are spiral and oblique with minimal overriding are the best candidates for nonsurgical treatment (Figure 3.83).
- The prognosis for fractures involving the greater tubercle and deltoid tuberosity is also very good with either conservative or surgical treatment.

Shoulder and Scapula

Bicipital (Intertubercular Bursa) Bursitis

Overview

- Inflammation of the intertubercular (bicipital) bursa can occur in horses of any age, breed, or sex and can be confused with other types of shoulder lameness.
- Bicipital bursitis can be septic or nonseptic in origin.

Anatomy

- The heavy, partly cartilaginous tendon of the biceps brachii muscle originates on the supraglenoid tubercle (SGT) of the scapula and occupies the intertubercle groove of the humerus.
- In addition to flexing the elbow, the biceps brachii fixes the elbow and shoulder in the standing position.

- An intertubercle bursa (bicipital bursa) lies between the bilobed biceps tendon and the M-shaped tubercles at the cranioproximal aspect of the humerus (Figure 3.37).
- Although uncommon, communication can exist between the shoulder joint and the bicipital bursa.

Imaging

- Radiography and ultrasonography are both usually required to characterize abnormalities within the bicipital bursa.
- Scintigraphy may be useful to detect early infected or actively remodeling bone adjacent to the bursal region when ultrasound and radiography appear normal.

Etiology

- Trauma to the cranial surface of the shoulder region is the most common cause of a primary bursitis.
- Falls or slips that result in flexion of the shoulder with extension of the elbow or stretching or tearing of the bursa or biceps tendon during the cranial phase of the stride with the limb in full extension may also occur.
- Infection, either from an open or penetrating wound or from hematogenous spread to the bursa, also may occur. Septic bicipital bursitis may be associated with the "joint ill" syndrome in foals.

Clinical Signs

- A history of trauma to the shoulder region is common and swelling over the cranial aspect of the shoulder may be evident in acute cases.
- Digital pressure applied over the biceps tendon and bursal region and manipulation of the shoulder region in flexion and extension usually result in a painful response.
- The lameness can be severe in acute cases and is often characterized by a shortened cranial phase of the stride, reduced carpal flexion, and a fixed shoulder appearance during movement. The horse is often reluctant to bear full weight on the limb.

- Generalized shoulder and pectoral muscle atrophy may be seen in more chronic cases and the severity of lameness can be variable.
- Intrasynovial anesthesia of the bursa is the best method to document the bursa as the site of the lameness.

Diagnosis

- Both radiography and ultrasonography of the shoulder region are often needed to completely assess the bicipital bursa. Generally, the mediolateral, craniomedial to caudolateral oblique, and flexed cranioproximal to craniodistal (skyline) radiographs are taken in adult horses.
- If a wound or draining tract is present, centesis with contrast material may help assess communication with the bursa.
- Ultrasound examination of the biceps tendon, bursa, and bicipital groove can be very informative, especially when radiographs appear normal. Ultrasound changes associated with bursitis have included edema or hemorrhage in the biceps tendon or bursa, disruption of the tendon architecture with peritendinous thickening, an irregular surface of the bicipital groove, and hyperechoic material in the bicipital bursa (Figure 3.85).

Treatment

- Noninfectious bursitis without evidence of bone or soft tissue pathology usually respond favorably to rest and a controlled exercise program, parenteral and/or topical NSAIDs, and intrasynovial medications.
- ESWT may benefit bicipital tendon lesions particularly those that are ossified.
- Ultrasound-guided intralesional treatment of tendon injuries may be performed with PRP, IRAP, stem cells, or other biologics.
- Bursitis from either a fracture, osteitis of the proximocranial aspect of the humerus (Figure 3.86), or sepsis generally requires surgery to resolve the problem. Incisional as well as endoscopic approaches to the bursa have been described, but bursoscopy is recommended.

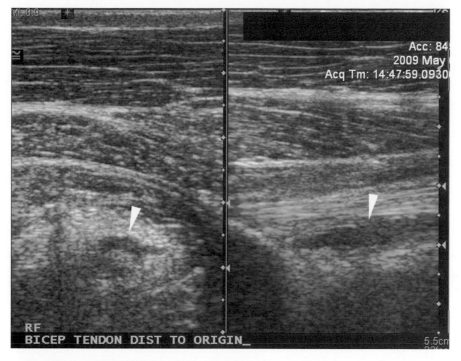

Figure 3.85 Core lesion of the medial branch of the biceps tendon just distal to the origin of the biceps brachii muscle (arrowheads). Courtesy of Jeremy Hubert.

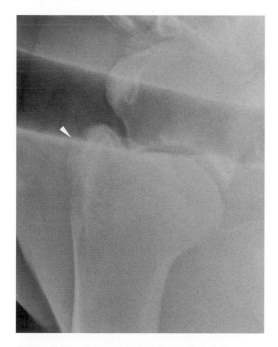

Figure 3.86 Osseous changes on the tubercles of the cranioproximal humerus (arrowhead). Infiltration of lidocaine into the bursa resolved the lameness in this case. Courtesy of Jeremy Hubert.

- Septic bursitis is treated similarly to other types and locations of intrasynovial sepsis.

Prognosis
- Acute cases of nonseptic bursitis in the absence of a fracture or tendon injury often respond favorably to conservative treatment.
- Conservative therapy for more chronic cases of nonseptic or septic bursitis appears less satisfactory.
- The prognosis is considered poor for horses with chronic septic bursitis, but surgical intervention is thought to improve the prognosis.

Osteochondrosis (OC) of the Scapulohumeral (Shoulder) Joint

Overview

- Shoulder OC is most frequently diagnosed in weanlings and yearlings 6–12 months of age but has been reported in horses up to eight years old.

- Males appear to be more commonly affected than females and no specific breed predilection has been identified.
- The condition is the most debilitating form of OC and when it is diagnosed in older yearlings, chronic secondary OA is usually present.
- Lesions may be located on the humeral head, glenoid of the scapula, or both the glenoid and humeral head (most common) and often affect a major part of the joint surface.

Anatomy

- The scapulohumeral joint is a ball-and-socket-type joint that is formed by the humeral head and the glenoid cavity of the scapula (Figure 3.37). The articular surface of the humeral head is about twice the surface area of the glenoid cavity.
- A large portion of both the proximal humerus (greater and lesser tubercles) and distal scapula (SGT) are extra-articular and serve as attachment sites for important tendons and muscles (Figure 3.37).
- Two elastic glenohumeral ligaments reinforce the joint capsule as they diverge from the SGT to the humeral tuberosities. However, much of the stability of the shoulder joint is provided by the surrounding musculature.
- Muscles around the joint restrict abduction and adduction and rotation of the joint is very limited.

Imaging

- Radiographs are necessary to definitively diagnose OC lesions in the shoulder and both joints should be radiographed because the lesions can be bilateral.
- Arthroscopy may occasionally be used as both a diagnostic and therapeutic tool when other imaging techniques are inconclusive.

Etiology

- In most cases, OC is considered developmental in origin. Overnutrition, imbalanced nutrition, and a genetic predisposition to rapid growth may all be contributory.
- Some SCLs of the glenoid may be associated with trauma and not OC, but this is difficult to document.

Clinical Signs

- Most cases present with a history of moderate-to-severe forelimb lameness with an insidious onset.
- Atrophy of the muscles associated with the shoulder region is a common finding in chronic cases.
- A smaller foot with a higher heel and excessive toe wear is also commonly observed in the foot of the affected limb and can be confused with a club foot.
- Direct, firm pressure with the thumb just cranial to the tendon of the infraspinatus muscle over the shoulder joint may elicit a painful response.
- The lameness is often characterized by a shortened cranial (extension) phase of the stride, a prominent shoulder lift, reduced carpal flexion, and limb circumduction may occur in severely affected horses. Upper limb extension/flexion is usually painful and increases the signs of lameness.
- Intrasynovial anesthesia can be used to localize the lameness to the shoulder region.

Diagnosis

- Radiographs are necessary to definitively diagnose the lesion. The most common radiographic findings include (Figure 3.87):
1) Flattening and indentation of the caudal aspect of the humeral head.
2) Alterations in the contour of the glenoid cavity with a subchondral cystic radiolucency.
3) Osteophytes at the caudal and cranial aspect of the glenoid cavity.
4) Subchondral bone sclerosis/lysis.

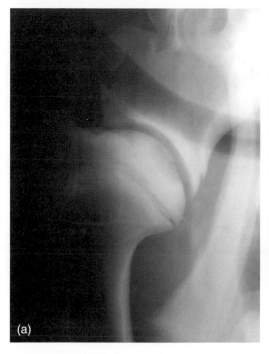 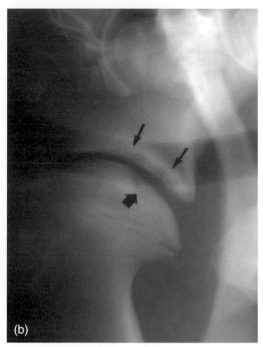

Figure 3.87 Radiographic manifestations of OCD of the shoulder. (a) The defect in the humeral head is the only lesion. (b) Defect in both the humeral head (large black arrow) and glenoid of the scapula (small black arrows). Courtesy of CW McIlwraith.

5) Remodeling of the humeral head and glenoid cavity.

- Arthroscopy may be needed to make a definitive diagnosis in cases in which the lameness is localized to the shoulder, but no lesion is identified radiographically.

Treatment

- Arthroscopic debridement of lesions is currently the recommended treatment for most horses. With very large lesions or those with severe degenerative changes, the prognosis is poor, and surgery is usually not recommended (Figure 3.88).
- Rest and confinement may be considered for horses not intended for athletic performance that have mild-to-moderate radiographic changes.
- Euthanasia may be required in horses with severe lameness and radiographic abnormalities with a very poor prognosis.

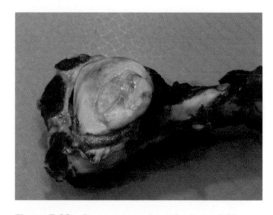

Figure 3.88 Postmortem view of a large OCD lesion of the caudal humeral head that had severe radiographic signs of OA.

Prognosis

- Generally, the prognosis for rest or surgery is considered guarded, but is dependent on the intended use of the horse and the severity of the OC lesion.

- Horses with mild-to-moderate OC lesions have the best prognosis and those with severe lesions usually remain lame.
- Currently, the prognosis is about 50–50 following arthroscopic debridement but depends on case selection.

Osteoarthritis (OA) of the Scapulohumeral (Shoulder) Joint

Overview

- Shoulder OA is an uncommon condition that can affect a variety of breeds, ages, and uses of horses. A higher incidence has been in Shetland ponies, miniature horses, and Falabella ponies, suggesting a possible congenital cause.
- Shoulder OA is often secondary to either a congenital, developmental, infectious, or traumatic cause.

Anatomy (Please refer to previous section on "Shoulder OC")

Imaging (Please refer to previous section on "Shoulder OC")

Etiology

- Shoulder OA can have multiple causes but is nearly always secondary.
- In younger horses, a developmental role due to OC may be the cause, whereas traumatic joint injury is more likely in older horses.
- Dysplasia of the glenoid cavity and/or chronic subluxation of the shoulder joint as is seen in some breeds of ponies may also predispose to OA.

Clinical Signs

- The signs of lameness are typical of shoulder lameness, and the degree depends on the severity and duration of the problem.
- Mild swelling may be apparent over the shoulder region in acute cases, but muscle atrophy is variable and may not reflect the chronicity or severity of the lameness.
- Upper limb manipulation (flexion, extension, adduction, and abduction) may also result in a painful response.
- Ponies with chronic shoulder subluxation and severe OA are often lame at the walk, usually "fix" the joint on each stride, and have atrophy of the shoulder musculature.

Diagnosis

- Radiography, ultrasound, nuclear medicine, and/or arthroscopy may be required to make a definitive diagnosis depending on the stage of the disease.
- Radiography often underestimates the full extent of the changes involving the glenoid cavity and the humeral head and subtle abnormalities can be difficult to interpret.
- Radiographic signs of significant shoulder OA include glenoid sclerosis/lysis, SCLs of the glenoid, alteration in the contour of the humeral head, osteophytes, enthesophytes, and shoulder subluxation (Figure 3.89).

Treatment

- Conservative treatment may be indicated in horses with mild lameness and minimal radiographic lesions. Treatment may involve controlled exercise, NSAIDs, and IA medications.
- Arthroscopic exploration may be necessary in horses that do not respond to other treatments to help both diagnose and the treat the primary problem.
- Horses/ponies with severe shoulder OA can be difficult to manage. IA corticosteroids are usually necessary to help control the pain.
- Arthrodesis of the shoulder can be successfully performed in ponies with severe OA.

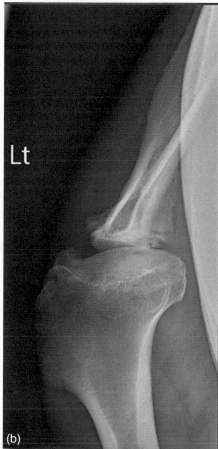

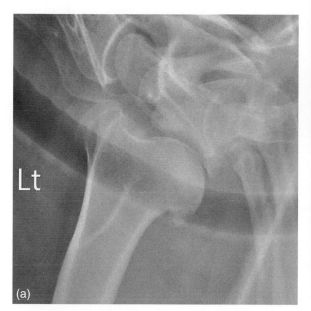

Figure 3.89 Radiographs of a subluxated left shoulder in a miniature horse that was lame at the walk. The humerus and scapula were positioned more laterally than normal (a), and the joint had significant radiographic signs of OA (b).

Prognosis

- The prognosis appears favorable for horses without significant radiographic lesions that respond favorably to conservative therapy and IA medications.
- Horses with obvious radiographic evidence of OA generally do not respond well to most any type of therapy.
- The prognosis for horses treated by arthroscopy appears good for mild lesions, provided that the OA does not progress.
- The prognosis for ponies/miniature horses with shoulder dysplasia does not appear

favorable although shoulder arthrodesis can successfully resolve the problem in select cases (Figure 3.89).

Suprascapular Nerve Injury (Sweeny)

Overview

- The term "sweeny" has been defined as atrophy of the shoulder muscles in horses and is a commonly used synonym for suprascapular nerve paralysis.

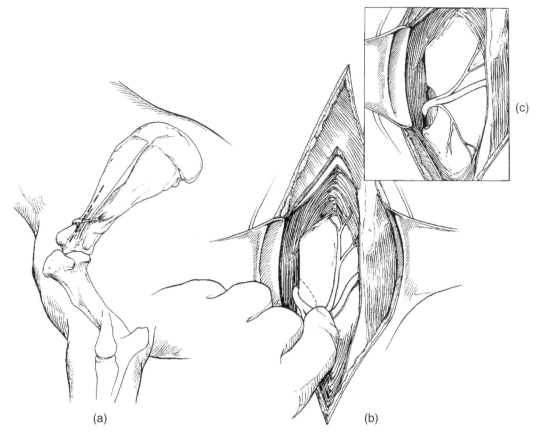

Figure 3.90 The suprascapular nerve courses over the cranial edge of the scapula (a) and is thought to be vulnerable to trauma (b & c). The dotted line is the location of the surgery site for the scapular notch procedure (a).

- Suprascapular nerve injury resulting in atrophy of the supraspinatus and infraspinatus muscles and shoulder joint instability can affect any age or breed of horse.
- The condition was originally reported to occur in draft breeds due to repeated trauma to the shoulder region from poorly fitted harness collars.
- Currently, "sweeny" is most commonly seen in horses as result of acute trauma to the shoulder region.

Anatomy

- The suprascapular nerve originates from the sixth and seventh cervical spinal segments and passes via the brachial plexus to innervate the supraspinatus and infraspinatus muscles.

- As the nerve reflects around the cranial edge of the scapula, it passes beneath a small but strong tendinous band and is susceptible to direct trauma and compression against the underlying bone (Figure 3.90).
- The infraspinatus and supraspinatus muscles provided lateral stability to the shoulder joint, and denervation of these muscles results in lateral luxation/subluxation of the shoulder (i.e. shoulder slip).

Imaging

- Radiography of the region should be obtained to rule out an underlying problem within the shoulder region.
- Electromyographic evaluation (EMG) of the supraspinatus and infraspinatus muscles is

necessary to confirm selective suprascapular nerve injury, although this is not routinely performed.

Etiology

- Trauma to the suprascapular nerve as it passes over the cranial thin border of the scapula is believed to be the cause.
- It has been suggested that chronic neuronal injury may make the suprascapular nerve more susceptible to acute trauma or that spontaneous development of the condition, without a traumatic insult, may be possible.
- Trauma to the suprascapular nerve may also occur secondary to surgical procedures in the shoulder region.

Clinical Signs

- The clinical signs vary, depending on the extent of the nerve damage and the duration of the condition prior to examination.
- Horses with acute injuries often exhibit severe pain and are reluctant to bear weight on the affected limb. As the pain subsides and the horse begins to bear weight, a pronounced lateral instability (excursion) of the shoulder joint (shoulder slip) during weight-bearing is observed.
- The outward excursion of the shoulder may cause intermittent stretching of the suprascapular nerve, leading to continued trauma and perpetuation of the paralysis.
- The progression of the condition depends on the amount of damage to the nerve and can range from temporary neuropraxia to complete severance and denervation.
- Horses with temporary neuropraxia may regain normal function within a few days to weeks, whereas those with true nerve damage will develop significant muscle atrophy as early as 10–14 days after injury (Figure 3.91).

Diagnosis

- A presumptive diagnosis of suprascapular nerve injury can be made from the clinical signs and the history of trauma.
- Radiographs of the region should be obtained to rule out a fracture, OA, or luxation of the shoulder joint.

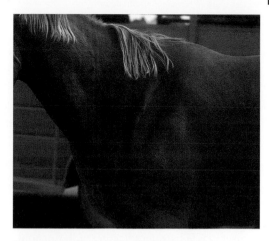

Figure 3.91 Prominent atrophy of the supraspinatus muscle is evident in this horse with suprascapular nerve injury.

- EMGs of the muscles can confirm selective suprascapular nerve injury but are not accurate until a minimum of seven days after injury.
- EMG findings of denervation of muscles supplied by other branches of the brachial plexus should prompt further evaluation of other neurologic problems.

Treatment

- Initial treatment is directed toward reducing inflammation in the region of the nerve. Stall rest, systemic and local NSAIDs, and topical cryotherapy are usually indicated.
- Conservative treatment consisting of confinement with or without injection of the shoulder joint may be used until shoulder joint stability returns.
- Based on peripheral nerve regeneration rates (1 mm/day), nerve function should return within 10–12 weeks. In one study, the mean time for resolution of the gait abnormality was 7.4 months and 7/8 horses evaluated had complete resolution.
- Surgical decompression or the "scapular notch procedure" may be considered in patients that continue to exhibit signs of suprascapular nerve dysfunction after 10–12 weeks. Entrapment of the suprascapular nerve by scar tissue between the overlying ligament and the cranial border of the scapula is thought to occur in these horses.

- Some surgeons suggest that faster resolution of the clinical signs can be obtained with surgical decompression earlier in the disease process (before 10 weeks).

Prognosis

- The prognosis for return to soundness is reported to be favorable for both conservative and surgical treatments. Seven of eight horses treated conservatively became sound and 18/20 horses treated surgically became sound in two different reports.
- A severe complication associated with the surgery is subsequent fracture of the glenoid.
- Horses that have severe muscle atrophy prior to surgery may not regain normal muscle mass.

Fractures of the Scapula/ Supraglenoid Tubercle (SGT)

Overview

- Scapular fractures can occur in all ages and breeds of horses, although young intact males appear more prone to sustain the fracture.
- Scapular fractures can also result in fatal musculoskeletal injuries in racing Quarter horses and Thoroughbreds.
- Fractures of the scapula can involve the spine, SGT, body, neck, and glenoid cavity.
- Fractures of the SGT are most common and are often simple, IA, and usually affect horses less than two years of age.

Anatomy

- The scapula is a thin, flat bone that helps form the shoulder joint distally and is attached to the withers via the dorsoscapular ligament and surrounding musculature (Figure 3.37).
- The spine of the scapula courses along the outer surface of the bone for about 2/3rd its most proximal length. Numerous muscles attached to the spine.
- The scapula is surrounded by extensive musculature that stabilizes the bone to the trunk

and essentially attaches the limb to the body of the horse.
- The SGT is the most cranial protuberance of the scapula and serves as the proximal attachment for the biceps brachii muscle and two glenohumeral ligaments that support the scapulohumeral joint (Figure 3.37).

Imaging

- Radiography can usually document most distal scapular fractures but some fractures through the body of the scapula can be difficult to image.
- Scintigraphy is necessary to document suspected stress and incomplete fractures.
- Ultrasonography can be used to diagnose some scapular fractures, especially those involving the scapular spine and superficial aspect of the scapula.

Etiology

- Fracture of the SGT is most frequently associated with trauma (falling or direct blows) to the cranial shoulder region.
- Overflexion of the shoulder leading to increased tension on the biceps brachii and coracobrachialis tendons that attach to the SGT also has been proposed as a cause.
- It has also been suggested that SGT fractures may result from a separation of the physis of the SGT in young horses.
- Scapular fractures resulting from racing or race falls at high speeds tend to be comminuted.
- Bone sequestra may also develop following fractures of the scapular spine, particularly when a penetrating wound is present.

Clinical Signs

- A history of trauma resulting in severe lameness that improves rapidly is common with fractures of the SGT.
- Swelling over the point of the shoulder, pain on palpation, and crepitus are usually present in acute cases of SGT fractures.
- Horses with an acute fracture of the scapular spine usually exhibit focal swelling, will often bear weight, and usually exhibit a mild-to-moderate lameness at exercise.

- Lameness severity may vary depending on fracture location and duration, but the cranial phase of the stride is often markedly shortened, and the horse may carry the limb more axially than normal.
- Horses with fractures of the body or neck of the scapula are usually reluctant to bear weight initially, have difficulty advancing the affected limb, and often have swelling over the fracture site (Figure 3.92).
- Varying degrees of muscle atrophy are usually apparent in chronic cases and upper limb flexion tests usually worsen the lameness.

Diagnosis

- Radiography is used to make a definitive diagnosis in most cases. Medial to lateral, ventrodorsal, and oblique cranial to caudal radiographic projections reveal most fractures of the scapula.
- Some fractures through the body of the scapula can be difficult to image because of the superimposition of the ribs and vertebrae over the scapula.
- The size and type of SGT fractures (simple vs. comminuted) can vary, but generally the fracture is displaced due to the pull of the biceps tendon (Figure 3.93).
- If a fracture is suspected but not observed, the horse can be re-radiographed in two weeks or scintigraphy can be performed.

Treatment

- Some minimally displaced nonarticular fractures of the scapular body and neck, stress fractures, and fractures of the spine may be treated conservatively with good results.
- Transverse fractures of the body and proximal neck can be surgically treated with internal fixation in young animals.
- Treatment options for SGT fractures include conservative management, removal, or internal fixation with lag screws or bone plates.
- Conservative management (confinement for three to four months) can be used in horses with nonarticular or minimally displaced SGT fractures.

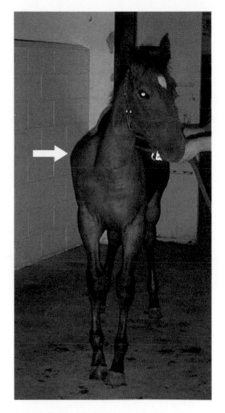

Figure 3.92 Prominent swelling located over the lateral right shoulder region of a young horse with a complete fracture of the body of the scapula. The foal was lame at the walk and carried the limb further axially than normal.

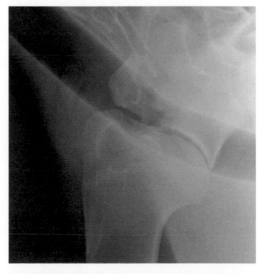

Figure 3.93 Fracture of the supraglenoid tubercle of the scapula with moderate displacement.

- Surgical excision of the SGT is best for horses with chronic or comminuted articular fractures. Removal of the fragment is thought to decrease the pain caused by movement of the fracture and prevent further joint damage.
- Internal fixation is recommended for large articular SGT fractures that can support plates and screws. The goal of surgery is to prevent secondary OA caused by joint incongruity.
- Bone plating combined with partial or complete transection of the biceps brachii tendon is currently the recommended surgical approach.

Prognosis

- Young horses with nonarticular simple or minimally comminuted fractures of the body and proximal neck have a good prognosis for soundness after application of internal fixation.

- In adults, nondisplaced fractures of the body or neck may heal satisfactorily with conservative therapy.
- Horses with complete fractures in the distal neck, articular fractures, and severely comminuted fractures all have a poor prognosis for return to performance.
- A good prognosis for return to performance can be expected for conservative management of horses that have nonarticular or minimally displaced articular fractures of the SGT.
- The prognosis following surgical excision of the fracture is considered to be better than for conservative management, but this depends on the fracture type and complications that may occur (i.e. suprascapular nerve injury).
- The prognosis for internal fixation appears best if a combination of internal fixation and complete transection of the biceps brachii tendon is used.

Bibliography

1 Adams MN, Turner TA: 1999. Endoscopy of the intertubercular bursa in horses. *J Am Vet Med Assoc* 214:221–225.

2 Anderson DE: 1995. Comminuted, articular fractures of the olecranon process in horses: 17 cases. *Vet Comp Orthop Traumatol* 8:141–145.

3 Anthenill LA, Stover SM, Gardner IA, et al.: 2007. Risk factors for proximal sesamoid bone fractures associated with exercise history and horseshoe characteristics in Thoroughbred racehorses. *Am J Vet Res* 68:760–761.

4 Arensburg L, Wilderjans H, Simon O, et al.: 2011. Nonseptic tenosynovitis of the digital flexor tendon sheath caused by longitudinal tears in the digital flexor tendons: A retrospective study of 135 tenoscopic procedures. *Equine Vet J* 43:660–668.

5 Bani Hassan E, Mirams M, Hrasem-Zadeh A, et al.: 2016. Role of subchondral bone remodeling in collapse of the articular surface of Thoroughbred racehorses with palmar osteochondral disease. *Equine Vet J* 48:228–233.

6 Barber SM, Penizzi L, Lang HM: 2009. Treatment of carpal metacarpal osteoarthritis by arthrodesis in 12 horses. *Vet Surg* 38:1006–1011

7 Barr AR, Sinnott MJ, Denny HR: 1990. Fractures of the accessory carpal bone in the horse. *Vet Rec* 126:432–434.

8 Barr ED, Pinchbeck GL, Clegg PD, et al.: 2009. Postmortem evaluation of palmar osteochondral disease (traumatic osteochondrosis) of the metacarpo/metatarsophalangeal joint in Thoroughbred racehorses. *Equine Vet J* 41:366–371. https://doi.org/10.2746/042516409X368372.

9 Barrett EJ, Rodgerson DH: 2014. Ultrasound assisted arthroscopic approach for removal of basilar sesamoid fragments of the proximal sesamoid bones in horses. *Vet Surg* 43:712–714.

10 Bassage LH, Richardson DW: 1998. Longitudinal fractures of the condyles of the third metacarpal and metatarsal bones in racehorses: 224 cases (1986–1995). *J Am Vet Med Assoc* 212:1757–1761.

11 Baxter GM, Doran RE, Allen D: 1992. Complete excision of a fractured fourth metatarsal bone in eight horses. *Vet Surg* 21:273–276.

12 Beinlich CP, Nixon AJ: 2005. Prevalence and response to surgical treatment of lateral palmar intercarpal ligament avulsion in horses: 37 cases (1990–2001). *J Am Vet Med Assoc* 226:760–766.

13 Beisser A, McClure S, Rezabek G, et al.: 2014. Frequency of and risk factors associated with catastrophic musculoskeletal injuries in Quarter Horses at two Midwestern racetracks: 67 cases (2000–2011). *J Am Vet Med Assoc* 245:1160–1168.

14 Bertone AL: 2004. Distal Limb: Fetlock and Pastern. *In:* Hinchcliff KW, Kaneps AJ, Goer RJ (eds) *Equine Sports Medicine and Surgery*, Oxford, Elsevier Science Ltd., 289–319.

15 Bischofberger AS, Furst A, Auer J, et al.: 2009. Surgical management of complete diaphyseal third metacarpal and metatarsal bone fracture: Clinical outcome in 10 mature horses and 11 foals. *Equine Vet J* 41:465–473.

16 Bleyaert H: 1998. Shoulder Injuries. *In:* White N, Moore J (eds) *Current Techniques of Equine Surgery and Lameness.* Philadelphia, WB Saunders and Co., 422–423.

17 Bleyaert HF, Madison JB: 1999. Complete biceps brachii tenotomy to facilitate internal fixation of supraglenoid tubercle fractures in three horses. *Vet Surg* 28:48–53.

18 Bramlage L: 1996. Fetlock Arthrodesis. *In:* Nixon AJ (ed) *Equine Fracture Repair*, Philadelphia. WB Saunders Co, 17–172.

19 Brokken MT, Schneider RK, Sampson SN, et al.: 2007. Magnetic resonance imaging features of proximal metacarpal and metatarsal injuries in the horse. *Vet Radiol Ultrasound* 48:507–517.

20 Brokken, MT, Schneider RK, Tucker RL: 2008. Surgical approach for removal of nonarticular base sesamoid fragments of the proximal sesamoid bones in horses. *Vet Surg* 37:619–624.

21 Brommer HB, Voermans M, Verra S, et al.: 2014. Axial osteitis of the proximal sesamoid bones and desmitis of the intersesamoidean ligament in the hindlimb of Friesian horses: Review of 12 cases (2002–2012) and post-mortem analysis of the bone-ligament interface. *BMC Vet Res* 10:272. https://doi.org/10.1186/s12917-014-0272-x.

22 Busschers, E, Richardson DW, Hogan PM, et al.: 2008. Surgical repair of mid-body proximal sesamoid bone fractures in 25 horses. *Vet Surg* 37:771–780.

23 Carmalt JL, Borg H, Naslund H, et al.; 2014. Racing performance in Swedish Standardbred trotting horses with proximal palmar/plantar first phalangeal (Birkeland) fragments compared to fragment free controls. *Vet J* 202:43–47.

24 Carmalt JL, Borg H, Naslund H, Waldner C: 2015. Racing performance in standardbred trotting horses with proximal palmar/plantar first phalangeal fragments relative to the timing of surgery. *Equine Vet J* 47:433–437.

25 Carpenter RS, Galuppo LD, Simpson EL, et al.: 2008. Clinical evaluation of the locking compression plate for fetlock arthrodesis in six Thoroughbred racehorses. *Vet Surg* 37:263–268.

26 Carrier TK, Estberg L, Stover SM, et al.: 1998. Association between long periods without high-speed workouts and risk of complete humeral or pelvic fracture in Thoroughbred racehorses: 54 cases (1991–1994). *J Am Vet Med Assoc* 212:1582–1587.

27 Carter BG, Schneider RK, Hardy J, et al.: 1993. Assessment and treatment of equine humeral fractures: Retrospective study of 54 cases (1972–1990). *Equine Vet J* 25:203–207.

28 Chesen AB, Dabareiner RM, Chaffin MK, et al.: 2009. Tendinitis of the proximal aspect of the superficial digital flexor tendon in horses: 12 cases (2000–2006) *J Am Vet Med Assoc* 234:1432–1436.

29 Colon JL, Bramlage LR, Hance SR, et al.: 2000. Qualitative and quantitative documentation of the racing performance of 461 Thoroughbred racehorses after arthroscopic removal of dorsoproximal first

phalanx osteochondral fractures (1986–1995). *Equine Vet J* 32:475.

30 Crabill MR, Chaffin MK, Schmitz DG: 1995. Ultrasonographic morphology of the bicipital tendon and bursa in clinically normal quarter horses. *Am J Vet Res* 56:5–10.

31 Crabill MR, Watkins JP, Schneider RK, et al.: 1995. Double plate fixation of comminuted fractures of the second phalanx in horses in 10 cases (1985–1993). *J Am Vet Med Assoc* 207:1458–1461.

32 Dabareiner RM, White NA, Sullins KE: 1996. Radiographic and arthroscopic findings associated with subchondral lucency of the distal radial carpal bone in 71 horses. *Equine Vet J* 28:93–97.

33 Dallap BL, Bramlage LR, Embertson RM: 1999. Results of screw fixation combined with cortical drilling for treatment of dorsal cortical stress fractures of the third metacarpal bone in 56 Thoroughbred racehorses. *Equine Vet J* 31:252.

34 Davis AM, Fan X, Shen L, et al: 2017. Improved radiological diagnosis of palmar osteochondral disease in the Thoroughbred racehorse. *Equine Vet J* 49:454–460.

35 Denny H, Barr A, Waterman A: 1987. Surgical treatment of fractures of the olecranon in the horse: A comparative review of 25 cases. *Equine Vet J* 19:319–325.

36 Derungs S, Fuerst A, Haas C, et al.: 2001. Fissure fractures of the radius and tibia in 23 horses: A retrospective study. *Equine Vet Educ* 13:313–318.

37 Doran R: 1996. Fractures of the Small Metacarpal and Metatarsal (Splint) Bones. *In:* Nixon AJ (ed): *Equine Fracture Repair.* Philadelphia, Saunders, 20–200.

38 Doyle PS, White NA: 2000. Diagnostic findings and prognosis following arthroscopic treatment of subtle osteochondral lesions in the shoulder joint of horses: 15 cases (1996–1999). *J Am Vet Med Assoc* 217:1878–1882.

39 Dubois M, Morello S, Rayment K, et al.: 2014. Computed tomographic imaging of subchondral fatigue cracks in the distal end of the third metacarpal bone in the Thoroughbred racehorse can predict crack micromotion in an ex-vivo model. *PLoS One* 9:7. https://doi.org/10.1371/journal.pone.0101230.

40 Dutton DM, Honnas CM, Watkins JP: 1999. Nonsurgical treatment of suprascapular nerve injury in horses: 8 cases (1988–1998). *J Am Vet Med Assoc* 214:1657–1659.

41 Dyson S, Denoix J: 1995. Tendon, tendon sheath, and ligament injuries in the pastern. *Vet Clin North Am Equine Pract* 11:217–233.

42 Dyson S: 1986. Shoulder lameness in horses: An analysis of 58 suspected cases. *Equine Vet J* 18:29–36.

43 Dyson S: 1985. Sixteen fractures of the shoulder region in the horse. *Equine Vet J* 17:104–110.

44 Dyson SJ, Arthur RM, Palmer SC, et al.: 1995. Suspensory ligament desmitis. *Vet Clin North Am Equine Pract* 11:177–184.

45 Dyson SJ: 1995. Proximal suspensory desmitis in the hindlimb. *Equine Vet J* 7:275–280.

46 Dyson SJ, Weekes JS, Murray RC: 2007. Scintigraphic evaluation of the proximal metacarpal and metatarsal regions of horses with proximal suspensory desmitis. *Vet Radiol Ultrasound* 48:78–85.

47 Dyson SJ: 1992. Some observations on lameness associated with pain in the proximal metacarpal region. *Equine Vet J Suppl* 6:43–46.

48 Dyson SJ: 2004. Medical management of superficial digital flexor tendinitis: A comparative study in 219 horses (1992–2000). *Equine Vet J* 36:415–19.

49 Dyson SJ, Murray RC: 2011. Management of hindlimb proximal suspensory desmopathy by neurectomy of the deep branch of the lateral plantar nerve and plantar fasciotomy: 155 horses (2003–2008). *Equine Vet J* 44:361–367.

50 Edinger J, Mobius G, Ferguson J: 2005. Comparison of tenoscopic and ultrasonographic methods of examination of the digital flexor tendon sheath in horses. *Vet Comp Orthop Traumatol* 18:209–214.

51 Fischer AT, Jr., Stover SM: 1987. Sagittal fractures of the third carpal bone in horses: 12 cases (1977–1985). *J Am Vet Med Assoc* 191:106–108.

52 Fiske-Jackson AR, Barker WHJ, et al.: 2013. The use of intrathecal analgesia and contrast radiography as preoperative diagnostic methods for digital flexor tendon sheath pathology. *Equine Vet J* 45:36–40.

53 Fiske-Jackson AR, Crawford AL, Archer RM, et al.: 2010. Diagnosis, management, and outcome in 19 horses with deltoid tuberosity fractures. *Vet Surg* 39:1005–1010.

54 Fjordbakk CT, Strand E, Milde AK, et al.: 2007. Osteochondral fragments involving the dorsomedial aspect of the proximal interphalangeal joint in young horses: 6 cases (1997–2006). *J Am Vet Med Assoc* 230:1498–1501.

55 Fortier LA, Nixon AJ, Ducharme NG, et al.: 1999. Tenoscopic examination and proximal annular ligament desmotomy for treatment of equine "complex" digital sheath tenosynovitis. *Vet Surg* 28:429–435.

56 Fugaro MN, Adams SB: 2002. Biceps brachii tenotomy or tenectomy for the treatment of bicipital bursitis, tendinitis, and humeral osteitis in 3 horses. *J Am Vet Med Assoc* 220:1508–1511.

57 Galuppo LD, Simpson EL, Greenman SL, et al.: 2006. A clinical evaluation of a headless, titanium, variable-pitched, tapered, compression screw for repair of nondisplaced lateral condylar fractures in Thoroughbred racehorses. *Vet Surg* 35:423–430.

58 Garret KS, Bramlage LR, Spike-Pierce DL, et al.: 2013. Injection of platelet- and leukocyte-rich plasma at the junction of the proximal sesamoid bone and the suspensory ligament branch for treatment of yearling Thoroughbreds with proximal sesamoid bone inflammation and associated suspensory ligament branch desmitis. *J Am Vet Med Assoc* 243:120–125

59 Goodrich LR, Nixon AJ, Conway JD, et al.: 2014. Dynamic compression plate (DCP) fixation of propagating medial condylar fractures of the third metacarpal/metatarsal bone in 30 racehorses: Retrospective analysis (1990–2005). *Equine Vet J* 46:695–700.

60 Goodship AE: 1993. The pathophysiology of flexor tendon injury in the horse. *Equine Vet Educ* 5: 23–29.

61 Grondahl AM, Gaustad G, Engeland A: 1994. Progression and association with lameness and racing performance of radiographic changes in the proximal sesamoid bones of young standardbred trotters. *Equine Vet J* 26:152–155.

62 Groom LJ, Gaughan EM, Lillich JD, et al.: 2000. Arthrodesis of the proximal interphalangeal joint affected with septic arthritis in 8 horses. *Can Vet J* 41:117–123.

63 Halper J, Kim B, Khan, A, et al.: 2006. Degenerative suspensory ligament desmitis as a systemic disorder characterized by proteoglycan accumulation. *BMC Vet Res* 12:2–12.

64 Hewes CA, White NA: 2006. Outcome of desmoplasty and fasciotomy for desmitis involving the origin of the suspensory ligament in horses: 27 cases (1995–2004). *J Am Vet Med Assoc* 229:407–412.

65 Hill AE, Gardner IA, Carpenter TE, et al.: 2016. Prevalence, location and symmetry of noncatastrophic ligamentous suspensory apparatus lesions in California Thoroughbred racehorses, and association of these lesions with catastrophic injuries. *Equine Vet J* 48:27–32.

66 Hogan PM, McIlwraith CW, Honnas CM, et al.: 1997. Surgical treatment of subchondral cystic lesions of the third metacarpal bone: Results in 15 horses (1986–1994). *Equine Vet J* 29:477–482.

67 Holcombe SJ, Schneider RK, Bramlage LR, et al.: 1995. Lag screw fixation of noncomminuted sagittal fractures of the proximal phalanx in racehorses: 59 cases (1973–1991) *J Am Vet Med Assoc* 206:1195–1199.

68 Honnas CM, Schumacher J, McClure SR, et al.: 1995. Treatment of olecranon bursitis in horses: 10 cases (1986–1993). *J Am Vet Med Assoc* 206:1022–1026.

69 Hopen LA, Colahan PT, Turner TA, et al.: 1992. Nonsurgical treatment of cubital subchondral cyst-like lesions in horses: Seven cases (1983–1987). *J Am Vet Med Assoc* 200:527–530.

70 Imboden I, Waldern NM, Wiestner T, et al.: 2008. Short term analgesic effect of extracorporeal shock wave therapy in horses with proximal palmar metacarpal/plantar metatarsal pain. *Vet J* 179: 50–59.

71 Jackson M, Furst A, Hassig M, et al.: 2007. Splint bone fractures in the horse: A retrospective study 1992–2001. *Equine Vet Educ* 19:329–335.

72 Jackson M, Kummer M, Auer J, et al.: 2011. Treatment of type 2 and 4 olecranon fractures with locking compression plate (LCP) osteosynthesis in horses: A prospective study (2002–2008). *Vet Comp Orthop Traumatol* 24:57–61.

73 James FM, Richardson DW: 2006. Minimally invasive plate fixation of lower limb injury in horses: 32 cases (1999–2003). *Equine Vet J* 38:246–251.

74 Jenner F, Ross MW, Martin BB, et al.: 2008. Scapulohumeral osteochondrosis. A retrospective study of 32 horses. *Vet Comp Orthop Traumatol* 21:406–412.

75 Joyce J, Baxter GM, Sarrafian TL, et al.: 2006. Use of transfixation pin casts to treat adult horses with comminuted phalangeal fractures: 20 cases (1993–2003). *J Am Vet Med Assoc* 229:725–730.

76 Kamm JL, Bramlage LR, Schnabel LV, et al.: 2011. Size and geometry of apical sesamoid fracture fragments as a determinant of prognosis in Thoroughbred racehorses. *Equine Vet J* 43:412–417.

77 Kane AJ, Stover SM, Gardner IA, et al.: 1996. Horseshoe characteristics as possible risk factors for fatal musculoskeletal injury of Thoroughbred racehorses. *Am J Vet Res* 57:1147–1151.

78 Kasashima Y, Kuwano A, Katayama Y, et al.: 2002. Magnetic resonance imaging application to live horse for diagnosis of tendinitis. *J Vet Med Sci* 64:577–582.

79 Kawcak CE, Barrett MF: 2016. Carpus. *In:* McIlwraith CW, Frisbie D, Kawcak CE, et al. (eds) *Joint Disease in the Horse.* St. Louis, MO, Elsevier, 318–331.

80 Kawcak CE, McIlwraith CW, Norrdin RW, et al.: 2000. Clinical effects of exercise on subchondral bone of carpal and metacarpophalangeal joints in horses. *Am J Vet Res* 61:1252–1258.

81 Kawcak CE, McIlwraith CW: 1994. Proximodorsal first phalanx osteochondral chip fragmentation in 336 horses. *Equine Vet J* 26:392–396.

82 Kay A: 2006. An acute subchondral cystic lesion of the equine shoulder causing lameness. *Equine Vet Educ* 18:316–319.

83 King JN, Zubrod CJ, Schneider RK, et al.: 2013. MRI findings in 232 horses with lameness localized to the metacarpo(tarso) phalangeal region and without a radiographic diagnosis. *Vet Radiol Ultrasound* 54:36–47.

84 Knox PM, Watkins JP: 2006. Proximal interphalangeal joint arthrodesis using a combination plate-screw technique in 53 horses (1994–2003). *Equine Vet J* 38: 538–542.

85 Kraus BM, Richardson DW, Nunamaker DM, et al.: 2004. Management of comminuted fractures of the proximal phalanx in horses: 64 cases (1983–2001) *J Am Vet Med Assoc* 224:254–263.

86 Kuemmerie JM, Auer JA, Rademacher N, et al.: 2008. Short incomplete sagittal fractures of the proximal phalanx in ten horses not used for racing. *Vet Surg* 37:193–200.

87 Lacitiqnola L, Crovace A, Rossi G et al.: 2008. Cell therapy for tendinitis, experimental and clinical report. *Vet Res Commun* Suppl 1: S33–38.

88 Lang HM, Nixon AJ: 2015. Arthroscopic removal of discrete palmar carpal osteochondral fragments in horses: 25 cases (1999–2013) *J Am Vet Med Assoc* 246:998–1004.

89 Le Roux C, Carstens A: 2018. Axial sesamoiditis in the horse: A review. *J S Afr Vet Assoc* 89:e1–e8.

90 Lescun TB, McClure SR, Ward MP, et al.: 2007. Evaluation of transfixation casting for treatment of third metacarpal, third metatarsal, and phalangeal fractures in horses: 37 cases (1994–2004). *J Am Vet Med Assoc* 230:1340–1349.

91 Levine DG, Richardson DW: 2007. Clinical use of the locking compression plate (LCP) in horses: A retrospective study of 31 cases (2004–2006). *Equine Vet J* 39:401–406.

92 Lischer CJ, Ringer SK, Schnewlin M, et al.: 2006. Treatment of chronic proximal suspensory desmitis in horses using focused electrohydraulic shockwave therapy. *Schweiz Arch Tierheilkd* 148:561–568.

93 Mackay R: 2006. Peripheral Nerve Injury. *In:* Auer JA, Stick J (eds) *Equine Surgery, Third Edition*. St Louis, Saunders, 685–686.

94 MacKinnon MC, Bonder D, Boston RC, et al.: 2015. Analysis of stress fractures associated with lameness in Thoroughbred flat racehorses training on different track surfaces undergoing nuclear scintigraphic examination. *Equine Vet J* 47:296–301.

95 MacLellan KN, Crawford WH, MacDonald DG: 2001. Proximal interphalangeal joint arthrodesis in 34 horses using two parallel 5.5 mm cortical bone screws. *Vet Surg* 30:454–459.

96 Malone ED, Les CM, Turner TA: 2003. Severe carpometacarpal osteoarthritis in older Arabian horses. *Vet Surg* 32:191–195.

97 Markel MD, Richardson DW: 1985. Noncomminuted fractures of the proximal phalanx in 69 horses. *J Am Vet Med Assoc* 186:573–579.

98 Marr CM, Love S, Boyd JS, et al.: 1993. Factors affecting the clinical outcome of injuries to the superficial digital flexor tendon in National Hunt and Point-2-Point racehorses. *Vet Rec* 132:476–479

99 Martin F, Richardson DW, Nunamaker DM, et al.: 1995. Use of tension band wires in horses with fractures of the ulna: 22 cases (1980–1992). *J Am Vet Med Assoc* 207:1085–1089.

100 McGhee JD, White NA, Goodrich LR: 2005. Primary desmitis of the palmar and plantar annular ligaments in horses: 25 cases (1990–2003). *J Am Vet Med Assoc* 226:83–86.

101 McIlwraith CW, Nixon AJ, Wright IM: 2015. *Diagnostic and Surgical Arthroscopy in the Horse, Fourth edition*. London, Elsevier.

102 McIlwraith CW, Yovich JV, Martin GS: 1987. Arthroscopic surgery for the treatment of osteochondral chip fractures in the equine carpus. *J Am Vet Med Assoc* 191:531–540.

103 McIlwraith CW: 2005. Diagnostic and Surgical Arthroscopy of the Phalangeal Joints. *In:* McIlwraith CW, Nixon AJ, Wright IM, (eds) *Diagnostic and Surgical Arthroscopy in the Horse*. Philadelphia, Elsevier, 347–364.

104 McLellan J, Plevin S: 2014. Do radiographic signs of sesamoiditis in yearling Thoroughbreds predispose the development of suspensory ligament branch injury? *Equine Vet J* 46:446–450.

105 Mez JC, Dabareiner RM, Cole RC, et al.: 2007. Fractures of the greater tubercle of the humerus in horses: 15 cases (1986–2004). *J Am Vet Med Assoc* 230:1350–1355.

106 Minshall GJ, Wright IM: 2014. Frontal plane fractures of the accessory carpal bone and implications for the carpal sheath of the digital flexor tendons. *Equine Vet J* 46:579–584.

107 Nixon A: 1996. Fractures of the Ulna. *In:* Nixon A (ed) *Equine Fracture Repair*, Philadelphia, WB Saunders, 222–230.

108 Nixon AJ, Schachter BL, Pool RR: 2004. Exostoses of the caudal perimeter of the radial physis as a cause of carpal synovial sheath tenosynovitis and lameness in horses: 10 cases (1999–2003). *J Am Vet Med Assoc* 224:264–270.

109 Nixon AJ: 1996. Fractures of the Humerus. *In:* Nixon A (ed) *Equine Fracture Repair.* Philadelphia, WB Saunders, 242–253.

110 Nixon AJ: 2006. Phalanges and the Metacarpophalangeal and Metatarsophalangeal Joints. *In:* Auer JA, Stick JA (eds) *Equine Surgery, Third Edition.* Philadelphia, Elsevier, 1217–1238.

111 Norris Adams M, Turner TA: 1999. Endoscopy of the intertubercular bursa in horses. *J Am Vet Med Assoc* 214:221–225.

112 Nunamaker DM, Nash RA: 2008. A tapered-sleeve transcortical pin external skeletal fixation device for use in horses: Development, application, and experience. *Vet Surg* 37:725–732.

113 Nunamaker DM: 1996. Metacarpal stress fractures. *In:* Nixon AJ (ed) *Equine Fracture Repair.* Philadelphia, WB Saunders, 195–199.

114 O'Brien T, Baker TA, Brounts SH, et al.: 2011. Detection of articular pathology of the distal aspect of the third metacarpal bone in thoroughbred racehorses: Comparison of radiography, computed tomography and magnetic resonance imaging. *Vet Surg* 40: 942–951.

115 O'Sullivan CB, Lumsden JM: 2003. Stress fractures of the tibia and humerus in Thoroughbred racehorses: 99 cases (1992–2000). *J Am Vet Med Assoc* 222: 491–498.

116 Olive J, Mair TS, Charles B: 2009. Use of standing low-field magnetic resonance imaging to diagnose middle phalanx bone marrow lesions in horses. *Equine Vet Educ* 21:116–123.

117 Olive J, Serraud N, Vila T, et al: 2017. Metacarpophalangeal joint injury patterns on magnetic resonance imaging: A comparison in racing Standardbreds and Thoroughbreds. *Vet Radiol Ultrasound* 58:588–597.

118 Owen KR, Dyson SJ, Parkin TD, et al.: 2008. Retrospective study of palmar/plantar annular ligament injury in 71 horses: 2001–2006. *Equine Vet J* 40:237–244.

119 Pankowski R, Grant BD, Sande R, et al.: 1986. Fracture of the supraglenoid tubercle: Treatment and results in five horses. *Vet Surg* 15:33–39.

120 Parente EJ, Richardson DW, Spencer P: 1993. Basal sesamoidean fractures in horses: 57 cases (1989–1991). *J Am Vet Med Assoc* 202:1293.

121 Parkin TD, Clegg PD, French NP, et al.: 2004. Risk of fatal distal limb fractures among Thoroughbreds involved in the five types of racing in the United Kingdom. *Vet Rec* 154:493–497.

122 Parkin TD, Clegg PD, French NP, et al.: 2006. Catastrophic fracture of the lateral condyle of the third metacarpus/metatarsus in UK racehorses – fracture descriptions and pre-existing pathology. *Vet J* 171:157–165.

123 Penizzi L, Barber SM, Lang HM, et al.: 2009. Carpal metacarpal osteoarthritis in 33 horses. *Vet Surg* 38:998–1005.

124 Penizzi L, Barber SM, Lang HM, et al.: 2011. Evaluation of a minimally invasive arthrodesis technique for the carpal metacarpal joint in horses. *Vet Surg* 40:464–472.

125 Perkins NR, Reid SW, Morris RS: 2005. Risk factors for injury to the superficial digital flexor tendon and suspensory apparatus in Thoroughbred racehorses in New Zealand. *N Z Vet J* 53: 184–192.

126 Peterson PR, Pascoe JR, Wheat JD: 1987. Surgical management of proximal splint bone fractures in the horse. *Vet Surg* 16:367–372.

127 Pinchbeck GL, Clegg PD, Boyde A, et al.: 2013. Pathological and clinical features associated with palmar/plantar osteochondral disease of the metacarpo/metatarsophalangeal joint in Thoroughbred racehorses. *Equine Vet J* 45:587–592. https://doi.org/10.1111/evj.12036.

128 Plevin S, McLellan J, O'Keeffe T: 2016. Association between sesamoiditis, subclinical ultrasonographic suspensory ligament branch change and subsequent

clinical injury in yearling Thoroughbreds. *Equine Vet J* 48:543–547.

129 Powell SE: 2012. Low field standing magnetic resonance imaging findings of the metacarpo/metatarsophalangeal joint of racing thoroughbreds with lameness localized to the region: A retrospective study of 131 horses. *Equine Vet J* 44:169–177.

130 Radcliffe RM, Cheetham J, Bezuidenhout AJ, et al.: 2008. Arthroscopic removal of palmar/plantar osteochondral fragments from the proximal interphalangeal joint in four horses. *Vet Surg* 37:733–740.

131 Rakestraw PC, Nixon AJ, Kaderly RE, et al.: 1991. Cranial approach to the humerus for repair of fractures in horses and cattle. *Vet Surg* 20:1–8.

132 Ramzan PL, Palmer L, Powell SE: 2015. Unicortical condylar fractures of the Thoroughbred fetlock: 45 cases (2006–2013). *Equine Vet J* 47:680–683.

133 Redding W, Pease A: 2010. Imaging of the shoulder. *Equine Vet Educ* 22:199–209.

134 Richardson DW: 1996. Fractures of the Proximal Phalanx. *In:* Nixon AJ (ed) *Equine Fracture Repair*, Philadelphia, WB Saunders, 117–128.

135 Riggs CM, Whitehouse GH, Boyde A: 1999. Pathology of the distal condyles of the third metacarpal and third metatarsal bones of the horse. *Equine Vet J* 31:140–148.

136 Rose PL, Seeherman H, O'Callaghan M: 1997. Computed tomographic evaluation of comminuted middle phalangeal fractures in the horse. *Vet Radiol Ultrasound* 38:424–429.

137 Russell TM, MacLean AA: 2006. Standing surgical repair of propagating metacarpal and metatarsal condylar fractures in racehorses. *Equine Vet J* 38: 423–427.

138 Sampson SN, Schneider RK, Tucker RL, et al.: 2007. Magnetic resonance imaging features of oblique and straight distal sesamoidean desmitis in 27 horses. *Vet Radiol Ultrasound* 48:303–311.

139 Sarrafian TL, Case JT, Kinde H, et al.: 2012. Fatal musculoskeletal injuries of Quarter Horse racehorses: 314 cases (1990–2007). *J Am Vet Med Assoc* 241:935–942.

140 Schnabel LV, Bramlage LR, Mohammed HO, et al.: 2006. Racing performance after arthroscopic removal of apical sesamoid fracture fragments in Thoroughbred horses age > or =2 years: 84 cases (1989–2002). *Equine Vet J* 38:446–451.

141 Schnabel LV, Bramlage LR, Mohammed HO, et al.: 2007. Racing performance after arthroscopic removal of apical sesamoid fracture fragments in Thoroughbred horses age <2 years: 151 cases (1989–2002). *Equine Vet J* 39:64–68.

142 Schneider JE, Adams OR, Easley KJ, et al.: 1985. Scapular notch resection for suprascapular nerve decompression in 12 horses. *J Am Vet Med Assoc* 187:1019–1020.

143 Schneider RK, Bramlage LR, Gabel AA, et al.: 1988. Incidence, location and classification of 371 third carpal bone fractures in 313 horses. *Equine Vet J* Suppl 20:33–42.

144 Schneider RK, Tucker RL, Habegger SR, et al.: 2003. Desmitis of the straight sesamoidean ligament in horses: 9 cases (1995–1997). *J Am Vet Med Assoc* 222:973–977.

145 Semevolos SA, Watkins JP, Auer JA: 2003. Scapulohumeral arthrodesis in miniature horses. *Vet Surg* 32:416–420.

146 Smith LC, Greet TR, Bathe AP: 2009. A lateral approach for screw repair in lag fashion of spiral third metacarpal and metatarsal medial condylar fractures in horses. *Vet Surg* 38:681–688.

147 Smith MR, Wright IM: 2006. Noninfected tenosynovitis of the digital flexor tendon sheath: A retrospective analysis of 76 cases. *Equine Vet J* 38:134–41.

148 Smith RK, Werling NJ, Dakin SG, et al.: 2013. Beneficial effects of autologous bone marrow-derived mesenchymal stem cells in naturally occurring tendinopathy. *PLoS One* 25:e75697.

149 Smith RK: 2008. Mesenchymal stem cell therapy for equine tendinopathy. *Disabil Rehabil* 30:1752–1758.

150 Smith S, Dyson SJ, Murray RC: 2008. Magnetic resonance imaging of distal sesamoidean ligament injury. *Vet Radiol Ultrasound* 49:516–528.

151 Snyder JR, Wheat JD, Bleifer D: 1986. Conservative management of metacarpophalangeal joint instability. *Proceedings Am Assoc Equine Pract* 32:357.

152 Southwood LL, McIlwraith CW: 2000. Arthroscopic removal of fracture fragments involving a portion of the base of the proximal sesamoid bone in horses: 26 cases (1984–1997). *J Am Vet Med Assoc* 217:236–240.

153 Southwood LL, Stashak TS, Fehr JE, et al.: 1997. Lateral approach for endoscopic removal of solitary osteochondromas from the distal radial metaphysis in three horses. *J Am Vet Med Assoc* 210:1166–1168.

154 Southwood LL, Trotter GW, McIlwraith CW: 1998. Arthroscopic removal of abaxial fracture fragments of the proximal sesamoid bones in horses: 47 cases (1989– 1997). *J Am Vet Med Assoc* 213:1016–1021.

155 Spike-Pierce DL, Bramlage LR: 2003. Correlation of racing performance with radiographic changes in the proximal sesamoid bones of 487 Thoroughbred yearlings. *Equine Vet J* 35:350–353.

156 Stephens PR, Richardson DW, Spencer PA: 1988. Slab fractures of the third carpal bone in Standardbreds and Thoroughbreds: 155 cases (1977–1984). *J Am Vet Med Assoc* 193:353–358.

157 Stewart S, Richardson D, Boston R, et al.: 2015. Risk factors associated with survival to hospital discharge of 54 horses with fractures of the radius. *Vet Surg* 44:1036–1041.

158 Sun TC, Riggs CM, Cogger N, et al.: 2019. Noncatastrophic and catastrophic fractures in racing Thoroughbreds at the Hong Kong Jockey Club. *Equine Vet J* 51:77–82.

159 Swor TM, Watkins JP, Bahr A, et al.: 2003. Results of plate fixation of type 1b olecranon fractures in 24 horses. *Equine Vet J* 35:670–67.

160 Tetens J, Ross MW, Lloyd JW: 1997. Comparison of racing performance before and after treatment of incomplete, midsagittal fractures of the proximal phalanx in Standardbreds: 49 cases (1986–1992) *J Am Vet Med Assoc* 210:82–86.

161 Tnibar M, Auer J, Bakkali S: 1999. Ultrasonography of the equine shoulder: Technique and normal appearance. *Vet Radiol Ultrasound* 40:44–57.

162 Torre K, Motta M: 1999. Incidence and distribution of 369 proximal sesamoid bone fractures in 354 Standardbred horses (1984–1995). *Equine Pract* 21:6–10.

163 Tull TM, Bramlage LR: 2011. Racing prognosis after cumulative stress-induced injury of the distal portion of the third metacarpal and third metatarsal bones in Thoroughbred racehorses: 55 cases (2000–2009). *J Am Vet Med Assoc* 238:1316–1322.

164 Vallance S, Case J, Entwistle R, et al.: 2012. Characteristics of Thoroughbred and Quarter Horse racehorses that sustained a complete scapular fracture. *Equine Vet J* 44:425–431.

165 Vatistas NJ, Pascoe JR, Wright IM, et al.: 1996. Infection of the intertubercular bursa in horses: Four cases (1978–1991). *J Am Vet Med Assoc* 208: 1434–1437.

166 Watkins JP: 2006. The Radius and Ulna. *In:* Auer JA, Stick JA (eds) *Equine Surgery, Third Edition.* Philadelphia, WB Saunders, 1267–1279.

167 Whitcomb MB: 2008. Ultrasonographic appearance and distribution of deep digital flexor injuries in the pastern region. *Proceedings Am Assoc Equine Pract* 54:452–454.

168 Wilderjans H, Boussauw B, Madder K, et al.: 2003. Tenosynovitis of the digital flexor sheath and annular ligament constriction syndrome caused by longitudinal tears in the deep digital flexor tendon: A clinical and surgical report of 17 cases in Warmblood horses. *Equine Vet J* 35:270–275.

169 Woodie JB, Ruggles AJ, Bertone AL, et al.: 1999. Apical fracture of the proximal sesamoid bone in Standardbred horses: 43 cases (1990–1996). *J Am Vet Med Assoc* 214:1653–1656.

170 Wright IM, McMahon PJ: 1999. Tenosynovitis associated with longitudinal tears of the digital flexor tendons in horses: A report of 20 cases. *Equine Vet J* 31: 12–18.

171 Wright IM, Minshall GJ: 2012. Clinical, radiological and ultrasonographic features, treatment and outcome in 22 horses with caudal distal radial osteochondromata. *Equine Vet J* 44:319–324.

172 Wright IM, Minshall GJ: 2018. Short frontal plane fractures involving the dorsoproximal articular surface of the proximal phalanx: Description of the injury and a technique for repair. *Equine Vet J* 50:54–59.

173 Wright IM, Smith MR: 2009. A lateral approach to the repair of propagating fractures of the medial condyle of the third metacarpal and metatarsal bone in 18 racehorses. *Vet Surg* 38:689–695.

174 Young DR, Nunamaker DM, Markel MD: 1991. Quantitative evaluation of the remodeling response of the proximal sesamoid bones to training-related stimuli in Thoroughbreds. *Am J Vet Res* 52:1350–1356.

175 Zamos DT, Parks AH: 1992. Comparison of surgical and nonsurgical treatment of humeral fractures in horses: 22 cases (1980–1989). *J Am Vet Med Assoc* 201:114–116.

176 Zekas LJ, Bramlage LR, Embertson RM, et al.: 1999. Characterization of the type and location of fractures of the third metacarpal/metatarsal condyles in 135 horses in central Kentucky (1986–1994). *Equine Vet J* 31: 304–308.

177 Zekas LJ, Bramlage LR, Embertson RM, et al.: 1999. Results of treatment of 145 fractures of the third metacarpal/ metatarsal condyles in 135 horses (1986–1994). *Equine Vet J* 31:309–313.

178 Zubrod CJ, Schneider RK, Tucker RL, et al.: 2004. Use of magnetic resonance imaging for identifying subchondral bone damage in horses: 11 cases (1999–2003). *J Am Vet Med Assoc* 224:411–418.

Revised from "Lameness of the Distal Limb" and "Lameness of the Proximal Limb" in *Adams and Stashak's Lameness in Horses, 7th Edition*, **by Ashlee E. Watts, Gary M. Baxter, Kyla F. Ortved, Matt Brokken, Alicia L. Bertone, Chris Kawcak, and Jeremy Hubert.**

4

Common Conditions of the Hindlimb

Distal Hindlimb and Foot

Overview

- Because of the anatomical and functional similarities between the distal forelimb and hindlimb in the horse, many of the same lameness conditions occur distal to the carpus and tarsus. However, the frequency of these conditions often differs.
- Despite these similarities, many lameness conditions almost exclusively occur in the distal forelimb (navicular syndrome/disease, bucked shins, etc.) or hindlimb (DDFT injuries) likely related to conformational and biomechanical differences.
- The reader is referred to Chapters 2 (Common Conditions of the Foot) and 3 (Common Conditions of the Forelimb) for further information on lameness conditions that affect the distal hindlimb and foot.

Anatomy

- The hind foot is somewhat smaller and more elongate than the fore foot and the angle of the toe is usually slightly greater.
- Within the hind pastern, the middle phalanx is narrower and longer and the proximal phalanx somewhat shorter than their counterparts in the thoracic limb (Figure 4.1).
- The suspensory apparatus of the hind fetlock and the configuration of the fetlock

(joint) are much the same as in the thoracic limb except that the dorsal articular angle of the fetlock is approximately 5° greater (slightly more "upright").

- MTIII is about 16% longer than MCIII and is more rounded in contour (Figures 3.37 and 4.1), and the rear splint bones have smaller articulating surfaces than their counterparts on the forelimb.
- The tendon of the long digital extensor muscle extends the length of MTIII analogous to the tendon of the CDE muscle along MCIII.
- The SDFT and DDFT in the hindlimb are similar to their counterparts in the distal forelimb but the inferior check ligament is often weakly developed or even absent in some horses within the hindlimb.
- The SL of the hindlimb is relatively thinner, more rounded, and longer than the ligament in the forelimb and may contain more muscle than the SL of the forelimb.

Imaging

- Imaging options for the distal hindlimb are the same as the forelimb in most cases.

Etiology

- The forelimb receives 60–65% of the weight of the horse and rider during locomotion, while the hindlimbs are used primarily to generate forward momentum.
- Lameness in the hindlimb in sport horses is often related to a rearward shift in weight

Manual of Equine Lameness, Second Edition. Gary M. Baxter.
© 2022 John Wiley & Sons, Inc. Published 2022 by John Wiley & Sons, Inc.
Companion website: www.wiley.com/go/baxter/manual

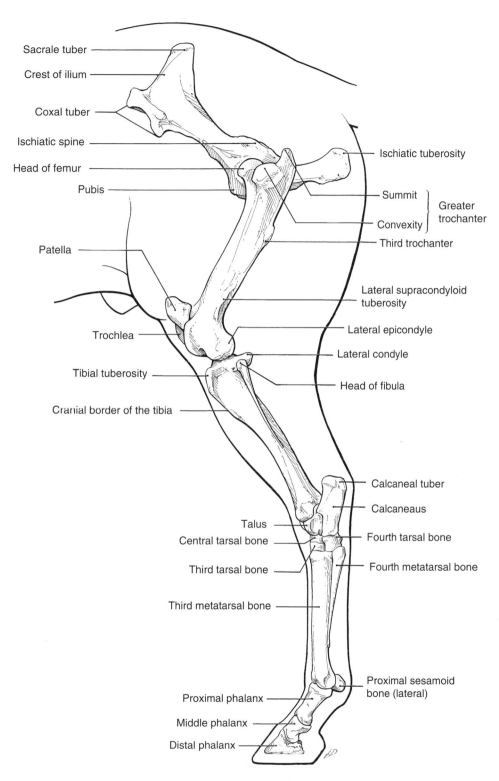

Sacrale tuber

Crest of ilium

Coxal tuber

Ischiatic spine

Head of femur

Pubis

Patella

Trochlea

Tibial tuberosity

Cranial border of the tibia

Talus

Central tarsal bone

Third tarsal bone

Third metatarsal bone

Proximal phalanx

Middle phalanx

Distal phalanx

Ischiatic tuberosity

Summit

Convexity

Greater trochanter

Third trochanter

Lateral supracondyloid tuberosity

Lateral epicondyle

Lateral condyle

Head of fibula

Calcaneal tuber

Calcaneaus

Fourth tarsal bone

Fourth metatarsal bone

Proximal sesamoid bone (lateral)

Figure 4.1   Bones of the left pelvic limb, lateral view. *Source*: Courtesy of J Daugherty.

distribution, which requires more impulsion from the hind end.

- Many types of injuries in the hindlimb are related to excessive propulsion, stopping, twisting, or slipping during exercise or from direct external trauma.
- Fewer repetitive, concussive type injuries (MCIII stress fractures, navicular syndrome, POD, etc.) will occur in the distal hindlimb compared with the forelimb.

Clinical Signs and Diagnosis

- The severity of clinical signs and degree of lameness are usually comparable for similar lameness conditions of the distal forelimb and hindlimb.
- The diagnosis is usually made in a similar manner regardless of forelimb vs. hindlimb.

Treatment and Prognosis

- Treatment options are usually similar for injuries of the distal forelimb or hindlimb.
- In general, the prognosis is often slightly improved for similar conditions in the distal hindlimb compared with the forelimb.

Tarsus

Distal Tarsal Osteoarthritis (OA)

Overview

- Distal tarsal OA is often referred to as "bone spavin" and is a common cause of tarsal lameness in performance horses in a variety of disciplines. It usually involves the DIT and TMT joint, occasionally the PIT joint.
- Horses with occult spavin, blind spavin, or tarsitis are described as having similar clinical features of distal tarsal OA but without radiographic abnormalities. Juvenile spavin is the term used to describe distal tarsal OA in horses less than three years old due to developmental lesions within the tarsal cuboidal bones.

- Chronic cases of distal tarsal OA often develop an enlargement over the medial or dorsomedial aspects of the joints.
- Distal tarsal OA is most frequently observed in jumping horses; dressage and event horses; horses that pull carts; and Western performance horses used for reining, roping, and cutting.
- Icelandic horses also appear to be prone to Distal tarsal OA.

Anatomy

- The bones of the tarsus include the talus, calcaneus, and the central, first and second (fused), third and fourth tarsal bones (Figure 4.1).
- Proximally, the trochlea of the talus articulates with the cochlear surface of the tibia forming the TC joint, which is responsible for nearly all of the movement of the hock.
- Three low-motion joints (PIT, DIT, and TMT) form the remainder of the tarsus with the distal row of tarsal bones articulating with the three metatarsal bones.
- There is a very close association between the TMT joint and the attachment of the SL on the plantar surface of MTIII and the distal row of tarsal bones.
- Extensive collateral ligaments span the TC and intertarsal joints (Figure 4.2).

Imaging

- Radiography and ultrasonography are considered the minimum imaging techniques to evaluate bone and soft tissue structures of the tarsus.
- Radiography is usually adequate to diagnosis the majority of horses with distal tarsal OA and those with OC of the TC joint.
- All of the advanced imaging techniques (scintigraphy, MRI, and CT) have applications in the tarsus and can be used to help with the diagnosis when necessary.

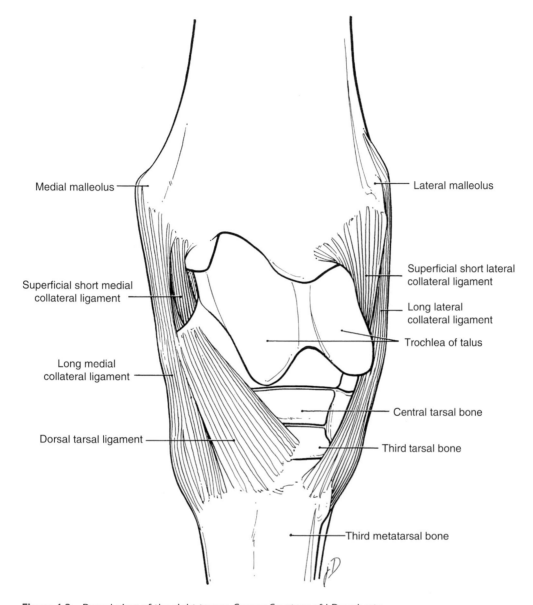

Figure 4.2 Dorsal view of the right tarsus. *Source*: Courtesy of J Daugherty.

Etiology
- Repetitive compression and rotation of the tarsal bones and excessive tension on the associated ligaments related to the type and intensity of exercise are thought to contribute to the disease.

- Increased torsional and shear forces on the distal tarsal joints can lead to excessive "wear and tear" on the joints.
- In some breeds such as the Icelandic horse, there appears to be a genetic component to development of distal tarsal OA.

- Sickle hock, cow-hocked, and very straight tarsal conformations are thought to cause greater stress on the medial aspect of the tarsus and contribute to the disease. The incidence of distal tarsal OA has been decreased in Dutch Warmbloods by selecting against these conformational traits.
- Congenital/developmental malformation of the tarsal cuboidal bones often contributes to the disease, as do specific traumatic injuries to the distal tarsus (Figure 4.3).

Clinical Signs

- There is usually a gradual onset of lameness or reduced performance, especially if affected bilaterally.
- The lameness is usually worse when the horse is first used, may warm out of the lameness initially but will often worsen with exercise as the disease progresses.
- The horse may have a history of a being stiff or jerky when circled to the affected side and refusal to perform discipline-specific maneu-

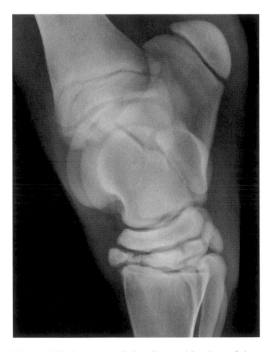

Figure 4.3 Lateromedial radiographic view of the tarsus of a foal showing collapse of the third tarsal bone. *Source*: Courtesy of Robert Hunt.

vers. A mild-to-moderate unilateral or bilateral hindlimb lameness is usually observed.
- Gait abnormalities that may be observed in horses with distal tarsal pain include reduced arc of the foot flight, reduced flexion of the hock, carrying the limb axially and then stabbing the limb outward (so-called J-step), and dragging the toe.
- Thickening or enlargement of the medial aspect of the hock may be observed visually in horses with advanced disease (Figure 1.37).
- Palpation of the medial aspect of the tarsus (with or without a visual enlargement) may elicit pain and be suggestive of distal tarsal OA (Figure 1.38).
- Tarsal flexion or full limb flexion tests usually worsen the lameness and should be performed bilaterally since the disease can affect both tarsi.
- Horses with distal tarsal OA often have other musculoskeletal abnormalities (back pain and forelimb foot pain) that must be investigated.
- IA anesthesia of one or both distal tarsal joints is usually the most specific and expedient method to document the site of the lameness.

Diagnosis

- The diagnosis is often made based on the combination of clinical findings, response to IA anesthesia, and radiographic abnormalities. Radiographs or clinical findings alone are not reliable as the only method of diagnosis.
- Radiographic signs of distal tarsal OA can be variable but may include:
  1) Periarticular osteophytes or enthesophytes ("spurs")
  2) Irregularity and lucency at the intertarsal joint margins
  3) Irregular width of the joint space and cysts in the subchondral bone
  4) Narrowing or loss of joint space
  5) Subchondral bone lysis or sclerosis
  6) Periosteal new bone production
  7) Varying degrees of ankylosis (Figure 4.4)

- Early radiographic evidence of OA usually begins on the dorsomedial surfaces of the TMT and DIT joints that progress dorsally.
- The correlation between the degree of lameness and the extent of radiographic abnormalities is poor. Therefore, some clinicians rely heavily on the clinical findings and even subtle radiographic lesions can support the diagnosis in the presence of appropriate clinical findings.
- Scintigraphy can be used to accurately detect distal tarsal inflammation and is useful when the diagnosis is complicated by multiple problems or difficulty blocking the joints (Figure 4.5).
- MRI may be necessary to help differentiate between a distal tarsal joint problem and PSD since lameness referable to the proximal SL in the hindlimb is often initially assumed to originate from the DT joints.

Treatment

- Horses with mild-to-moderate lameness and radiographic changes usually respond favorably to a short period of reduced activity, systemic NSAIDs, corrective shoeing, IA medication, and a change in the work program. Horses with minimal radiographic abnormalities may not require repetitive IA treatment.
- Most clinicians recommend some form of IA medication (corticosteroid +/- HA, ACS, or PSGAGs) to subdue the inflammatory changes within the distal tarsal joints. Many clinicians use TA in horses with minor signs of OA and MPA in horses with more advanced signs of OA.
- Hoof management is aimed at reducing the rotation/shear forces at the tarsus by easing break-over, rolling/squaring the toe, elevating the heel, and extending the branches of the shoe slightly beyond the end of the heels.

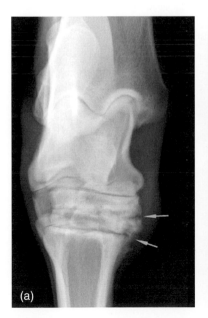
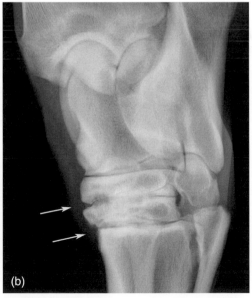

Figure 4.4 (a) Radiographic changes of OA of the distal tarsal joints can vary considerably including periarticular osteophyte formation, (b) subchondral lysis and sclerosis, periosteal new bone (arrows), and narrowing of joint spaces. The dorsolateral-plantaromedial oblique radiograph on the right revealed significant subchondral bone lysis of the DIT joint and other changes in the TMT joint that were causing significant lameness. *Source*: Courtesy of Rich Redding.

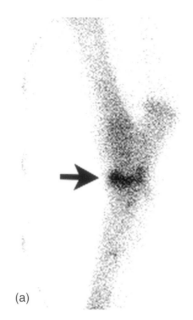

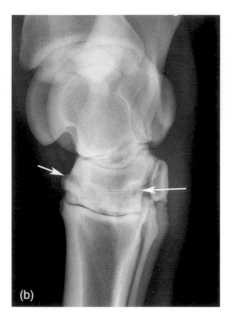

(a)

(b)

Figure 4.5 Lateral scintigram (a) and radiograph (b) of the tarsus of a horse with distal tarsal OA. There is diffuse uptake within the distal tarsal joints and joint space narrowing and lysis within the DIT joint (arrows) visible on the radiograph. *Source*: Courtesy of Rich Redding.

- Bisphosphonates [tiludronate (Tildren$_R$) and clodronate (Osphos$_R$)] and ESWT may also be used to treat horses that do not respond to more traditional therapies.
- Horses with advanced OA are the most problematic to treat. Some may respond to the same treatment as described for horses with less severe disease but may require more frequent IA treatment and a change in career.
- Joint ankylosis or arthrodesis may be required in severe disease if other treatments fail. Exercise-facilitated ankylosis (with or without corticosteroids) is not successful in most cases and spontaneous ankylosis rarely occurs.
- Methods to induce chemical arthrodesis in the distal tarsal joints include IA monoiodacetate (MIA) and 70% ethanol. MIA is currently not recommended. Ethanol (3 mL of 70%) is the best option and has been shown to cause arthrodesis experimentally and improvement in clinical signs clinically.
- Methods to surgically arthrodese the distal tarsal joints include IA laser treatment, IA

drilling, and IA drilling plus stabilization with a small bone plate. Variable success rates have been reported with these techniques.

Prognosis
- The prognosis for horses with distal tarsal OA often depends on the severity of lameness and radiographic abnormalities, and the intended use of the horse.
- Horses with mild disease often have a good prognosis, whereas horses with more advanced disease usually have a guarded prognosis. A more accurate prognosis can usually be made after the response to the initial therapy is known.
- Many horses can be successfully managed throughout their athletic career with consistent (biannual to annual) IA corticosteroids combined with good farriery.
- Horses with advanced disease requiring arthrodesis techniques have approximately a 50–50 chance of returning to athletic use regardless of the technique used.

Osteochondritis Dissecans (OCD) of the TC Joint/Bog Spavin

Overview

- Synovitis and fluid accumulation within the TC joint is a common finding in young horses and is referred to by laypeople as "bog" spavin.
- Young horses of any breed with effusion of the TC joint should be suspected of having OCD as this is the most likely cause.
- Other causes of bog spavin may include OA of the TC and PIT joints, traumatic injuries, poor conformation, and infection.
- Many horses with OCD are not lame and the lesion may be found on routine radiographs taken before a sale or as an incidental finding.
- Tarsocrural OCD is quite common in Standardbreds but is found in nearly all breeds.
- Typical sites for OCD fragmentation include the distal intermediate ridge of the tibia (DIRT), lateral trochlear ridge, medial malleolus, and medial trochlear ridge. Lesions in more than one location can be found in the same TC joint.

Anatomy (Please refer to previous section on "Distal Tarsal OA")

Imaging (Please refer to the previous section on "Distal Tarsal OA")

Etiology

- OCD is a developmental abnormality that is defined as a focal disturbance of endochondral ossification with a multifactorial etiology.
- The most commonly cited contributing factors are heredity, rapid growth, anatomic conformation, trauma, and dietary imbalances.
- Trauma within the TC joint may be difficult to differentiate from true OCD lesions because traumatic events can destabilize a pre-existing OCD fragment.
- Other factors that may contribute to TC effusion include traumatic injuries to the joint and/or collateral ligaments, OA, poor conformation, and infection.

Clinical Signs

- Non-painful effusion of the TC joint is by far the most common presenting complaint (Figure 1.34).
- If periarticular or regional edema or swelling beyond the TC joint is present, another problem should be suspected such as trauma to the tarsus.
- Lameness may be absent or mild; severe lameness is not consistent with OCD lesions.
- Many horses are sound at a walk and trotting in hand but may display lameness at faster speeds or when put into work.
- Hindlimb flexion tests usually increase the severity of the lameness, especially if the joint effusion is severe.

Diagnosis

- The diagnosis is usually confirmed with a complete radiographic examination of the tarsus. A slightly oblique DP view may be necessary to highlight a lesion of the medial malleolus (Figure 4.6).
- The radiographic abnormalities may include fragmentation, irregular or flattened contour of the subchondral bone surface, subchondral bone lucency and/or sclerosis, a partially ossified "flap," or multiple loose bodies within the joint (Figure 4.7).
- The opposite tarsus should be radiographed because approximately half of affected horses have similar contralateral lesions.
- OC lesions found before the age of five months may resolve with time, but most lesions detected after five months typically will persist.
- Ultrasonography can be useful in cases where OC is suspected, but the radiographs are inconclusive.
- A small percentage of horses may not have lesions apparent with routine imaging techniques and may require arthroscopy to make a definitive diagnosis.

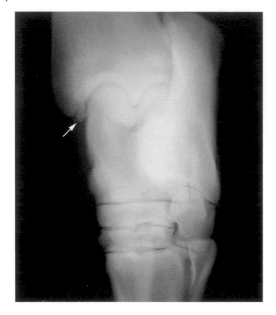

Figure 4.6 Dorsolateral-plantaromedial radiograph of the tarsus demonstrating a medial malleolar OCD lesion (arrow). The fragment is often located on the axial surface of the medial malleolus adjacent to the medial trochlear ridge.

Treatment

- Most horses benefit from arthroscopic removal of the OCD fragment. Lesion location or type has not been correlated to differences in outcome.
- Horses with small lesions, with minimal effusion, and without lameness may not require surgery, particularly if they are pleasure horses or light-use horses.
- Prolonged effusion of the TC joint before surgery usually increases the chance that the bog spavin will persist after fragment removal.
- Horses with radiographic lesions but no clinical signs may not require surgery, but clinical signs can always appear during training if the fragment becomes dislodged.
- In general, lesions in foals should not be operated until they are seven to eight months of age.

Prognosis

- The prognosis for athletic activity after surgical removal of OCD lesions is good and

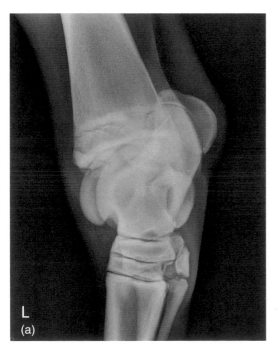

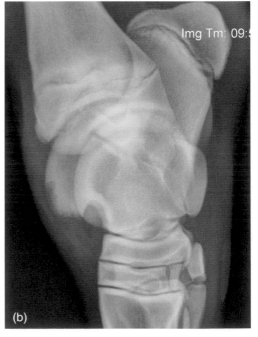

Figure 4.7 Dorsomedial plantarolateral radiographs demonstrating OCD lesions of the distal intermediate ridge (a) of the tibia (DIRT) and the lateral trochlear ridge (b) of the talus. *Source:* Image (b) courtesy of Wayne McIlwraith.

effusion resolves in 89% or racehorses and 74% of nonracehorses. Lesion location and unilateral vs. bilateral lesions do not appear to alter the prognosis.

- Effusion appears to be less likely to resolve following surgery on lateral trochlear ridge or medial malleolus lesions.
- Superficial cartilage fibrillation does not alter the prognosis, but more severe cartilage degeneration or erosion decreases the success of surgery.

Slab/Sagittal Fractures of the Small Tarsal Bones

Overview

- Slab fractures of the central and third tarsal bones occur most often in racing disciplines or other high-speed events.
- Fractures of the third tarsal bone are more common in TB and STB racehorses and are normally found on the dorsal and dorsolateral aspects of the bone.
- The central tarsal bone tends to fracture along the dorsomedial aspect, whereas the third tarsal bone is most often affected dorsally or dorsolaterally.
- Small tarsal bone fractures from external trauma are more likely to involve both bones and be comminuted.

Anatomy

- The central and third tarsal bones are located on top of one another on the dorsal aspect of the tarsus between MTIII distally and the talus proximally (Figures 4.1 and 4.2).
- The small tarsal bones together with the distal tarsal joints (PIT, DIT, and TMT) are stabilized by a thick layer of ligamentous tissue that includes the dorsal tarsal ligament (Figure 4.2).
- The dorsal aspect of the tarsal region is also stabilized by the extensor bundle composed of the tendons of insertion of tibialis cranialis and peroneus tertius (PT).

- The small tarsal bones (central and third) are subjected to axial compression, torsional, and tensile forces during exercise.

Imaging

- Diagnosis of central and third tarsal bone fractures can usually be confirmed with radiography but often requires multiple oblique projections to define the fracture.
- Scintigraphy can be utilized to demonstrate active bone remodeling associated with the fracture if a fracture is suspected but cannot be seen on radiographs.
- CT is ideally suited to more accurately define the fracture(s), especially if surgical repair is warranted.

Etiology

- Their main function of the small tarsal bones is to absorb concussion and neutralize twisting forces associated with exercise. When these bones are subjected to the even greater stress of racing speeds, fracture can occur.
- Slab fractures are felt to be exercise-induced injuries in racehorses and result from accumulated bone damage on the dorsal aspect of the central and third tarsal bones.
- Small tarsal bone fractures in nonperformance horses are usually due to some type of specific trauma and are more likely to involve both bones and be comminuted.
- Abnormal cuboidal bone formation in young horses may be a predisposing factor to the formation of slab fractures of the small tarsal bones.

Clinical Signs

- Horses typically present with a history of acute onset of severe lameness that diminishes relatively quickly.
- There can be little indication of a potential slab fracture and horses may present for routine lameness evaluation.
- Fractures of the third tarsal bone do not usually cause TC joint effusion, whereas effusion is common with slab fractures of the central tarsal bone.

- Heat and pain on palpation over the dorso-lateral aspect of the distal row of tarsal bones may be appreciated in acute cases.
- Most horses are very positive to the tarsal flexion test.

Diagnosis

- Radiography is required to confirm the diagnosis, but some fractures (non-displaced) can be difficult to document on radiographs (Figure 4.8).
- Several oblique projections at different angles around the tarsus may be necessary to identify fragmentation and the specific position of these fractures.
- Radiographic evidence of OA usually appears with tarsal bone fractures of long duration.
- With localization of the source of the lameness and no definitive radiographic lesion, scintigraphy or CT may be needed to document the problem.
- CT also can be helpful to determine if a fracture is a single slab that is repairable or comminuted and not repairable (Figure 4.8b).

Treatment

- Acute fractures should be repaired with lag screws as early as possible to facilitate reduc-tion and prevent degenerative changes in the joint(s). Fluoroscopy or CT guidance can facilitate efficient, accurate placement of the screw(s).
- Conservative treatment (prolonged stall rest) has also been utilized successfully with some horses returning to athletic use.
- Comminuted fractures are usually not candidates for surgical repair.

Prognosis

- A combined 22 of 28 horses treated with surgery in several different reports have returned to athletic performance.
- The presence of OA at the time of surgery diminishes the prognosis for athletic function and horses with central tarsal bone fractures tend to do worse than those with third tarsal bone fractures.
- With conservative therapy, 10 of 12 horses raced successfully in one report.

Subluxation/Luxation of the Tarsal Joints

Overview

- Subluxation/luxation of all four tarsal joints has been reported, but the PIT joint is most commonly affected.

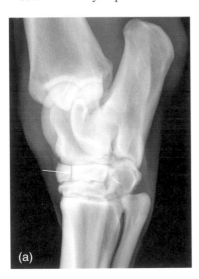
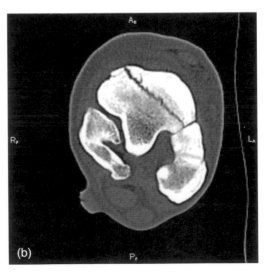

Figure 4.8 Tarsal radiograph (a; arrow) and CT (b) demonstrating a slab fracture of the central tarsal bone. These slab fractures are not always easily seen on radiographs and CT can help characterize the fracture. *Source*: Courtesy of Rich Redding.

- Substantial ligamentous damage around the tarsal joints must occur concurrently to permit subluxation/luxation of these joints.
- Subluxation/luxation of the tarsal joints is rarely open.
- The soft tissue injuries and fractures that accompany TC joint luxation are often so significant and incapacitating that salvage of the horse is frequently not possible.

Anatomy

- A long collateral ligament (CL) and three short collateral ligaments bind each side of the equine tarsus (Figure 4.2).
- The long lateral CL extends from the lateral malleolus caudal to the groove for the tendon of the lateral digital extensor, attaching distally to the calcaneus, fourth tarsal bone, talus, MTIV, and MTIII.
- The long medial CL extends from the medial malleolus and divides into two layers that attach to the distal tarsal bones, talus, MTII, and MTIII at both deep and superficial locations.
- The three short collateral ligaments both medially and laterally further stabilize all four of the tarsal joints.

Imaging

- Radiography can usually document most tarsal subluxations/luxations. Some may reduce spontaneously but can usually be demonstrated with a stressed DP radiograph.
- Ultrasonography may be used to document the severity of the CL injuries.

Etiology

- A severe wrenching or twisting action that may occur from a sudden slip or fall is believed to be the cause.
- Kicks from other horses and entrapment in fixed objects such as fences or cattle guards also have been implicated.

Clinical Signs

- Signs are usually quite obvious, with heat, pain, and swelling of the tarsus occurring in acute cases.
- The lameness is usually severe but usually improves with time. A limb deformity may be seen concurrently.
- On palpation, the limb is usually more moveable distal to the luxation, mostly in a medial-to-lateral direction.
- Luxation of the TC joint is the most severe; the tibia is usually displaced distally and cranially, making it very difficult to reduce.

Diagnosis

- The exact location and extent of damage should be verified with radiographs.
- The DP view is usually the most informative to evaluate luxation/subluxation of the distal tarsal joints (Figure 4.9b).
- Stress radiography may be necessary to document the exact location of the instability in the distal tarsal joints (Figure 4.9).

Treatment

- Tarsal luxations in the absence of significant fractures can be treated with a full-limb cast for two to three months. To minimize complications of a full-limb cast, the limb can be maintained in a cast for four to six weeks if the CLs are intact and six to eight weeks if they are not.
- Re-luxation of the distal tarsal joints can occur after cast removal and may require internal fixation.
- Internal fixation with a bone plate or transarticular screws may be required to achieve adequate stabilization if the subluxation/luxation is unstable. It is usually recommended to arthrodese the distal tarsal joints at the same time.

Prognosis

- The prognosis is reasonably good for simple luxation of the distal tarsal joints without fracture; however, the prognosis decreases if a fracture is present.

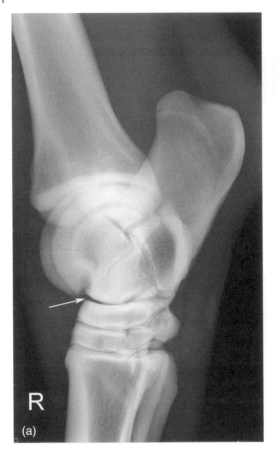
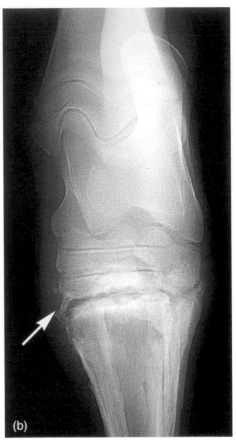

Figure 4.9 A stressed lateromedial radiograph (a) used to help demonstrate opening of the joint surface in this horse with a PIT joint luxation. This horse was maintained in a full-limb cast. *Source*: Image (a), courtesy of Rich Redding. Dorsoplantar radiograph (b) of a foal with luxation of the medial aspect of the TMT joint (arrow). A medial plate was used to stabilize the luxation and arthrodese the distal tarsal joints.

- Successful use of cast immobilization alone and internal fixation of distal tarsal and TC luxations have been reported.

Fractures of the Tibial Malleoli

Overview

- Fractures of the lateral malleolus are more common and typically smaller than those involving the medial malleolus.
- A larger portion of the medial malleolus is intra-articular and therefore more likely to contribute to secondary damage within the TC joint.

- Many fractures of the lateral malleolus affect the most dorsal portion where the short CL attaches, but some affect the entire malleolus through to the caudal compartment of the TC joint.
- Fragment removal should not compromise the stability of the TC joint, provided that the long CLs are not affected.
- These fractures can be closed or open.

Anatomy

- The tibial malleoli and the distal end of the tibial form interdigitating grooves for the lateral and medial trochlear ridges of the talus to glide during flexion and extension of the TC joint (Figure 4.2).

- Portions of both the medial malleolus and lateral malleolus of the distal tibia lie within the TC joint.
- A greater proportion of the medial malleolus is intra-articular, and the lateral malleolus is largely invested in the joint capsule and CL.
- The long medial and lateral CLs originate on the medial malleolus and lateral malleolus, respectively (Figure 4.2).
- Fractures of the medial or lateral malleolus may or may not involve the long CLs depending on the location of the fracture.

Imaging

- Fractures of the tibial malleoli are best demonstrated with DP radiographs. Multiple radiographic projections may be necessary to assess the extent of bony change(s).
- Ultrasonography of the affected CL is critical to assess its degree of damage to prevent fur-

ther injury that may occur on recovery from general anesthesia.

Etiology

- The tibial malleoli are usually fractured by direct trauma or avulsion of the CLs.
- The majority of horses acquire these injuries in a fall or from being kicked, with the lateral malleolus affected most frequently.

Diagnosis

- Radiographs usually confirm the diagnosis. The fractures are usually demonstrated best on DP or oblique radiographs (Figure 4.10a).
- Concurrent CL injury is common and should be confirmed with ultrasonography.
- Ultrasonography is a very useful tool to determine the exact location of the fragment(s) and to assess the extent of injury to other structures (Figure 4.10b).

Treatment

- Surgical removal with arthroscopy is indicated when the fragments are small or com-

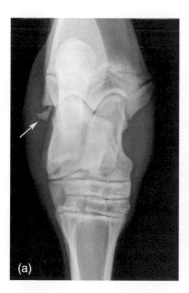
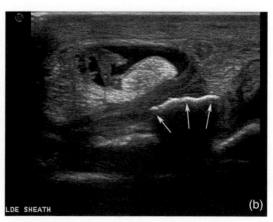

Figure 4.10 The DP radiographic projection on the left (a) demonstrates displacement of the lateral malleolar fragment due to the pull of the collateral ligament. The ultrasound image (b) demonstrates the fragment (arrows) and effusion within the lateral digital extensor tendon sheath because of their close anatomical position. *Source*: Courtesy of Rich Redding.

minuted, especially if the fracture is open. The fragment will usually need to be dissected from the CL, but this usually does not affect the stability of the TC joint.

- Marginally sized fragments of the lateral malleolus (>3 cm) are best repaired with lag screws but may split during the convalescent period and require removal.
- Three of four horses with lateral malleolar fractures treated by stall rest returned to athletic activity.
- Some large medial malleolus fractures can be repaired with lag screws (Figure 4.11) or treated conservatively.

Prognosis

- Overall good results are reported after removal of relatively small fragments from either the medial or lateral malleoli. Many of these fragments can be removed arthroscopically with minimal dissection into the joint capsule.
- A 50% return to performance following surgical repair with internal fixation of lateral malleolar fractures has been reported.
- The size of the fragment and concurrent CL damage greatly affect the prognosis.

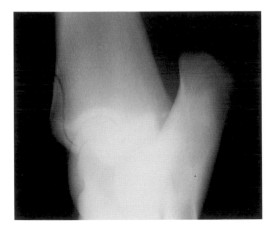

Figure 4.11 Oblique radiograph of a horse that had been kicked on the medial aspect of the tarsus. This articular fracture of the medial malleolus was repaired with lag screws.

Tarsal Collateral Ligament (CL) Injuries

Overview

- The stability of a TC joint is a product of the congruency of the joint surfaces, the integrity of the joint capsule, and the strength of the CLs.
- Injuries to the tarsal CLs typically accompany other bone or joint conditions in the tarsus and are infrequently a primary problem.
- Injuries to both the long and short CLs of the tarsus have been described.

Anatomy (Please refer to previous sections on "Tarsal Luxation and Tibial Malleoli Fractures")

Imaging (Please refer to previous sections on "Tarsal Luxation and Tibial Malleoli Fractures")

Etiology

- CL injury of the TC joint most often occurs due to some form of traumatic injury.
- Twisting and torquing of the tarsus while the lower limb is fixed to the ground is also thought to contribute to CL injuries.
- Increasing tensile stress (and probably the rate at which it is loaded) within the CL may lead to fractures of the malleoli together with CL injuries.

Clinical Signs and Diagnosis

- Physical exam findings usually include tarsal swelling with edema and/or fibrosis localized over the medial or lateral CL regions. With chronicity, a generalized firm enlargement of the entire tarsus may occur (Figure 4.12).
- The presence of TC effusion often occurs but the amount can be quite variable and palpable pain directly over the CL is not a consistent finding.
- Lameness varies from mild to severe, depending on the degree of CL damage and concurrent injury.

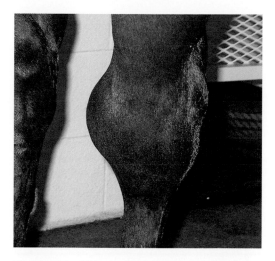

Figure 4.12 This young horse had a history of previous trauma to the tarsus. Part of the swelling was firm and painful to palpation, but there was also effusion within the TC joint.

- Hindlimb proximal limb flexion usually significantly worsens the lameness.
- The diagnosis is usually made with a combination of radiographic and ultrasonographic examinations. Stress radiographs may be helpful in some cases.
- Injuries to the CLs within the TC joint may be difficult to accurately assess with standard imaging techniques and may require arthroscopic exploration.

Treatment and Prognosis
- Initial treatment of acute injuries involves stall rest, cold water therapy, and topical and systemic NSAIDs.
- Concurrent injuries such as malleolar fractures should be addressed to prevent chronic irritation and reinjury to the CLs.
- Arthroscopy permits direct visualization and debridement of torn fibers of the short CLs and is recommended when necessary.
- Rehabilitation will require increasing periods of controlled exercise determined by an improving ultrasonographic appearance of the injured structure.

- Prognosis depends on the severity of injury and effective treatment and rehabilitation.
- Horses with moderate injuries that develop periosteal new bone formation have been able to return to full athletic function, although some residual enlargement of the tarsus is likely to persist.

Capped Hock/Calcaneal Bursitis

Overview
- Swelling at the point of the hock (calcaneal tuber) is usually attributable to damage to the subcutaneous calcaneal bursa (capped hock) or to problems within the intertendinous calcaneal bursa (ICB) located beneath the SDFT.
- The subcutaneous bursa (SCB) at the tarsus is analogous to the bursa at the point of the olecranon and may communicate with the ICB in about one-third of horses.
- The ICB is a true synovial cavity and problems within this anatomic structure are much more problematic than those within the SCB.

Anatomy
- The tendinous complex of the SDFT, biceps femoris and semitendinosus muscles, attaches to the point and sides of the calcaneal tuber. The SDFT courses over the calcaneal tuber and is attached to the bone both medially and laterally (Figures 1.42 and 4.13).
- The calcaneal tendon of the gastrocnemius lies deep to the SDFT at the tarsus and inserts on the plantar surface of the calcaneal tuber. The gastrocnemius tendon together with the SDFT form the common calcaneal tendon and bursa.
- The calcaneal bursa includes both the gastrocnemius calcaneal bursa (GCB) and the ICB since they nearly always communicate.

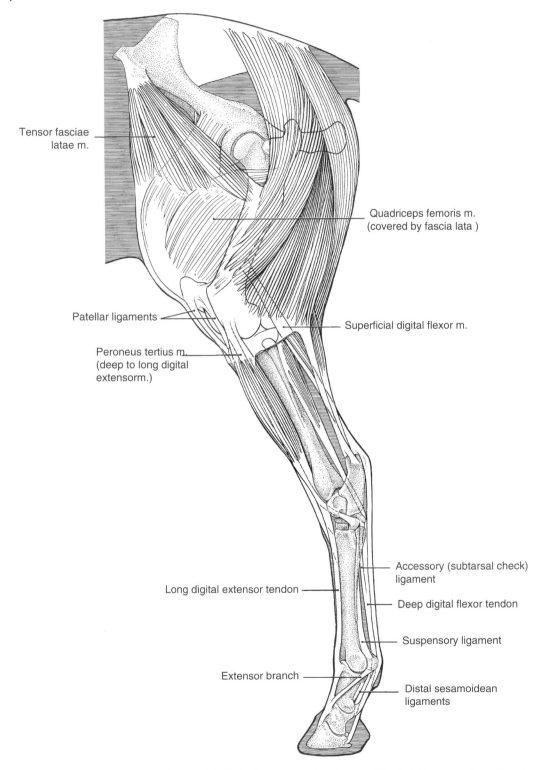

Tensor fasciae
latae m.

Quadriceps femoris m.
(covered by fascia lata)

Patellar ligaments

Superficial digital flexor m.

Peroneus tertius m.
(deep to long digital
extensorm.)

Accessory (subtarsal check)
ligament

Long digital extensor tendon

Deep digital flexor tendon

Suspensory ligament

Extensor branch

Distal sesamoidean
ligaments

Figure 4.13 Stay apparatus of the pelvic limb. Please note that the term "fibularis" is currently preferred over "peroneus" (fibular rather than peroneal), although both are widely used. The SDF muscle and tendon courses over the calcaneal tuber forming the calcaneal bursa and is attached to the calcaneal tuber both medially and laterally.

- A SCB also lies between the skin and the SDFT and can communicate with the true synovial ICB in about a third of limbs.
- The ICB extends approximately 9–10 cm proximally and 6–7 cm distally to the calcaneal tuber and is a true synovial cavity similar to the bicipital bursa.

Imaging

- A combination of radiography and ultrasonography is usually necessary to evaluate the structures surrounding the calcaneus.
- A flexed, proximoplantar to distoplantar tangential (skyline) radiographic view of the calcaneus is advantageous to evaluate the calcaneal tuber.

Etiology

- Direct trauma to the point of the hock from a kick or the horse hitting a hard object such as a stall wall, fence, etc., is the most common cause of a capped hock. These injuries may or may not be associated with a wound.
- Nonseptic calcaneal bursitis is usually secondary to luxation of the SDFT from the calcaneal tuber, damage to the attachment of gastrocnemius tendon to the tuber calcanei, and nonseptic osteolytic lesions within the calcaneus (Figure 4.14).
- Septic calcaneal bursitis is nearly always secondary to penetrating wounds that enter the calcaneal bursa. Secondary osteomyelitis within the calcaneal tuber is not uncommon.

Clinical Signs

- A capped hock (nonseptic) is usually characterized by a soft, fluctuant swelling located directly at the point of the hock (Figure 4.15). Lameness may or may not be present, depending on the time since injury, but is usually minimal after a few days.
- Horses with nonseptic calcaneal bursitis usually have palpable effusion within the bursa (above or below the calcaneal tuber) and the point of the hock is usually enlarged compared with the opposite calcaneus (Figure 1.36). These horses are often painful to direct palpation of the bursa, lame at the trot, and very positive to tarsal flexion.

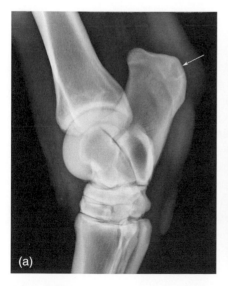 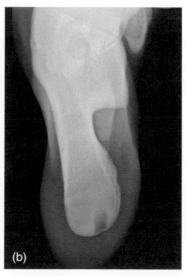

Figure 4.14 Well-circumscribed osteolytic or osseous cyst-like lesion (arrow) on the calcaneal tuber at the insertion of the GT may be indicative of an enthesopathy and calcaneal osteitis (a). A flexed, proximoplantar to distoplantar tangential (skyline) radiographic projection can often help better identify the boney lesion (b). *Source*: Courtesy of Rich Redding.

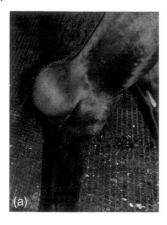 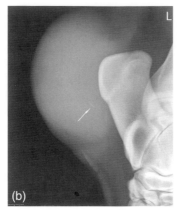 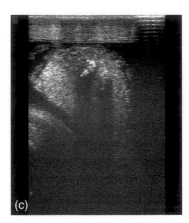

Figure 4.15   Clinical (a) and radiographic (b) appearance of a horse with swelling at the point of the hock (capped hock). Ultrasound (c) revealed a radiodense object within the swelling that can also be seen on the lateral radiograph (arrow). *Source*: Courtesy of Rich Redding.

- Horses with septic calcaneal bursitis are usually very lame, have severe swelling around the point of the hock, resent firm palpation of the bursa, and usually have purulent drainage from a previous penetrating injury.

Diagnosis

- The diagnosis of a capped hock can is usually based on clinical findings alone but both radiography and ultrasound can be useful to confirm the diagnosis (Figure 4.15).
- Wounds that involve the plantar surface of the calcaneal tuber should be carefully evaluated to ensure that they do not involve the deeper ICB.
- A definitive diagnosis of the cause of non-septic calcaneal bursitis usually requires a combination of radiography and ultrasonography.
- Horses with chronic calcaneal bursitis should be evaluated for osteolytic lesions on the tuber calcanei associated with the insertion of the gastrocnemius tendon ("gastrocnemius enthesitis"; Figure 4.14).
- Endoscopy of the bursa is recommended as a diagnostic tool if other imaging results are inconclusive.
- The diagnosis of septic bursitis is determined similarly to other sites of synovial

infection and includes a combination of plain and contrast radiography, ultrasonography, aspiration of synovial fluid, and culture.

Treatment
Capped Hock

- Small swellings over the tuber calcanei may merely be a cosmetic concern and not require treatment. Methods to prevent further trauma to the tuber calcanei are suggested to prevent the capped hock from worsening.
- Larger swellings can be treated with topical and systemic NSAIDs combined with bandaging and confinement.
- Other options include aseptic drainage and injection of corticosteroids or iodinated contrast agents. Counterpressure with bandaging is recommended for at least two weeks but can be difficult in this high-motion area.
- Surgical drainage using Penrose drains or complete removal of the bursa is rarely recommended due to the problems with wound healing in this location.

Nonseptic Calcaneal Bursitis

- The treatment often depends on the initiating cause but is often similar to other types of synovial/bursa inflammation.

- Acute bursitis without a defined cause is often treated with intrasynovial medications combined with a short period of rest and rehabilitation.
- Known causes of calcaneal bursitis such as osteolytic lesions within the calcaneus and abnormalities within the GT or SDFT should be debrided endoscopically.
- Endoscopy can be useful as both a diagnostic and therapeutic tool.

Septic Calcaneal Bursitis
- Superficial wounds to the SCB usually resolve with routine wound care and have an excellent prognosis.
- Wounds that involve the ICB should be treated aggressively in the acute stage to prevent chronic synovial infection.
- Horses with septic calcaneal bursitis should be treated with a combination of synovial lavage (endoscopy), local and parenteral antibiotics including IV regional perfusion, and NSAIDs.

Prognosis
- The prognosis for horses with a capped hock is usually very good unless it becomes chronic and fibrotic.
- Based on a very limited number of cases, horses with nonseptic calcaneal bursitis, including those with osteolytic lesions of the calcaneus, have a guarded prognosis for athletic activity.
- Horses with septic calcaneal bursitis tend to have a fair to guarded prognosis for athletic use because of the high motion required in this area during limb flexion.

Luxation of the SDFT from the Calcaneus

Overview
- A wide, flat, fibrous retinaculum arising from the SDFT attaches the tendon to the calcaneal tuber laterally and medially (Figures 1.42 and 4.13).
- Luxation of the SDFT from the calcaneal tuber occurs when one of its fascial attach-

ments (usually medial retinaculum) completely ruptures.
- This condition can be misdiagnosed as a capped hock or calcaneal bursitis, but careful evaluation usually reveals the SDFT has displaced laterally (Figure 4.16).
- Occasionally, the condition can occur bilaterally or can occur concurrently with a fracture of the calcaneus. They are rarely open.

Anatomy (Please refer to previous section on "Calcaneal Bursitis/Capped Hock")

Imaging (Please refer to previous section on "Calcaneal Bursitis/Capped Hock")
Etiology
- Trauma is the cause in most cases.
- Dislocation of the SDFT has been reported to occur as a racing injury, from simply bucking, or from unknown trauma.

Clinical Signs
- Heat, pain, and swelling at the point of the hock are usually present in acute cases.
- Lameness can be severe in the acute stage but usually improves quickly. Some horses with chronic dislocation may not be lame at presentation but have swelling around the tuber calcanei.

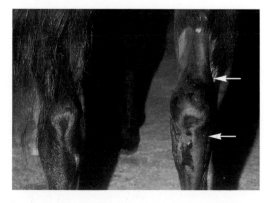

Figure 4.16 Caudal view of the tarsi in a horse with severe swelling within the right calcaneal bursa and evidence of lateral luxation of the right SDFT from the tuber calcanei (arrows).

- As the acute swelling subsides, the dislocation becomes more easily appreciated both visually and with palpation (Figure 4.16). The SDFT can usually be manually replaced over the tuber calcanei and then reluxates laterally when the tarsus is flexed.
- The tendon may remain completely luxated (stable luxation) or can reduce and then displace while walking (unstable luxation). Horses with actively luxating tendons may become quite distressed.
- Flexion of the tarsus is usually painful to the horse.

Diagnosis
- The diagnosis can usually be made based on clinical findings (Figure 4.16).
- Radiographs should be taken to rule out a fracture.
- Ultrasonography can be used to determine the extent of damage to the medial retinaculum and to document the severity of the concurrent calcaneal bursitis.

Treatment
- Treatment often depends on the degree of luxation and intended use of the horse.
- Partial dislocation of the SDFT should be treated conservatively with a three to four-month period of confinement and rehabilitation.
- Some clinicians feel that horses with complete luxation can do well without surgery while others recommend surgery. Too few numbers have been reported to determine which is best.
- Surgical options include debridement and repair of the torn fascia together with reinforcement of the suture line with mesh, or repair of the torn fascia and placing screws in the lateral aspect of the calcaneus to prevent re-luxation of the tendon. The limb is immobilized in a cast or sleeve cast for several weeks.
- Endoscopy of the bursa to debride the torn retinaculum and damaged fibrocartilage is recommended by some instead of surgical repair.

Prognosis
- The prognosis for breeding soundness or light pleasure riding is good with conservative treatment.
- Very few cases have been treated surgically but the results have often been disappointing.
- Some horses can perform normal work with the altered appearance and movement of the tendon at the calcaneal tuber.
- Some horses with a permanently luxated SDFT can, with conservative management, return to useful work.

Tarsal Sheath Tenosynovitis (Thoroughpin)

Overview
- Thoroughpin is a morphologic description of swellings of the tarsal sheath that occur from a variety of problems and with varying degrees of inflammation (Figure 1.35).
- True idiopathic tenosynovitis of the tarsal sheath can occur and is often bilateral and most likely related to limb conformation.
- Potential causes for tarsal sheath tenosynovitis include damage to the lateral digital flexor tendon (LDFT), sustentaculum tali, or calcaneus and infection from penetrating injuries.

Anatomy
- On the medial aspect of the tarsus, the tarsal fascia thickens into a flexor retinaculum, bridging the groove on the sustentaculum tail of the calcaneus to form the tarsal canal or sheath (Figure 4.17).
- The tarsal sheath contains the principal tendon of the DDF muscle (Figure 4.17) that is referred to as the LDFT.
- The tendon's synovial sheath, the tarsal sheath, extends from 5 to 8 cm proximal to the medial malleolus to the proximal fourth of the metatarsus (Figure 4.18).

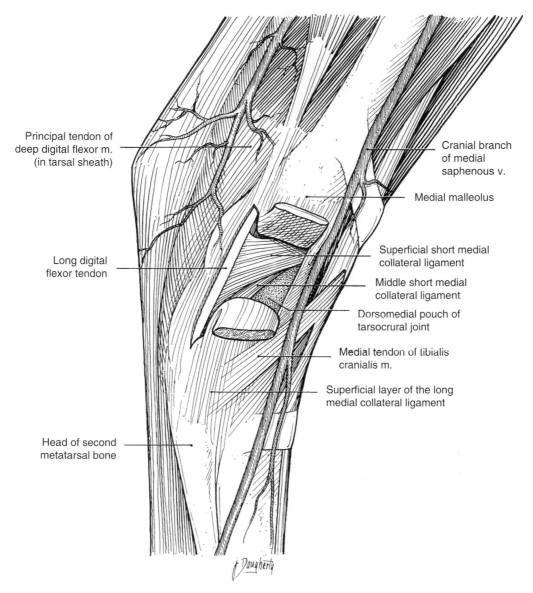

Principal tendon of
deep digital flexor m.
(in tarsal sheath)

Cranial branch
of medial
saphenous v.

Medial malleolus

Long digital
flexor tendon

Superficial short medial
collateral ligament

Middle short medial
collateral ligament

Dorsomedial pouch of
tarsocrural joint

Medial tendon of tibialis
cranialis m.

Superficial layer of the long
medial collateral ligament

Head of second
metatarsal bone

Figure 4.17 Medial view of the left tarsus. The long medial collateral ligament has been cut and reflected. The principal tendon of the deep digital flexor muscle can be seen within the tarsal sheath medial to the calcaneus within the sustentaculum tali. *Source*: Courtesy of J Daugherty.

Imaging

- Radiography and ultrasonography are usually both necessary to evaluate the tarsal sheath.
- MRI can be utilized to further define abnormalities within the LDFT but is usually unnecessary.
- Endoscopy of the tarsal sheath can be both a useful diagnostic and therapeutic tool.

Etiology

- Some horses have effusion within the tarsal sheath for what is thought to be no apparent reason and is referred to as idiopathic thoroughpin.
- Previous trauma to the sustentaculum tali, such as kick injuries to the medial aspect of the tarsus, is a likely contributing factor.

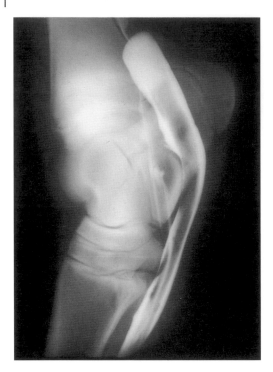

Figure 4.18 Iodinated contrast material has been injected into the tarsal sheath, showing the proximal and distal limits of this synovial cavity on the medial aspect of the tarsus.

- Damage to the LDFT can occur from exercise, direct trauma or secondarily from an exostosis of the sustentaculum tali.
- Penetrating injuries to the tarsal sheath may lead to infectious tenosynovitis similar to any synovial structure. Osteomyelitis of the sustentaculum tali is not an uncommon finding in many of these horses.

Clinical Signs

- Horses with idiopathic tenosynovitis have effusion within the tarsal sheath but no apparent lameness or performance limitations. The effusion is typically located on the medial aspect of the tarsus and courses up and down the leg in the direction of the tarsal sheath but may also be visible and palpable from the lateral aspect of the tarsus (Figure 4.19).
- Horses with nonseptic tenosynovitis often present for lameness and swelling of the medial aspect of the tarsus (Figure 1.35). Most horses are grade 2 to 3/5 lame and are positive to a tarsal flexion test. Intrasynovial anesthesia of the tarsal sheath usually improves the lameness.
- Horses with infection of the tarsal sheath are usually non-weight-bearing lame and are painful to digital pressure applied to the sheath. Effusion within the sheath may be difficult to determine in some horses because of diffuse swelling of the entire tarsus.

Diagnosis

- A presumptive diagnosis of tarsal sheath tenosynovitis can usually be made based on the clinical finding of effusion within the sheath (Figures 1.35 and 4.19).
- Clinically significant abnormalities within the sheath should be suspected in horses that are lame, positive to tarsal flexion, or improve with intrasynovial anesthesia of the sheath.
- Radiographs of the tarsus including a skyline view of the sustentaculum tali are recommended. The 45° dorsomedial-plantarolateral oblique projection is also helpful.
- Contrast radiography or a fistulogram may be helpful to document synovial involvement in horses with penetrating wounds of the tarsal sheath.
- Fractures, osteomyelitis, and proliferative exostosis of the sustentaculum tali are common radiographic abnormalities seen (Figure 4.20).
- Ultrasound should be performed to document abnormalities within the LDFT and sheath. Common findings include synovial proliferation, adhesions, fibrous masses, and fibrillation and architectural changes in the LDFT.
- Aspiration of synovial fluid from the sheath should be performed in horses with suspected sepsis or osteomyelitis of the sustentaculum tali to help document the presence of infection.

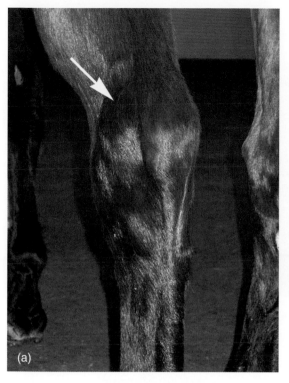
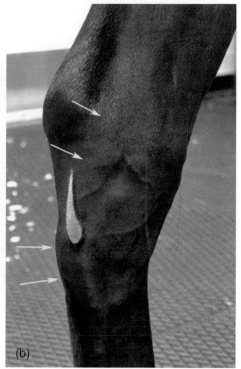

Figure 4.19 Thoroughpin can involve the lateral (a; arrow) or medial aspect of the tarsus (b; arrow). *Source*: Image (b) courtesy of Rich Redding.

Treatment

- True idiopathic tenosynovitis without lameness can be treated with benign neglect or intrasynovial medications combined with bandaging to prevent recurrence.
- Persistent idiopathic effusion also may be treated with intrasynovial atropine, but predisposing causes should be ruled out before resorting to this treatment.
- Horses with fractures, exostosis, or osteomyelitis of the sustentaculum tali are usually best treated surgically. This is especially true for open fractures and osteomyelitis with secondary infection of the sheath (Figure 4.20a).
- Endoscopy is the preferred surgical technique as lesions of the tarsal sheath, LDFT, and fragmentation of the sustentaculum tali are visible with tenoscopy and can be addressed directly with this technique.
- Horses with penetrating injuries or infection within the tarsal sheath are best treated with a combination of endoscopic lavage and debridement, parenteral and intrasynovial antimicrobials, and IV regional limb perfusion.

Prognosis

- Horses with idiopathic synovitis have a very good prognosis except for the cosmetic blemish.
- Horses with small fractures of the sustentaculum tali can do very well, provided damage to the LDFT is minimal (Figure 4.20).
- Chronic changes associated with fracture of the sustentaculum tali have been associated with a poor prognosis for return to athletic soundness.
- The overall prognosis for recovery from a septic tarsal sheath is only fair to guarded but is thought to be improved if no radiographic changes are present.
- The majority of horses with fractures or infection of the sustentaculum tali that are

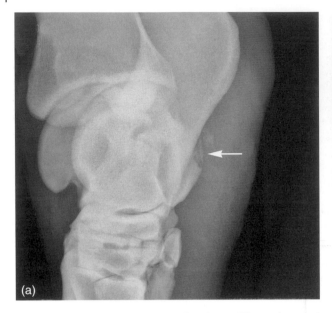
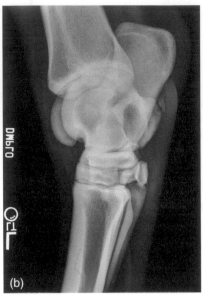

Figure 4.20 (a) Oblique radiographs of two different horses demonstrating an acute, open (a; arrow) and chronic, closed (b) fracture of the sustentaculum tali.

treated surgically should be able to return to performance, but the prognosis is variable based on many other factors.

Rupture of the Peroneus Tertius (Fibularis Tertius)

Overview

- The PT crosses both the stifle and tarsal joints surfaces and greatly contributes to the both the flexion and extension of these joints.
- When the PT is ruptured, the stifle flexes but the tarsus fails to flex as it should (Figure 4.21).
- The muscle or tendon can rupture anywhere along its course and an avulsion fracture at its origin in the extensor fossa of the femur can occur in young horses.

Anatomy

- The PT is a strong muscular band of tissue that lies between the long digital extensor and the tibialis cranialis muscle on the cranial aspect of the hindlimb.

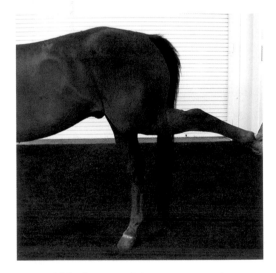

Figure 4.21 Rupture of the peroneus tertius disrupts the reciprocal apparatus, allowing extension of the tarsus and fetlock with the stifle flexed.

- The PT arises from the extensor fossa of the lateral femoral condyle and inserts with two distinct tendons to the tarsus and is tendinous over its entire length (Figures 1.42 and 4.13).

- The PT together with the superficial flexor muscle make up the reciprocal apparatus in the hindlimb and functions to passively flex the TC joint when the stifle joint is flexed (Figures 1.42 and 4.13).

Imaging

- Ultrasonography and radiography are usually necessary to document the site and severity of rupture.

Etiology

- Rupture of the PT is usually due to overextension of the hock joint. This may occur if the limb is entrapped and the horse struggles violently to free the limb.
- Rupture also may occur during the exertion of a fast start, when tremendous power is transferred to the limb. Examples include jumping and barrel racing.
- It also is a complication of full limb cast application to the hindlimb.

Clinical Signs

- With complete rupture, the stifle joint flexes as the limb advances and the tarsal joint moves forward with very little flexion.
- The portion of the limb below the hock tends to hang limp, giving the appearance that it is disconnected from the upper limb when carried forward.
- Swelling of the distal cranial aspect of the crus near the TC joint may be present in some adult horses, but lesions in the mid-crus seem to be more common and often are not associated with significant swelling.
- If the limb is lifted from the ground, a dimpling in the tendon of Achilles can be produced by extending the hock; the hock can be extended without extending the stifle (Figure 4.21).
- If the origin of the PT fractures from the femur, femoropatellar effusion is usually present and the gait deficit is similar. This is more common in young horses.

Diagnosis

- The diagnosis can usually be made based on the clinical findings.
- Radiographs of the stifle should be performed to document an avulsion fracture if femoropatellar joint effusion is present.
- Ultrasound can be used to better document the location and severity of the rupture.

Treatment

- Complete rest is the best treatment currently available. The horse should be placed in a box stall and kept quiet for at least four to six weeks and then limited exercise for the next two months.
- Most cases heal and eventually regain normal limb action. Some horses can return to normal work.
- Some horses will not regain a normal gait and the limb will appear "loose" or "sloppy" compared with the normal limb.

Prognosis

- The prognosis is guarded for athletic performance and can be difficult to predict.
- In one report, 71% of horses returned to their previous level of exercise with a mean rehabilitation period of 41.5 weeks. Performance horses were 11 times less likely to return to their intended use.
- Prognosis has been reported to be favorable when rupture occurs in the tibial region and poor if the rupture occurs at the point of origin from the extensor fossa of the lateral femoral condyle with any associated fracture.
- As with most soft tissue injuries, reinjury can occur.

Stringhalt

Overview

- Stringhalt is an involuntary hyperflexion of the hock when the horse moves that can affect one or both hindlimbs.

- The severity of the hyperflexion may vary from barely perceptible to the fetlock contacting the ventral abdomen.
- Two forms of stringhalt occur: a unilateral spontaneous form (North American stringhalt) of unknown cause (may be associated with trauma) and a bilateral form (Australian stringhalt) presumably caused by toxic plants or mycotoxins that reside on plants.

Anatomy and Imaging

- The extensor muscles (long and lateral digital extensors) on the cranial aspect of the tarsus are responsible for flexing the tarsus during movement.
- The hyperreflexia associated with stringhalt is thought to primarily involve the lateral digital extensor muscle tendon unit.
- Imaging is usually not beneficial in making the diagnosis. Radiography of the tarsus should be performed to determine if previous trauma could be a contributing factor.

Etiology

- One form of stringhalt affects isolated horses and is usually unilateral. It may follow an injury to the hindlimb.
- A small percentage of horses with stringhalt may have a history of previous injury to the dorsoproximal metatarsal extensor structures that healed by second intention.
- Australian stringhalt has been restricted to Australia and New Zealand and commonly occurs in outbreak proportions. It is usually bilateral and is thought to be due to certain toxic weeds including *Taraxacum officinael*, *Malva parviflora,* or *Hypochaeris radicata* (a dandelion), or mycotoxins that reside on the plants.
- A condition similar to Australian stringhalt has been reported in northern California, Washington, and southern Chile under similar conditions.

- The pathologic effect is thought to be a peripheral axonopathy in combination with a neurogenic myopathy with the plant-associated form of stringhalt.
- The pathophysiology of the hyperflexion remains unknown but is thought to be a hyperreflexia of the lateral digital extensor muscle unit.

Clinical Signs

- Signs of the disease are quite variable; some horses show a very mild flexion of the hock during walking, whereas others show a marked jerking of the foot toward the abdomen.
- The hyperflexion also may not occur with every step and is usually less prominent at the trot or canter.
- The signs are usually exaggerated when the horse is backed and may occur intermittently for unknown reasons.
- Most affected horses have a nervous disposition, which may play a part in the etiology and other peripheral neuropathies may occur concurrently.

Diagnosis

- For either form, the characteristic gait is usually enough to make the diagnosis.
- The condition must be differentiated from fibrotic myopathy and intermittent upward fixation of the patella (UFP).

Treatment

- The usual treatment for North American unilateral stringhalt is lateral digital extensor myotendonectomy (Figure 4.22). The success of this surgery is unpredictable.
- Spontaneous recovery of affected horses is uncommon but has been reported.
- For horses with Australian stringhalt, the majority of horses recover spontaneously without treatment once they are removed from pasture. Often, recovery can be protracted, from several weeks to one year.

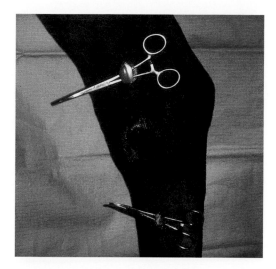

Figure 4.22 Lateral digital extensor myotenectomy illustrating the proximal and distal incision sites to perform this procedure.

- Pharmacological therapies that have been used include mephenesin, phenytoin, and baclofen, but their efficacy is unknown.

Prognosis
- For North American stringhalt, the prognosis ranges from guarded to favorable. Most horses show some improvement after surgery, but the degree of improvement is not predictable.
- For Australian stringhalt, the prognosis is similar. Many horses recover after removal from the pastures, whereas others do not.

Tibia and Crus

Tibial Stress Fractures

Overview
- Tibial stress fractures occur predominantly in young racehorses (primarily two-year-olds) during training before the horses have actually raced.

- These fractures tend to occur in either the caudolateral cortex in the distal metaphysis or diaphysis (Figure 4.23) or the proximal caudolateral cortex.
- They are usually unilateral but can occur bilaterally with one leg more severely affected.

Anatomy

- The crus or true leg is the region of the hindlimb containing the tibia and fibula and extends from the TC joint to the femorotibial joints.
- The tibia is one of the major weight-bearing bones of the hindlimb and extends obliquely downward and backward within the crus (Figures 4.1 and 4.13).
- The tibia is a tubular bone with a triangular-shaped cross section proximally changing to an oval shape as it courses distally.
- The proximal articular surface of the tibia is roughly triangular in shape with the tibial tuberosity protruding from the center of the triangle providing attachment for the patellar ligaments (Figure 4.1).
- The tibia is covered by muscle and tendon on the cranial, lateral, and caudal aspects but the medial surface is without muscle covering and easily palpated under the skin.
- The primary axis of tension strain in the tibia occurs on the cranial surface, while the caudal surface experiences compressive strains.

Imaging
- Scintigraphy is usually the imaging modality of choice to detect tibial stress fractures.
- Radiography may be able to detect some incomplete fractures and is usually diagnostic for complete fractures of the tibia.
- Large plates should be utilized to obtain radiographs of the entire length of the tibia and specific oblique projections can be performed of specific areas of interest.

Etiology
- Repetitive stresses leading to cyclic fatigue of the bone is the cause of stress fractures in horses that work at speed.
- Continued work at speed can cause catastrophic separation (complete tibia fracture) of incompletely healed stress fractures.

Clinical Signs
- An acute hindlimb lameness that gradually improves with inactivity and recurs with exercise is often observed.
- The lameness can be variable but is often moderate in severity with a shortened cranial phase of the stride and a stabbing hindlimb gait.
- There are usually no palpable abnormalities but occasionally deep palpation of the tibia at the typical locations for stress fractures may be painful.
- Local anesthesia is usually not helpful and is contraindicated to avoid repeated jogging of the horse.

Diagnosis
- The diagnosis usually involves a combination of radiology and scintigraphy.
- With acute fractures, scintigraphy is often required to document the lesion (Figure 4.23) as radiographs may be normal.
- If radiographically apparent, a small linear crack in the tibia may be all that is visible unless a healing callus is present (Figure 4.24).
- Oblique views may help demonstrate the presence of an endosteal and/or periosteal callus suggestive of a fracture.
- Repeat radiographs can be used to assess healing of the fracture but repeat scintigraphy may also be used.

Treatment
- An initial period of stall rest (4–12 weeks) followed by a controlled exercise program is the typical treatment.
- Time to return to racing is variable depending on the severity of the stress reaction and

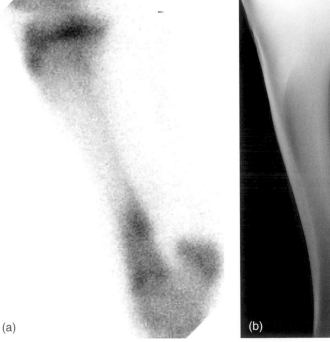
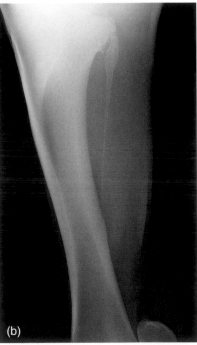

(a)

(b)

Figure 4.23 Lateral scintigram (a) showing a mild IRU in the distal tibia with the corresponding radiographic projection (b) demonstrating a periosteal callus and fracture. *Source*: Courtesy of Ryan Carpenter.

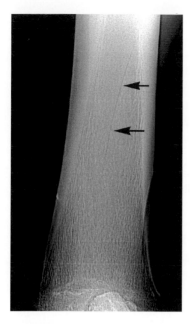

Figure 4.24 Radiograph demonstrating an incomplete tibial fracture (arrows).

should be based on a combination of clinical and imaging findings.

- Complete healing should be documented if possible before allowing the horse to return full exercise.

Prognosis

- The prognosis for return to racing is usually very good to excellent and the risk of recurrence is low.
- Returning horses to training too soon may predispose to complete fracture of the tibia.

Diaphyseal and Metaphyseal Tibial Fractures

Overview

- Both complete and incomplete fractures can occur in the tibia, but complete fractures are more common.
- Most complete fractures of the tibial shaft have a spiral configuration and/or are comminuted.
- Most fractures in older horses are highly comminuted due to the highly brittle nature

of the bone and affected horses are usually euthanized because of the poor prognosis with any form of treatment (Figure 4.25).

- In general, the smaller the patient, the better the prognosis for successful treatment.
- Open fractures are not uncommon because of the sparse soft tissue coverage on the medial aspect of the tibia.

Anatomy (Please refer to previous section on "Tibial Stress Fractures")

Imaging (Please refer to previous section on "Tibial Stress Fractures")

Etiology

- The cause of most complete tibial fractures is external trauma (e.g. kick, fall, pivot, or bad step).

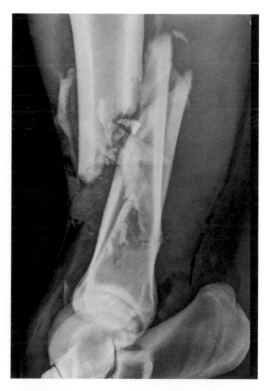

Figure 4.25 Injuries that impart significant energy to the tibia often cause the bone to shatter, especially in older horses. *Source*: Courtesy of Rich Redding.

- Complete fractures may occur subsequent to stress or incomplete fractures at any location in the tibia.
- Incomplete tibial fractures can occur from external trauma or subsequent to exercise as part of the stress fracture complex (Figure 4.24).
- Midshaft tibial fractures can occur from falls during a race or spontaneously for no apparent reason.

Clinical Signs

- Complete fracture of the tibia is characterized by a non-weight-bearing lameness, marked soft tissue swelling, angular deformity of the limb, and palpable crepitus.
- Craniomedial overriding of the proximal fragment coupled with valgus angulation frequently results in an open fracture due to the lack of soft tissue covering the medial aspect of the tibia.
- Horses with incomplete fractures usually present with severe lameness but typically do not have soft tissue swelling or angular deformity.

Diagnosis

- The obvious instability, swelling, and pain in the tibial region usually make a tentative diagnosis obvious.
- Radiographs are required to define the fracture configuration and to formulate a treatment plan or recommend euthanasia (Figure 4.25).
- Some incomplete or non-displaced fractures of the tibia may be difficult to diagnose, and several oblique projections may be needed to demonstrate the fracture (Figure 4.24).
- If no fracture can be identified, scintigraphy can be performed, or the horse should be confined, and the radiographs repeated in several days.

Treatment

- Euthanasia is advised for adult horses with severely comminuted fractures that cannot be stabilized, especially if they are open.

- Conservative management of cross-tying the horse in the stall can be used to treat some incomplete or minimally displaced tibial fractures. Horses with shorter (3–7 cm) visible fissure lines are more likely to survive (fractures do not displace) than those with longer (12–15 cm) spiral fissure lines (Figure 4.24).
- Incomplete fissure fractures of the distal metaphysis may benefit from a full-limb cast that is applied in the sedated standing horse in a normal weight-bearing position.
- The decision to use internal fixation on non-displaced tibial fractures can be difficult. Fractures traversing much of the length of the tibia probably should be repaired with internal fixation.
- Any form of external coaptation to treat displaced tibial fractures can be difficult, regardless of the size of the horse, and is generally not recommended.
- Internal fixation using 1 or 2 plates is usually the best treatment option in young horses with displaced tibial fractures. Simple, closed, oblique, or spiral fractures are the best candidates for surgical repair.

Prognosis

- The prognosis for a fractured tibia in an adult horse is extremely poor.
- Incomplete, non-displaced fractures usually heal with stall rest, but complete separation may still occur even after several weeks.
- The prognosis for successful repair of tibial fractures in young horses with internal fixation is reported to be about 60–70% but depends on the fracture type, its duration, and the treatment selected.

Tibial Tuberosity/Crest Fractures

Overview

- The physis of the tibial tuberosity is partially ossified at birth and forms a fibrocartilage union with the epiphysis during the second year of life.

- The tibial tuberosity is relatively broad and the area of the insertion of the lateral patellar ligament protrudes prominently and is usually involved with the fracture.
- Fractures are usually in the frontal plane, can be articular or nonarticular, frequently displace proximally, and can be open.

Anatomy

- The large cranial eminence of the proximal aspect of the cranial tibia is called the tibial tuberosity (Figures 4.1 and 4.13).
- This tuberosity has a prominent groove that serves as the site for attachment of the middle patellar ligament and is flanked by rough areas for attachment of the medial and lateral patellar ligaments (Figure 4.26).
- The cranial border of the proximal tibia distal to the groove for the middle patellar ligament is referred to as the tibial crest.
- The tibial tuberosity is a supplementary center of ossification that is completely ossified between 36 and 42 months of age.
- The three patellar ligaments also serve as the site of insertion for the quadriceps femoris muscle group onto the tibial tuberosity.
- The physis of the tibial tuberosity is partially ossified at birth and forms a fibrocartilage union with the epiphysis during the second year of life.

Imaging

- Radiography is used to document the location and configuration of the fracture.
- Ultrasonography can be used to evaluate concurrent injuries to the patella ligaments.

Etiology

- Most tibial crest fractures occur from direct trauma, such as a kick, or from hitting a jump or fence. It is a common injury in sport horses.
- Horses may occasionally avulse a fragment from the tuberosity due to sudden quadriceps tension. Displacement is in the proximal and

cranial direction and quadriceps integrity usually remains intact.

Clinical Signs

- The severity of the clinical signs depends on the size and duration of the fracture.
- Most horses are acutely lame with the typical signs of inflammation localized to the proximal tibial region. Swelling can be significant, and crepitus is usually palpable.
- Horses with small nonarticular fractures usually improve quickly but focal swelling of the tibial crest usually remains.
- Large fractures can cause considerable lameness and if the middle patellar ligament is compromised, the stifle may be "dropped," and the horse may not be willing or able to fix the limb in extension.
- An open wound may be present, especially with kick injuries, and must be taken into account when planning treatment.

Diagnosis

- The lateromedial radiograph usually demonstrates the fracture but an oblique Cd35″L-CrMO radiographic view may provide additional information (Figure 4.27).
- The most common fracture is a nondisplaced, nonarticular fracture. Fractures that extend at or caudal to the intercondylar eminence are usually articular.
- Secondary osteomyelitis of the fracture may be present with chronic open fractures (Figure 4.28).
- Ultrasound is useful to detect concurrent soft tissue injury and identify which patellar ligament insertions are involved with the fracture.

Treatment

- Non- or minimally displaced fractures can heal following stall rest and cross-tying for several weeks. Traction by the patellar ligaments may distract the fragment and prolong the healing time.
- Small fractures not involving the insertion of the middle patellar ligament can be removed, especially if they are open or infected

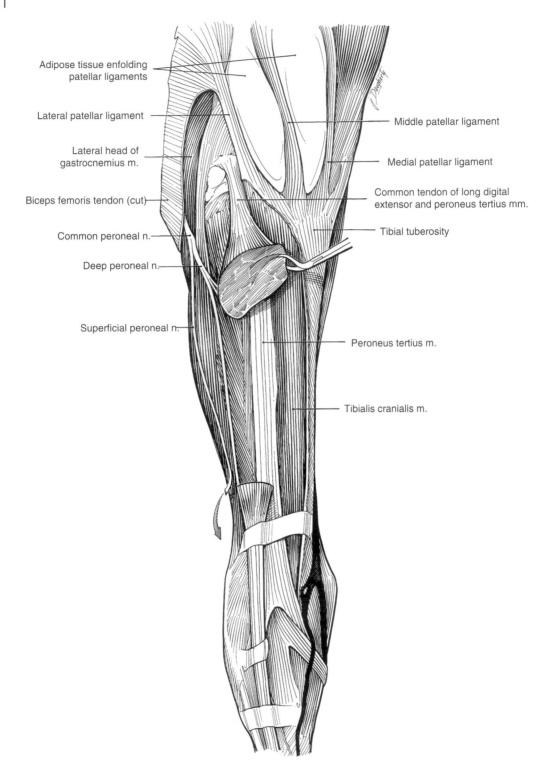

Adipose tissue enfolding patellar ligaments

Lateral patellar ligament

Lateral head of gastrocnemius m.

Biceps femoris tendon (cut)

Common peroneal n.

Deep peroneal n.

Superficial peroneal n.

Middle patellar ligament

Medial patellar ligament

Common tendon of long digital extensor and peroneus tertius mm.

Tibial tuberosity

Peroneus tertius m.

Tibialis cranialis m.

Figure 4.26 Dorsal view of the right stifle, crus, and tarsus. The long digital extensor muscle belly has been removed, along with the terminal parts of the superficial fibular (peroneal) nerve (arrow). The tibial tuberosity and the three patellar ligaments are visible on the cranial aspect of the stifle. *Source*: Courtesy of J Daugherty.

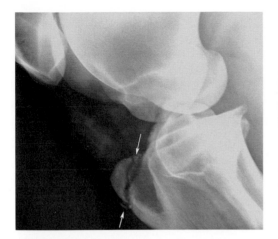

Figure 4.27 Fractures of the tibial tuberosity most often occur in mature sport horses usually due to a direct impact of the stifle on a fence or jump. Some non-displaced fragments (arrows) may heal with stall confinement. *Source*: Courtesy of Rich Redding.

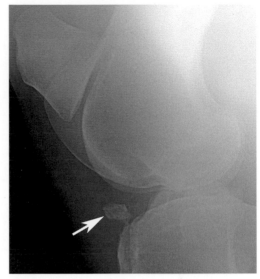

Figure 4.28 This small, chronic fracture of the lateral tibial tuberosity was removed because it was contributing to chronic drainage.

(Figure 4.28). If left, these fractures tend to take a very long time to heal and may cause lameness.

- Unstable, displaced, or articular fractures should be repaired with internal fixation using the tension-band principle. Application of a bone plate improves the repair when the fragment is large and/or unstable.

Prognosis

- Horses with nondisplaced nonarticular fractures have a very good prognosis with conservative treatment (14 of 17 horses became sound in one report).
- The recovery rate for surgically repaired tibial tuberosity fractures also is generally good, provided stable fixation can be accomplished.
- Horses tend to have a very good prognosis following removal of small tuberosity fractures regardless of whether they are open or closed.

Fractures of the Proximal Tibial Physis

Overview

- Young horses are at increased risk to develop fractures through a physis and fractures of

the proximal tibial physis have been observed in foals up to eight months of age.

- The fracture is nearly always a Salter Harris Type II fracture with the metaphyseal fragment located laterally (Figure 4.29).
- The fracture is rarely open or articular and concurrent soft tissue injuries are uncommon.

Anatomy (Please refer to previous section on "Tibial Tuberosity Fractures")

Imaging (Please refer to previous section on "Tibial Tuberosity Fractures")

Etiology

- The injury usually occurs from direct trauma (e.g. kick) while the limb is bearing weight, or from bending while having the limb somehow entrapped or when the mare steps on the recumbent foal's uppermost hindlimb.
- The forces apply pressure in a valgus direction, causing medial tension to separate the physeal cartilage. The epiphysis and bone fragment displace laterally due to the "ramp" defect left in the proximal lateral metaphysis (Figure 4.29).

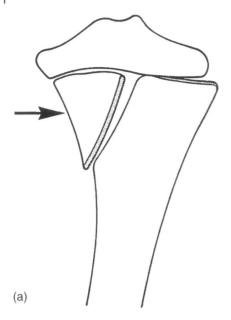
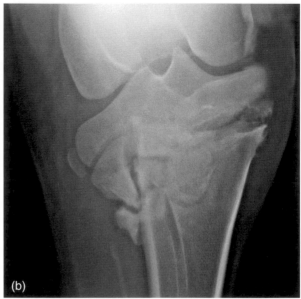

(a)

(b)

Figure 4.29   Line illustration (a) and caudocranial radiograph (b) of the stifle demonstrating a Salter-Harris Type II fracture of the proximal tibial physis. The metaphyseal component is always lateral (arrow) and usually involves approximately one-third of the distance across the physis.

Clinical Signs

- The affected limb usually assumes a "stifle" valgus position (the distal limb is deviated outward distal to the stifle).
- Lameness is usually severe initially and improves with time. Swelling and pain typical of a fracture are often palpable. Crepitus is usually difficult to detect.

Diagnosis

- Radiographs are required to confirm the diagnosis. The caudal-cranial view is the most informative, revealing the displacement of the epiphysis and metaphyseal component (Figure 4.29b).
- Most fractures are considerably displaced, and the epiphysis is usually tilted.

Treatment

- Surgical repair with a bone plate placed on the medial aspect of the tibia is the treatment of choice. The fixation may be further improved by the placement of a tension band along the tibial crest.

- No external coaptation is used after surgery and the implants should be removed in eight to 10 weeks to help prevent the development of a permanent ALD.
- Conservative management has been used successfully to treat non-displaced tibial physeal fractures in a small number of horses but is usually not recommended.

Prognosis

- The prognosis is generally favorable for fracture repair, barring complications such as failure of the fixation, ALD, infection, or wound dehiscence.
- The smaller and younger the foal, the better the prognosis.
- The prognosis for athletic activity following successful fixation is about 50%.

Gastrocnemius Disruption in Foals and Adults

Overview

- Disruption of the gastrocnemius muscle can cause dysfunction of the reciprocal apparatus and can be a source of lameness in the adult or the neonate.

- In foals, the injury is usually severe and can cause recumbency and an inability to stand (Figure 4.30).
- Disruption of the SDF muscle in the caudal crus has also been reported in adult horses and may present in a similar manner to damage to the gastrocnemius muscle.

Anatomy

- Descending from their origins on the supracondyloid tuberosities of the femur, the two heads of the gastrocnemius enclose the round, mostly tendinous superficial digital flexor in the caudal crus.
- The superficial digital flexor muscle is part of the caudal component of the reciprocal apparatus of the hindlimb and is closely associated with the gastrocnemius muscle and tendon (Figures 4.13).

- Disruption of either the gastrocnemius muscle and tendon or the SDF muscle and tendon can result in similar postural changes in the hindlimb.

Imaging

- Ultrasonography is the primary imaging tool to confirm the site and severity of the muscular damage and associated hematoma formation.

Etiology

- The condition is recognized in neonates following both normal deliveries and dystocias, but larger foals appear to be predisposed to the condition.
- Disruption in both foals and adults can be partial or total.
- In adult horses, the injury usually involves the origin of the muscle, and is caused by forceful extension of the hindlimb. Total disruption is uncommon.

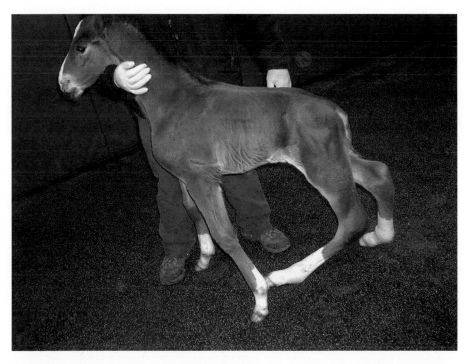

Figure 4.30 Excessive flexion of the hock in a foal with rupture of the left gastrocnemius muscle. *Source:* Courtesy of Robert Hunt.

- Ultrasonography is the primary imaging tool to confirm the site and severity of the muscular damage and associated hematoma formation.

Clinical Signs and Diagnosis

- With a complete tear of the muscle, the foal is unable to extend the limb, which will collapse with weight-bearing and the excessive flexion of the hock with the stifle in a fixed position, resulting in a typical, crouched position (Figure 4.30).
- With partial rupture, there is moderate flexion of the tarsus, but the foal can still bear weight on the limb.
- Affected adult horses may have a gait abnormality characterized by lateral rotation of the point of the calcaneus and medial rotation of the toe.
- The diagnosis is usually made based on the history and characteristic stance in foals and can be confirmed with ultrasound.
- The diagnosis is more difficult in adult horses with only partial disruptions and may require a combination of scintigraphy and radiography to evaluate the origin of the gastrocnemius muscle on the distal aspect of the femur.

Treatment and Prognosis

- Splinting of the limb is usually required in foal. Bandages must be changed frequently to prevent focal pressure necrosis, adequately support the limb, and support ambulation while healing occurs.
- In adults with an extended period of rest followed by a gradual return to exercise can be successful in returning the horse to soundness.
- Prognosis for future soundness in foals is good with conservative treatment.
- Horses with partial disruption of the gastrocnemius have a reasonable chance to return to athletic function.

Stifle – Femoropatellar Region

Femoropatellar OCD

Overview

- Femoropatellar OCD is a common cause of stifle effusion and lameness in young horses (Figures 4.31 and 1.44).
- Thoroughbreds are commonly affected but it can occur in all breeds.
- The majority of affected horses are yearlings (<2 years old) with twice as many males as females affected, and they typically are the better individuals in the herd.
- The most common site for femoropatellar OCD is the lateral trochlear ridge of the femur.
- Half or more of affected horses have bilateral lesions.

Anatomy

- The stifle is the region including the stifle joint (femorotibial joints plus the femoropatellar joint) and surrounding structures.
- The synovial space of the stifle is partitioned into three distinct sacs: the femoropatellar

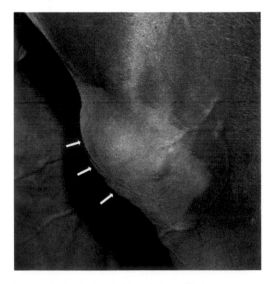

Figure 4.31 Lateral view of the stifle in a horse with severe femoropatellar effusion (arrows).

joint sac and the right and left femorotibial joint sacs.

- The patella and the two trochlear ridges of the distal femur comprise the femoropatellar joint (Figure 4.1).
- The articular surface of the patella is much smaller than the trochlear surface of the femur and the medial trochlear ridge is much larger than the lateral trochlear ridge (Figure 4.32).
- Contact between the patella and the wide groove between the trochlea changes as the patella moves on its larger gliding surface during flexion of the stifle joint.

Imaging
- Radiography is the initial imaging tool to evaluate the stifle in most cases.

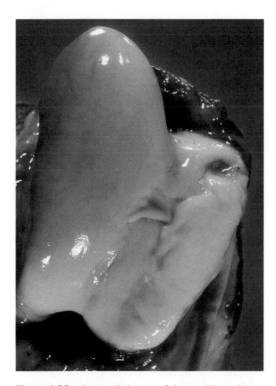

Figure 4.32 Anatomic image of the trochlear ridges of the distal femur. The medial trochlear ridge (left) is much larger than the lateral ridge. A very large OCD lesion is present on the lateral trochlear ridge. Lesion size is thought to correlate with prognosis.

- Ultrasonography can be helpful to evaluate both intra-articular and periarticular structures and is used mostly within the femorotibial joints.
- Specially designed CT and MRI units can be used to image the stifle of most horses depending on their size, but their use is not considered routine.

Etiology
- OCD is a developmental abnormality that is defined as a focal disturbance of endochondral ossification with a multifactorial etiology.
- The most commonly cited contributing factors are heredity, rapid growth, anatomic conformation, trauma, and dietary imbalances.
- Trauma within the joint may be difficult to differentiate from true OCD lesions because traumatic events can destabilize a pre-existing OCD fragment.

Clinical Signs
- Femoropatellar OCD usually causes visible joint effusion (Figure 4.31) and variable hindlimb lameness.
- The lameness may be so mild that joint effusion is the main presenting complaint but hindlimb flexion is usually positive in horses with clinically significant OCD.
- Horses presenting after training has begun generally have less severe lesions than horses presenting at an earlier age.
- Some weanlings may present with joint effusion, lameness, and no radiographic abnormalities.
- Infrequently, bilaterally affected horses may be extremely lame and may have difficulty rising from recumbency.

Diagnosis
- LM radiographs of the stifle usually demonstrate a flattened defect in the proximal portion of the lateral trochlear ridge of the femur. Ossification within the defect is variable and loose bodies may be present (Figure 4.33).

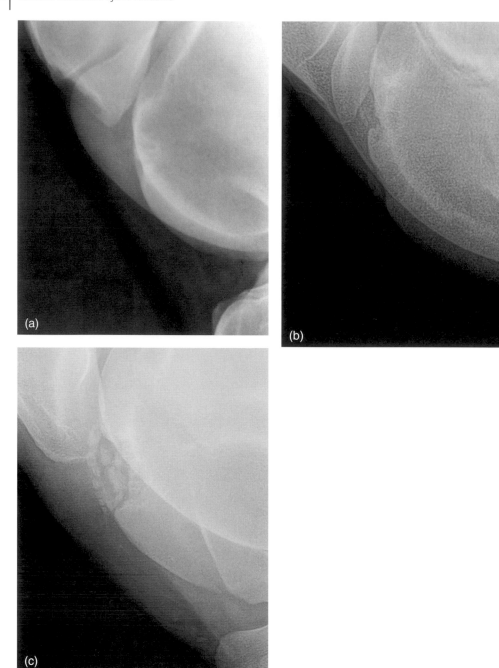

Figure 4.33 Radiographs of three cases of OCD of the lateral trochlear ridge of the femur in the femoropatellar joint. (a) A small defect in the lateral trochlear ridge without obvious fragmentation within the defect (treated conservatively). (b) A fragment within a defect. (c) Multiple fragments in a more severe lesion. *Source*: Courtesy of C.W. McIlwraith.

- Caudolateral to craniomedial oblique films may provide more information about the severity of lateral trochlear ridge defects.
- Other locations for OCD lesions in the stifle include the medial trochlear ridge, the trochlear groove, the articular surface of the patella, or in any combination.
- Secondary abnormalities of the patella can usually be observed in the LM view and typically contribute to a worse prognosis.
- Ultrasound can be used as an adjunct to radiographs because the trochlear surfaces of the distal femur are readily imaged using ultrasound.

Treatment

- Surgical management is the mainstay of treatment for OCD in young athletic horses.
- Some OCD lesions may resolve over time in foals less than one year of age. Stall confinement is recommended to protect the articular surface, and both systemic and IA biological therapies may be beneficial. IA corticosteroids are contraindicated.
- Weanlings and short yearlings can present with effusion and lameness, but no radiographic lesions and conservative therapy is indicated unless clinical signs persist.
- Arthroscopic surgery is indicated when it is obvious that the lesion will not heal with conservative therapy and in horses beyond a year of age with persistent clinical signs.
- When clinical signs are present in adults, surgical debridement produces better results than conservative therapy.
- Arthroscopic reattachment of OCD cartilage flaps has been reported in select horses but is not performed routinely.

Prognosis

- The prognosis for athletic activity following arthroscopic surgery for femoropatellar OCD is generally very good.
- Increasing OCD lesion size has a negative effect on outcome and may increase the risk of developing a surgical site infection.

- A recent study also suggests that OCD lesions of the femoropatellar joint limited future performance of affected horses compared with OCD lesions at other locations.
- Horses with lateral trochlear ridge lesions and patellar lesions usually have a reduced prognosis.

Fractures of the Patella

Overview

- Several configurations of patellar fractures including sagittal, transverse, comminuted, basilar (proximal), and distal fragmentation of the patella can occur in the horse.
- Most patellar fractures are articular and involve the medial aspect of the bone (Figure 4.34).
- Patellar fractures may be accompanied by severe soft tissue trauma involving the patellar ligaments and joint capsule of the stifle joint.
- Open fractures associated with kick injuries are not uncommon.

Anatomy

- The patella is a sesamoid bone intercalated in the termination of the quadriceps femoris muscle with the three patellar ligaments, constituting the tendon of insertion (Figure 4.13).
- Deep to the skin, three patellar ligaments descend from the patella, converging to their attachments on the tibial tuberosity (Figures 4.26 and 4.13).
- An extensive pad of adipose tissue is interposed between the ligaments and the joint capsule of the femoropatellar joint, and the adipose tissue enfolds the ligaments.
- The base, cranial surface, and medial border of the patella, and the parapatellar fibrocartilage and femoropatellar joint capsule serve as attachments for the insertions of the quadriceps femoris muscle (Figure 4.13).

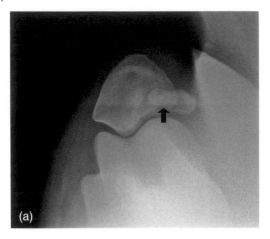
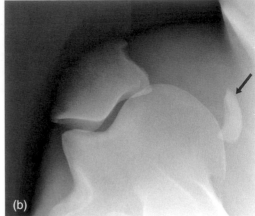

Figure 4.34 Cranioproximal to craniodistal (skyline) projections showing a typical medial patellar fracture fragment (a; arrow) and a large displaced sagittal fracture (b; arrow). Arthroscopic removal is indicated in (a). Arthroscopy was attempted in (b) but an arthrotomy was necessary for removal.

Imaging

- Radiography is the imaging technique of choice to document a suspected patella or other type of IA fracture of the femoropatellar joint. A cranioproximal to craniodistal (skyline) projection is usually necessary to document the fracture.
- Ultrasonography is primarily used to determine secondary damage to the patellar ligaments or other soft tissue injuries in the area.

Etiology

- Direct trauma to the patella while the stifle joint is in a semi-flexed position is the usual cause. Horses that jump can strike jumps or the fracture can occur from a kick to the cranial aspect of the stifle.
- The prominence of the medial trochlear ridge may be a point of contact causing a relative higher incidence of fractures toward the medial side of the patella.
- Fragmentation of the distal patella may occur following a MPL desmotomy if horses are returned to work too soon or may be due to trauma secondary to temporary patellar instability (Figure 4.35).

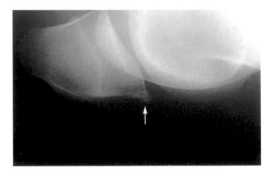

Figure 4.35 Flexed lateromedial radiograph of the stifle demonstrating fragmentation of the apex of the patella (arrow).

Clinical Signs

- Most horses present with an acute onset of moderate-to-severe lameness and a painful swelling associated with the cranial aspect of the stifle.
- Femoropatellar effusion is usually present but significant soft tissue swelling may obscure its detection.
- Flexion of the stifle joint will usually elicit a painful response and exacerbate the lameness.
- Weight-bearing may be difficult with compromise of the quadriceps or from pain and the horse may stand with the limb partially flexed without locking the stifle (Figure 4.36).

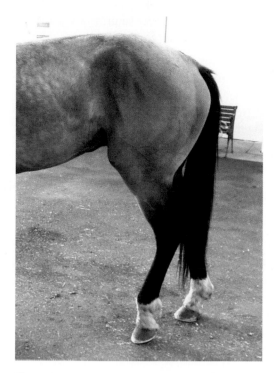

Figure 4.36 Typical stance of a horse with a patella fracture. This horse had been kicked and there was a wound over the cranial aspect of the stifle.

- Horses with smaller fractures may present for routine lameness evaluation but typically have effusion of the femoropatellar joint and are positive to stifle flexion.
- Comminuted patellar fractures that compromise the middle patellar ligament and/or quadriceps muscle may cause an inability of the horse to support weight on the limb.

Diagnosis
- Radiographs are required to document the type and extent of the fracture. Routine lateromedial and caudocranial projections usually demonstrate transverse or comminuted fractures; the caudolateral-to-craniomedial oblique projection accentuates the apex (distal border) of the patella.
- Smaller medial fragments may not be visible on routine radiographs and may require a cranioproximal to craniodistal (skyline) projection (Figure 4.34).

- Ultrasound is useful to identify patellar ligament disruption or other lesions that may not be radiographically visible such as medial fibrocartilage separation.

Treatment
- Nonarticular or small medial or basilar fragments may heal with rest and anti-inflammatory therapy.
- Horses with intra-articular fractures seldom remain sound when returned to work and stable fragments may displace when horses return to sustained work.
- With adequate quadriceps stability, fragments approximating one-third of the patellar substance can be successfully removed, and arthroscopy is recommended (Figure 4.34).
- Fragmentation of the distal patella secondary to medial patellar ligament (MPL) desmotomy is best treated with arthroscopic debridement.
- Internal fixation should be considered for displaced fractures with sizeable fragments and transverse fractures. Successful internal fixation of transverse distracted, and longitudinally displaced fractures of the patella have been reported.
- Horses with highly comminuted fractures and/or those with compromise of the middle patellar ligament or quadriceps function are candidates for euthanasia.

Prognosis
- The prognosis following removal of articular medial fragments is considered very good (16 of 19 horses returned to work in one study).
- The prognosis for debridement of distal patellar fragmentation is also very good if secondary articular cartilage damage is minimal.
- The prognosis remains fair to guarded for horses undergoing internal fixation of complicated fractures.
- Horses with severely comminuted fractures are likely to remain lame but some may

attain breeding soundness with prolonged confinement.

Upward Fixation of the Patella (UFP)

Overview

- UFP occurs when the MPL becomes caught over the medial trochlear ridge.
- With the MPL fixed in this position, the hindlimb cannot be flexed, and the horse assumes a posture with the affected limb extended in a caudally abducted position with the fetlock flexed due to the reciprocal apparatus (Figure 4.37).
- Intermittent "catching" of the MPL occurs more commonly and is considered a less severe stage of UFP.
- UFP appears to be common in ponies and miniature horses but can occur in all breeds of horses.

Anatomy (Please refer to previous section on "Patella Fractures")

Imaging (Please refer to previous section on "Patella Fractures")

Etiology

- Horses that have exceptionally straight hindlimbs are considered to be prone to UFP. To support this, hyperextension of the limb by walking a horse downhill usually exacerbates UFP.
- Body type is strongly inherited and therefore it is likely that the tendency for UFP could be congenital.
- Loss of quadriceps muscle tone due to reduced work or debilitation functionally "lengthens" the MPL, allowing it to catch over the medial trochlear ridge. This is observed in young horses beginning training with insufficient muscle tone and in horses abruptly taken out of training and confined to a stall.

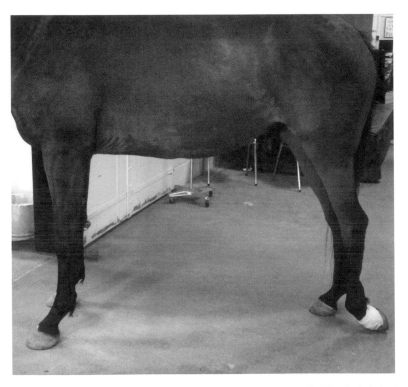

Figure 4.37 A horse with severe upward fixation of the patella. The limb is locked in extension causing the horse to drag its left hindlimb.

- Higher medial hoof wall and elongated toes have been reported to cause hyperextension of the stifle and outward rotation of the limb, contributing to UFP.
- Craniodorsal luxation of the coxofemoral joint predisposes to UFP by causing excessive straightening of the hindlimb.

Clinical Signs

- With acute UFP, the hindlimb is locked in extension and the stifle cannot be flexed. When the horse is forced to move forward with the limb locked, it drags the front of the hoof on the ground (Figure 4.37). The condition may correct itself or remain locked for several hours or even days.
- Intermittent UFP is described as intermittent "catching" of the patella as the horse walks or jogs contributing to a jerking gait. Walking the horse downhill, backing it, or moving it in a tight circle usually exacerbates the signs. When the MPL releases, the hindlimb usually jerks up quickly, mimicking stringhalt.
- Usually both hindlimbs are potentially affected, but unilateral UFP can occur.
- Palpation of the limb when locked in extension reveals tense patellar ligaments and the patella locked above the medial trochlear ridge of the femur.
- Lameness usually is not present unless the condition is very chronic.

Diagnosis

- The diagnosis is usually based on the characteristics of the gait and limb posture.
- When the limb is in a normal position, the predisposition to UFP can be evaluated by forcing the patella upward and outward with the hand. If the limb can be manually locked in extension for one or more steps, it is predisposed to UFP.
- Radiographs of the stifle should be taken to eliminate conditions that may predispose to UFP, but radiographic abnormalities are uncommon.

Treatment

- Horses with a persistent UFP that repeatedly reoccurs after manually unlocking the patella often require an MPL desmotomy to resolve the problem.
- Less severely affected horses respond to controlled conditioning to increase quadriceps strength and tone, which tightens the MPL.
- Shortening the toe and lowering the medial hoof wall sufficient to move break-over medial to the toe may help alleviate UFP in some horses.
- Other treatments for UFP include "tightening" the MPL by splitting the ligament in multiple locations or injecting counterirritants (2% iodine in almond oil or ethanolamine oleate). This results in substantial thickening of the MPL, presumably causing a functional shortening and tightening of the MPL.
- Estrogen therapy (1 mg of estradiol cypionate IM for every 45 kg of body weight (i.e. 11 mg/500 kg) once weekly for three to five weeks) has also been recommended.
- If all treatments fail to correct the UFP, an MPL desmotomy can be performed. Fragmentation of the distal patella is a risk but is less likely to occur in horses that have persistent UFP compared with those that do not.
- A logical progression of treatment after conditioning and ensuring correct shoeing is counterirritant injection, MPL splitting, and then a MPL desmotomy.

Prognosis

- The prognosis is very good for horses that respond to a conditioning program and maintain that level of fitness.
- Most horses do well following injection of a counterirritant or MPL splitting procedure.
- Horses that require an MPL desmotomy also have a very good prognosis and are unlikely to have complications if they receive a 60- to 90-day convalescence following surgery.

Stifle – Femorotibial Region

Subchondral Cystic Lesions (SCLs) of the Stifle

Overview

- SCLs within the stifle are nearly always located on the medial femoral condyle but can occasionally occur on the lateral femoral condyle and the proximal tibia.
- SCLs of the medial femoral condyle can occur in several different configurations and sizes and is one of the most difficult lameness conditions in the horse to resolve (Figure 4.38).
- The presence of concurrent OA in the medial femorotibial (MFT) joint is usually associated with a reduced prognosis.

Anatomy

- The femoral condyles of the distal femur articulate lie within the medial and lateral femorotibial joints within the stifle.
- Two fibrocartilaginous menisci intervene between the femoral condyles and tibial plateau creating individual medial and lateral femorotibial joint spaces.
- In addition to the support rendered by medial and lateral collateral ligaments, the femur and tibia are joined by the two cruciate ligaments that cross one another in the intercondyloid space between the two synovial sacs of the femorotibial joints (Figure 4.39).
- The femorotibial joints are major weight-bearing surfaces within the stifle and many clinical problems occur within the MFT joint.

Imaging

- Radiography is used to document most SCL's within the stifle.
- Ultrasonography is routinely used to characterize damage to the menisci, ligaments, and periarticular structures.

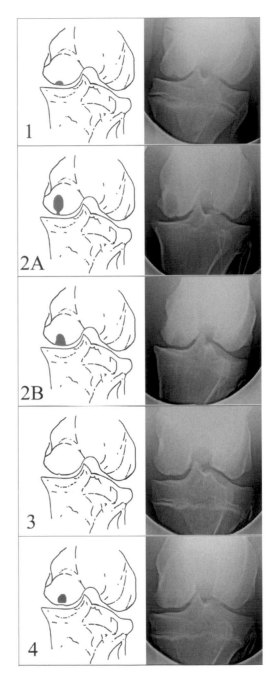

Figure 4.38 Grades of subchondral cystic lesions (SCLs). *Source*: Reprinted with permission from Wallis TW, Goodrich LR, McIlwraith CW, et al.: 2008. Arthroscopic injection of corticosteroids into the fibrous tissue of subchondral cystic lesions of the medial femoral condyle in horses: A retrospective study of 52 cases (2001–2006). *Equine Vet J* 40:461–467.

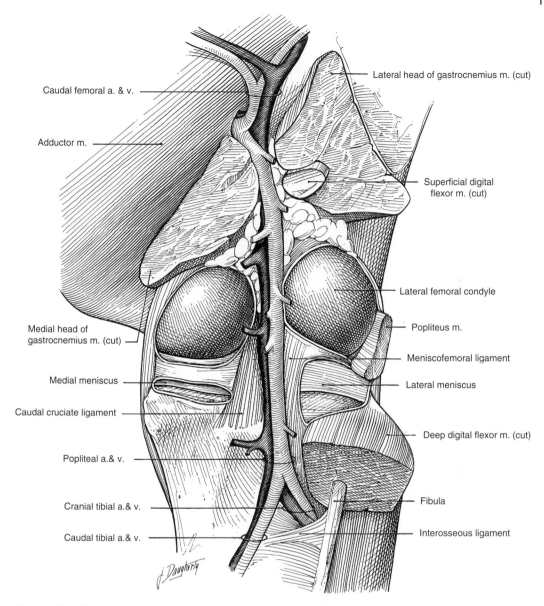

Caudal femoral a. & v.

Adductor m.

Medial head of gastrocnemius m. (cut)

Medial meniscus

Caudal cruciate ligament

Popliteal a.& v.

Cranial tibial a.& v.

Caudal tibial a.& v.

Lateral head of gastrocnemius m. (cut)

Superficial digital flexor m. (cut)

Lateral femoral condyle

Popliteus m.

Meniscofemoral ligament

Lateral meniscus

Deep digital flexor m. (cut)

Fibula

Interosseous ligament

Figure 4.39 Deep dissection of the caudal aspect of the right stifle. The joint capsule of the femorotibial joints has been opened exposing the medial and lateral menisci and the caudal cruciate and meniscofemoral ligaments. *Source*: Courtesy of J Daugherty.

- Cross-sectional imaging (CT and MRI) can be used to image the stifle when appropriate imaging machines are available.
- Arthroscopy is often used for both diagnostic and therapeutic purposes in the femorotibial joints.

Etiology

- Many SCLs in the stifle are developmental in origin and are considered a type of developmental orthopedic disease (DOD) because they occur in young horses and are often bilateral (Figure 4.40a).

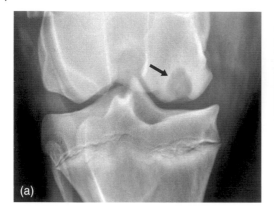 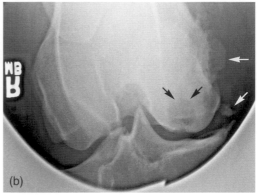

Figure 4.40 Caudal-cranial radiographs of the stifle in a yearling filly (a) and of an eight-year-old Quarter horse mare (b). There are minimal radiographic abnormalities in the MFT joint other than the SCL in (a) compared with multiple abnormalities in (b) (black arrows indicate a SCL; top white arrow indicates osteophyte production along the femur; bottom white arrow indicates mineralization of the medial meniscus). SCL in (a) is likely developmental in origin vs. the SCL in (b) is likely due to trauma.

- There is also both clinical and experimental evidence that SCLs can occur after trauma to the subchondral bone on weight-bearing articular surfaces. The SCL is usually unilateral, and concurrent abnormalities such as OA or meniscal problems are often present in the MFT joint (Figure 4.40b).
- Tissues from postmortem cystic material were found to have significant osteoclastic function on bone that may be responsible for enlargement and persistence of the SCL.

Clinical Signs

- The clinical presentation of horses with SCLs can vary from no lameness with the lesion being an incidental finding on radiographs to severe, debilitating lameness with multiple abnormalities within the MFT joint.
- Most horses with stifle SCLs become lame around the beginning of training, and a mild-to-moderate degree of lameness is usually present.
- Effusion may or may not be present within the MFT joints and the femoropatellar joints and horses are usually positive to upper limb flexion.
- In older horses that have been in training and competition, it is important to perform

IA analgesia of the MFT joint to document the significance of a SCL.

Diagnosis

- Radiography is the standard method of imaging for an accurate diagnosis. The caudo-cranial view is usually most diagnostic, but most SCLs can also be seen on a flexed lateral radiograph of the stifle.
- At minimum, a caudo-cranial view of the opposite stifle should always be obtained.
- A variety of shapes and sizes of lesions can be found. A grading scheme (Types 1 to 4) has been developed to help describe the different shape, size, depth, and articular involvement of the SCLs of the medial femoral condyle (Figure 4.38).
- The radiographic appearance of SCLs can change over time and should be monitored, especially in young horses.
- Concurrent radiographic signs of OA such as periarticular osteophytes and joint space narrowing are often seen in older horses. The caudoproximal to craniodistal oblique projection made at 10° from horizontal is the best projection to assess joint space width in the MFT joint.
- Ultrasound is used to evaluate the articular surface, joint effusion, debris, and

changes that may occur in the meniscus and MFT joint. SCLs typically show an irregularity on the condylar surface and thickening of the articular cartilage (Figure 4.41).

Treatment

- Conservative therapy (confinement, IA, and systemic medications) can be used in horses less than one year of age or in SCLs that are either small, have a small articular component, or may show limited communication between the SCL and the joint surface (intact subchondral bone plate).
- Continued lameness and/or SCL enlargement are indications for surgical treatment.

- Surgical treatment options include debridement of the cyst contents, injection of the cystic lining with corticosteroids, grafting of the debrided cyst with various products, and transcystic screw placement.

Prognosis

- The overall prognosis is approximately 56–77% of horses returning to their intended use with surgery regardless of the technique used.
- Horses in which more than 15 mm of the surface of the joint is involved have a reduced prognosis.
- Horses older than three years of age have a lower chance of soundness and return to work regardless of the treatment option.

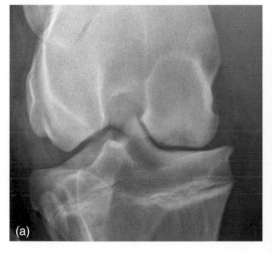
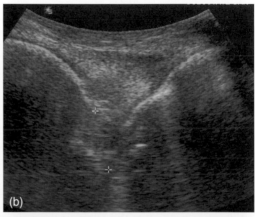
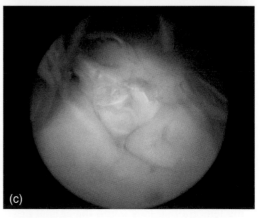

Figure 4.41 Radiograph (a), ultrasound (b), and intraoperative (c) images demonstrating an SCL that involved a large percentage of the articular surface. Note the joint space narrowing on the radiographic image (a), and the presence of the SCL as demonstrated by a defect in the subchondral bone on the ultrasonographic image (b). Thickening of the articular cartilage can be seen arthroscopically (c). *Source:* Courtesy of Chris Kawcak.

- Damage to the menisci and/or meniscal ligament or articular cartilage indicative of OA can further reduce the prognosis of affected horses.
- Horses with unilateral lesions have an improved prognosis compared with those with bilateral lesions.

Meniscal Injuries

Overview

- Horses of any breed and use are susceptible to meniscal lesions, especially horses that jump.
- Western performance and sport horses have a high incidence of stifle problems, and consequently are predisposed to secondary meniscal lesions.
- Although both lateral and medial meniscal lesions occur, damage to the medial meniscus is far more common.

Anatomy

- The medial and lateral menisci are fibrocartilaginous spacers that intervene between the femoral condyles and tibial plateau (Figures 1.43 and 4.39).
- The menisci are crescent-shaped, being thicker peripherally and thinner along the concave edge, and their proximal surfaces are concave to accommodate the convexity of the femoral condyles.
- Distally the menisci conform to the peripheral parts of the articular surfaces of the tibial condyles.
- Cranial and caudal ligaments anchor each meniscus to the tibia, and a meniscofemoral ligament attaches the caudal aspect of the lateral meniscus to the caudal surface of the intercondyloid fossa of the femur (Figure 4.39).
- The menisci act as shock absorbers within the femorotibial joints, and the cranial ligament of the medial meniscus is a common location for injury.

Imaging

- Meniscal damage can usually be documented with ultrasonography of the stifle.
- Arthroscopy is often helpful to both diagnose and debride meniscal injuries but much of the menisci and femorotibial joints cannot be viewed with the arthroscope.
- CT and MRI can be used to document meniscal injuries when appropriate cross-sectional imaging machines are available.

Etiology

- Meniscal lesions can be acute or chronic in nature.
- Acute damage can occur with a bad step or some sort of accident that leads to shifting or shear forces between the femur and tibia.
- Degenerative lesions of the meniscus seem to coincide with OA within the joint.
- It is not uncommon to see concurrent lesions in other structures such as the cruciate ligaments, articular cartilage, and medial femoral condyle.

Clinical Signs

- Lameness and other clinical signs can be acute or insidious in onset.
- Lameness is usually moderate in severity and worsens with exercise and upper limb flexion tests.
- MFT or femoropatellar joint effusion is present in about 50% of cases but most affect horses respond to IA anesthesia.
- Horses with severe lameness and evidence of chronic OA of the MFT joint should be suspected to have a concurrent medial meniscal injury (Figure 4.40).

Diagnosis

- Radiographs of the stifle can be normal in acute cases of primary meniscal damage.
- Chronic damage to the meniscus may lead to joint space narrowing, mineralization of the meniscus, and OA within the MFT joint (Figure 4.40).

- Horses with meniscal damage appear to be prone to develop new bone formation at the medial intercondylar eminence of the tibia (Figure 4.42).
- Ultrasonographic findings can include characterization of an abnormal size, thickness, variability in echogenicity, location of the meniscus, prolapsing of the meniscus medially and overt meniscal tearing.
- It is important to image the meniscus in both weight-bearing and non-weight-bearing stances to better demonstrate the tear (Figures 4.43).
- Arthroscopy can be both a diagnostic and treatment tool for some meniscal lesions.
- CT arthrography and MRI of the stifle can provide improved imaging of the meniscus but are not readily available.

Treatment

- Treatment usually involves arthroscopic surgery and debridement of the disrupted meniscal fibers that can be seen. "Looseness" of the meniscus as assessed by probing may be associated in some cases with damage and protrusion of the meniscus.

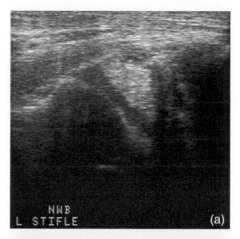
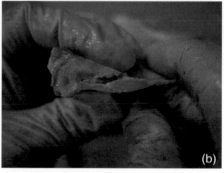

Figure 4.43 (a) Ultrasonographic image of a severe meniscal tear that correlated well with the gross appearance (b). *Source*: Courtesy of Laurie Goodrich.

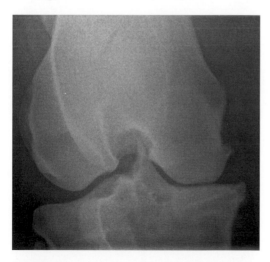

Figure 4.42 A caudal-cranial radiographic image showing osteophytes on the medial aspect of the tibia and the intercondylar eminence, which are common in many types of diseases involving the femorotibial joints. *Source*: Courtesy of Chris Kawcak.

- Lack of a visible lesion does not indicate the absence of meniscal damage because much of the meniscus is not visible with the arthroscope.
- The lesions have been graded based on arthroscopic findings: Grade I = axial tearing through the cranial ligament of the medial meniscus and into the meniscus, Grade II = same as Grade I but with torn tissue and visible extent of the damage, Grade III = severe tear that extends beneath the femoral condyle.
- The majority of lesions are either Grade I or Grade II (approximately 80% in one study) and many horses have concurrent articular cartilage damage.

- A tear or lesion in the body of the meniscus may also be treated by extracapsular injection of biologics into the lesion(s) or into the joint.

Prognosis

- Overall, approximately 50% of the horses with meniscal lesions may become sound after surgery.
- Sixty percent of horses with Grade I injury became sound compared with 65% of those with Grade II and 10% of those with Grade III in one report.
- The prognosis for lesions of the medial meniscus is worse than for lateral meniscal lesions.
- Horses with small lesions that can be debrided can do relatively well, although horses with significant tearing carry a poor prognosis.

Collateral/Cruciate Ligament Injury

Overview

- The medial collateral and cranial cruciate ligaments are most commonly injured in the horse.
- Most injuries are seen in adult horses.
- Combinations of injuries that involve the medial CL, cruciate ligament, and medial meniscus are possible.

Anatomy (Please refer to sections on "SCLs and Meniscal Injuries")

Imaging (Please refer to sections on "SCLs and Meniscal Injuries")

Etiology

- An acute traumatic event in which the limb was stressed in an abnormal direction is usually the cause, but this is often presumed.
- Mechanically induced tearing of the cranial cruciate ligament caused 9 of 15 limbs to fail in the ligament, 5 failed at the tibial insertion, and 2 failed at the femoral origin.
- Partial degeneration of the cranial cruciate ligament may occur in jumpers and racehorses.

Clinical Signs

- Clinical signs are usually acute and severe; however, minor injuries cause more subtle signs.
- Horses with cruciate injuries often present for an acute lameness, with significant stifle effusion and response to flexion.
- Horses with complete rupture of the medial collateral can show significant lateral movement of the distal limb and a palpable widening of the MFT joint space on the medial aspect of the stifle.
- A tibial thrust test in the caudal direction may worsen the lameness, but this is not considered specific for cranial cruciate ligament damage.

Diagnosis

- Often, radiographic findings are normal; however, the MFT joint may distract on a stressed caudocranial view (Figure 4.44).

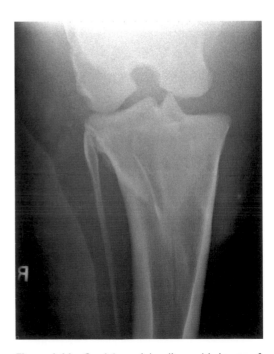

Figure 4.44 Caudal-cranial radiographic image of a stifle with a ruptured medial collateral ligament. Notice the widened joint space medially. *Source*: Courtesy of Chris Kawcak.

- Radiographs are usually unremarkable with cruciate ligament injuries unless the origin of the ligament avulses from the intercondylar fossa, a midbody tear shows dystrophic mineralization, or a medial tibial eminence fragment is present (Figure 4.45).
- A medial tibial eminence fragment is not pathognomonic for cranial cruciate ligament damage because a fracture at the apex of the eminence may not involve the ligament.
- Ultrasound is usually the primary method of diagnosis for medial CL injuries but is more variable for the cranial cruciate ligament because it is difficult to image.
- MRI is available in limited locations and probably provides the best chances of acquiring an accurate diagnosis for cruciate ligament injuries.
- Arthroscopic surgery is currently the best method to accurately diagnose cranial cruciate ligament damage.

Treatment

- Horses with partial tears of the medial CL are treated conservatively. This may include rest, IA, and topical anti-inflammatories, and ESWT or biological therapies injected into the site of ligament damage or IA.

- Horses with a complete rupture of the CL should be confined a stall for a minimum of eight to 12 weeks.
- Osteochondral fragments from the tibial eminence associated with cruciate damage can be removed and the damaged ligament debrided arthroscopically.
- Large intercondylar eminence fractures can also be repaired with internal fixation.

Prognosis

- Overall, the prognosis depends on the extent of damage to the ligament but is often considered poor to return to athletic use.
- Some horses with cruciate ligament injuries have returned to work but most with complete tearing are usually only pasture sound.
- Mild injuries to the ligament can be successfully treated in most horses.

Synovitis/Capsulitis/OA of the Femorotibial Joints

Overview

- Exercise-induced damage to the femorotibial joints in performance horses usually affects the MFT joint.

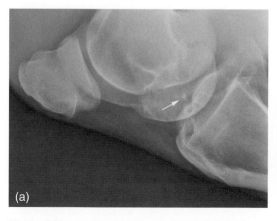 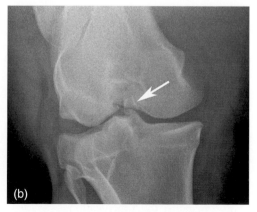

Figure 4.45 (a) Flexed lateromedial radiographic image that demonstrates fragmentation of the intercondylar eminence of the tibia (arrow). The fragment was attached to the cranial cruciate ligament but was loose during arthroscopic examination. (b) A caudal to cranial radiograph demonstrating fragmentation of the intercondylar eminence of the tibia (arrow) that was not associated with a cranial cruciate ligament injury and was removed arthroscopically.

- MFT joint synovitis is diagnosed commonly in Western performance horses, especially young cutting horses.
- Articular cartilage damage on the medial femoral condyle in performance horses is thought to predispose to OA within the MFT joint.
- Chronic MFT joint OA is usually a sequela to many types of intra-articular injuries (Figures 4.40 and 4.42).

Anatomy (Please refer to section on "SCLs and Meniscal Injuries")

Imaging (Please refer to section on "SCLs and Meniscal Injuries")

Etiology

- Horses that undergo chronic repetitive stress to the hindlimbs, such as young Western performance horses, are susceptible to synovitis of the MFT joint. This situation is similar to racehorses that develop synovitis in their fetlock and carpal joints.
- The primary source of synovitis usually is not apparent in many horses.
- Acute or chronic trauma to the stifle of any type that leads to IA trauma can contribute to OA in any of the stifle joints.
- The cause of cartilage lesions on the medial femoral condyles is thought to be chronic repetitive trauma although some feel they may be developmental in origin.

Clinical Signs

- Horses with synovitis of the femorotibial joints may not be lame but have mild-to-moderate effusion in the MFT joint (Figure 1.45). These horses may show some response to flexion and have a gait that can be described as "stiff."
- Horses with mild OA or synovitis secondary within the MFT joint usually have a history of mild lameness, lack of performance, or a short response to IA medication.
- Adult horses with medial femoral condyle lesions may or may not have effusion, are usually positive to hindlimb flexion, and respond to IA analgesia.

- Horses with significant OA of the MFT joint are usually very lame with loss of muscle mass, effusion of the MFT joint, and thickening of the MFT joint capsule.
- Although a history of predisposing injury and disease of the stifle is usually noted, some horses may develop chronic MFT OA insidiously without a notable injury.

Diagnosis

- All diagnostic techniques, including arthroscopy, can be negative in cases of primary synovitis/capsulitis.
- Flattening and sclerosis of the medial femoral condyle are subtle radiographic abnormalities that may suggest osteochondral damage but its clinical significance on performance is limited.
- Osteophytes on the medial tibial plateau are often an early sign of MFT OA (Figure 4.42).
- Advanced OA of the MFT joint is evidenced by osteophytes on the tibial plateau, intercondylar eminence, and medial femoral condyle, with or without joint space narrowing (Figure 4.40).
- Other diagnostics that can provide useful information include ultrasonography and arthroscopy.
- Arthroscopy is best technique to evaluate articular cartilage damage that is often found on the medial femoral condyle.

Treatment

- Horses with synovitis usually respond well to IA medication, topical anti-inflammatories, systemic medication, and ESWT.
- Rest or a reduction in training is often recommended and young horses or those with mild clinical signs typically respond well to this.
- Failure to respond to medication or recurrence of lameness is often the key finding that leads to more intensive imaging and possibly diagnostic arthroscopy.
- Arthroscopic findings in horses with femoral condyle disease usually include focal or generalized articular cartilage

lesions. Articular cartilage fibrillation, erosion, or subchondral bone lysis may also be present.

- Treatment of OA of the MFT joints is the same as for other joints except that arthrodesis is not an option. Intermittent IA medication and controlled exercise appear to help.
- Arthroscopic surgery may help reduce the progression of chronic OA by removing debris and fibrillated articular cartilage, but the disease process is likely to progress.

Prognosis

- Horses with synovitis are easily managed medically as long as a primary disease process is not present. This is some concern that chronic, persistent synovitis can lead to secondary damage to the articular cartilage, which may predispose to the onset of OA in the future.
- The prognosis for OA of the femorotibial joints depends on the severity and appears no different than for other joints in the horse.
- Severe OA can lead to significant lameness making it difficult for the horse to stand, with a questionable quality of life.

Femur and Coxofemoral Region

Fibrotic Myopathy

Overview

- Fibrotic myopathy refers to fibrosis with or without ossification of the muscle tissue in the crus that can involve the semitendinosus, semimembranosus, gracilis, or biceps femoris muscles (Figure 4.46).
- It is typical for the semitendinosus to be involved, but any of the gaskin muscles can be affected.
- The fibrosis and adhesions limit the action of the semitendinosus muscle, causing an abnormal gait characterized by a "slapping" down of the foot at the end of the cranial phase of the stride.

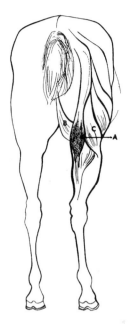

Figure 4.46 Drawing depicting the muscles in the fibrotic area in the gaskin of a horse affected with fibrotic myopathy. (a) Semitendinosus. (b) Semimembranosus. (c) Biceps femoris.

- The lesions are nearly always unilateral and Quarter Horses mares appear to be particularly prone to the condition.

Anatomy

- The main muscle mass on the caudal aspect of the thigh and hip is that of the semimembranosus with the semitendinosus, with the caudal division of the biceps femoris related to it laterally and the gracilis medially (Figure 4.46).
- The thick, roughly three-sided belly of the semimembranosus ends on a flat tendon that attaches to the medial femoral epicondyle.
- The semitendinosus muscle sweeps to its insertion on the cranial and medial border of the tibial and then distally toward its tarsal insertion (Figure 1.43).
- A prominent longitudinal groove marks the site of the intermuscular septum between the semitendinosus and the biceps femoris muscles.

Imaging

- Ultrasonography can be used to help document muscle damage once the initial swelling resolves.
- Nuclear scintigraphy and thermography may also be used to help document focal inflammation within the gaskin musculature.
- Radiography is typically not helpful in making the diagnosis unless ossification of the damaged muscles occurs.

Etiology

- The cause of the fibrosis is nearly always trauma, but the severity can range from a single severe acute injury to repetitive microdamage to the muscles due to exercise.
- Involved muscles may be injured during sliding stops in rodeo work, from slipping, getting the hindlimb caught in a fixed object or a halter, and from being kicked.
- The lack of muscle compliance and adhesions between the involved muscles that occurs with healing contribute to the gait abnormality. Ossification is believed to be a more severe progression from the fibrosis.
- Neurogenic atrophy of the affected muscles associated with a peripheral neuropathy has also been suggested as a potential cause.

Clinical Signs

- With acute injuries, lameness in the injured limb together with swelling and pain on palpation of the gaskin region are common findings. A gait abnormality is usually not present in the early stages.
- As the injury starts to heal, an area of firmness with a variable pain response can be palpated over the affected muscles on the caudal surface of the limb usually concentrated over the semitendinosus.
- With chronicity, the swelling and pain often subside, and the classic gait abnormality develops gradually as the muscle fibrosis continues. Lameness may or may not be present.
- In the cranial phase of the stride, the foot of the affected hindlimb is suddenly pulled caudally 3–5 inches just before contacting the ground. The gait abnormality is most noticeable when the horse walks.
- An area of firmness/fibrosis can often be palpated over the affected muscles on the caudal surface of the affected limb at the level of the stifle (Figure 4.47).

Diagnosis

- The diagnosis is usually based on the characteristic gait abnormality together with palpation of abnormal musculature within the gaskin region.
- Ultrasonography can be used to determine the severity of the muscle injury and whether ossification is present.
- The diagnosis can be more difficult in the acute stages due to the amount of swelling and pain that can occur in the gaskin region.

Treatment

- Treatment is often based on chronicity of the lesion. The more acute the lesion, the more the clinician should attempt to minimize the formation of a fibrotic scar.
- Preventing permanent fibrosis of the muscles is the goal with acute injuries. Icing, systemic and topical NSAIDs, and restricted exercise are important to reduce the inflammation and prevent further muscle injury.
- Physical therapy exercises to stretch the gaskin muscles will help prevent adhesions and shortening of the muscle-tendon unit and should be initiated as soon as the horse can tolerate it. Initially, the hindlimb can be stretched cranially and caudally working in deep massage of the affected muscle once the horse can handle it.
- Hand walking should start on a hard surface over the first few weeks, but range of motion exercises should be added in as soon as possible. This could include walking them part time in arena footing, followed by walking them over logs, progressing to cavelettis or an underwater treadmill, if available.

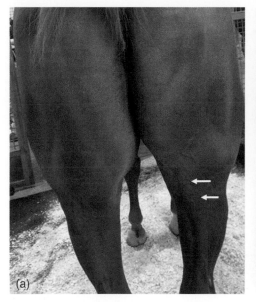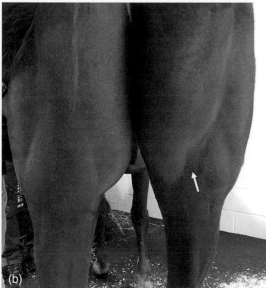

Figure 4.47 Images of the adult horse that sustained an acute muscle injury. (a) Six months after injury. (b) One and a half years after injury. Note that the thickened area of fibrous tissue in image (a) (arrows) is more distal than the final fibrous tissue after 1.5 years. This horse had multiple treatments to minimize the development of scar tissue. *Source*: Courtesy of Troy Trumble.

- Surgical treatment for fibrotic myopathy consists of either a semitendinosus tenotomy at the level of its insertion on the proximal medial tibia (requires general anesthesia) or a semitendinosus myotomy performed at the site of the fibrosis on the caudal aspect of the limb.
- With the myotomy, the incision is made directly over the affected semitendinosus muscle, which is transected using a blunt bistoury (Figure 4.48).

Prognosis
- Some immediate improvement may be evident with the myotomy, but it usually takes three to seven days for the maximum effect.
- With the standing myotomy technique, 83% of horses were able to perform at their pre-injury level, although the restrictive gait pattern did not resolve in all horses.
- Results for the tenotomy procedure are based on few cases (four of six improved) but the procedure is generally considered to be beneficial.
- The prognosis for successful surgery in horses affected by neurogenic atrophy/fibrosis of the muscles is considered poor.

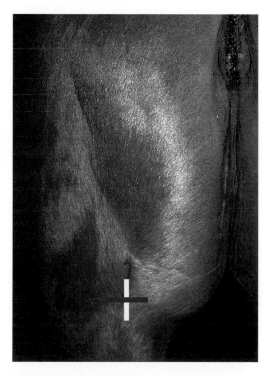

Figure 4.48 Caudal thigh region where the myotomy procedure is performed to correct fibrotic myopathy. The skin incision is made vertically (white line), and the fibrotic muscle is transected with a bistoury horizontally (red line).

- The overall effectiveness of preventing the characteristic gait deficit by treating acute cases is currently unknown.

Trochanteric Bursitis (Whirlbone Lameness)

Overview

- Trochanteric bursitis is inflammation of the bursa beneath the tendon of the accessory gluteal muscle (deep portion of the gluteus medius muscle) as it passes over the greater trochanter of the femur.
- In many cases, the bursitis is secondary to a concurrent source of chronic lameness in the same limb, particularly distal tarsitis.
- Trochanteric bursitis occurs in horses racing on small tracks, where the turns are close together, and in horses working on their hindlimbs that are frequently exercised in soft, deep arenas.

Anatomy

- On the lateral aspect of the hip, the smaller deep part of the gluteus medius, the gluteus accessorius, has a distinct flat tendon that plays over the convexity of the greater trochanter on its way to attach on the crest distal to the trochanter. The large trochanteric bursa lies between the tendon and the cartilage covering the convexity.
- The trochanter is covered with cartilage and the trochanteric bursa is interposed between it and the tendon.
- The tendon of the gluteus medius muscle also may be involved in the inflammatory response, as well as the cartilage over the trochanter.

Imaging

- Imaging the trochanteric bursa is difficult. Scintigraphy can be used to identify if the bursa as inflamed but is not used routinely.
- Ultrasonography can be helpful in identifying the bursa as being fluid-filled and can aid in centesis of the bursa.

Etiology

- Lameness may be caused by bruising as a result of the horse falling on the affected trochanter or by strain during racing or training.
- Short heels and long toes in the hindfeet seem to predispose to this lameness.
- Chronic forelimb lameness may contribute to the bursitis by causing the horse to place more strain on the hindlimbs.
- When the etiology is severe trauma, such as a direct kick, the cartilage or the bone of the trochanter may be fractured, causing persistent lameness.

Clinical Signs and Diagnosis

- Pain may be evident when pressure is applied over the greater trochanter on the affected side.
- At rest, the limb may remain flexed and as the horse moves, more weight may be placed on the inside of the foot causing it to wear more than the outside aspect.
- The horse tends to travel "dog fashion" since the hindquarters move toward the sound side because the stride of the affected limb is shorter than that of the sound side.
- If the condition becomes chronic, atrophy of the gluteal muscles can occur.
- The condition is difficult to differentiate from conditions of the hip joint and may be confused with distal tarsal lameness.
- Injection of a local anesthetic into the bursa is helpful to document the bursa as contributing to the lameness.

Treatment and Prognosis

- Since the bursitis is usually secondary to another lameness, it is important to address the primary source of lameness.
- Rest and systemic NSAIDs treatment are usually beneficial as is local ESWT and heat applied to the bursa.
- Injection of the bursa with corticosteroids appears to be the most effective treatment.
- The prognosis is usually associated with the prognosis of the primary source of lameness,

but most horses can return to soundness within four to six weeks.

- The prognosis is guarded to unfavorable with severe bursal injuries and recurrence is not uncommon when the horse returns to work.

Diaphyseal and Metaphyseal Femoral Fractures

Overview

- Fractures of the femur are relatively common in horses, especially young horses.
- In young animals, fractures often involve the proximal or distal growth plate, and diaphyseal fractures are usually oblique and spiraling.
- Adult horses often sustain irreparable comminuted fractures of the femoral shaft.
- Treatment of femoral fractures (internal fixation or confinement) is usually only recommended in young horses weighing less than 200–300 kg.

Anatomy

- The femur is a large, long bone in the thigh region between the stifle and the hip that is surrounded by heavy musculature.
- The femur serves as a point of origin and insertion for a large number of muscles that are important for the performance of the horse.
- The head of the femur inserts into the acetabulum of the pelvis to create a ball-and-socket-type articulation and the distal femur contributes to a hinge joint in the stifle.
- The femur is a major weight-bearing bone that can be very difficult to repair.

Imaging

- Radiography remains the best initial method to document femoral fractures in horses and is necessary for an accurate prognosis. The femur can be difficult to radiograph even in younger horses, and both standing and recumbent views may be necessary.

- Scintigraphy, particularly for less severe or more chronic injuries, may help localize femoral lesions not amenable to radiographic imaging.

Etiology

- Foals frequently sustain femoral fractures during initial handling or during halter breaking.
- In one study, causes included a fall, severe adduction, external trauma, being caught in a fence, and having the mare step on the foal.
- A severe traumatic event such as a fall is often the cause in adult horses.
- Femoral condylar avulsion fractures can occur in horses that had been cast with a sideline for castration without sedation and osteoporosis may contribute to femoral fractures in older horses.

Clinical Signs

- The obvious sign is non-weight-bearing lameness.
- When viewed from the side, the affected limb may appear slightly shortened with the hock held higher than the opposite hindlimb, and it may be externally rotated.
- Fractures of the distal femoral metaphysis may have swelling around the stifle, mimicking a stifle injury.
- Obvious swelling in the mid-femoral region is usually present with diaphyseal fractures (Figure 4.49).
- Manipulation of the limb often reveals crepitus and laxity of the limb whenever there is a complete diaphyseal fracture.

Diagnosis

- A tentative diagnosis can usually be made based on the severity of lameness, laxity of the limb, moderate-to-severe swelling, and the presence of crepitus.
- Radiographs are important to demonstrate the exact location and configuration of the fracture because these factors affect the treatment options and prognosis.

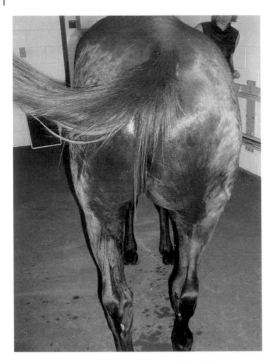

Figure 4.49 Caudal view of an adult with severe swelling of the femoral region associated with a diaphyseal femoral fracture. Notice that the horse is sweating and non-weight-bearing on the right hindlimb. *Source*: Courtesy of Troy Trumble.

- For the distal one-third of the femur, standing views will usually identify the fracture, but for the proximal two-thirds of the femur, particularly in adults, a recumbent position is required to obtain quality radiographs (Figure 4.50).
- When radiographs are not possible or advisable, ultrasound may be able to demonstrate cortical disruption of the diaphysis and fractures of the capital physis.

Treatment

- Treatment of femoral shaft fractures depends on the age of the animal and the type and location of the fracture. Euthanasia is indicated for most adult horses that have sustained femoral shaft fractures.
- Diaphyseal fractures have been treated with stall rest in foals weighing up to approximately 200 kg, but malunion is a risk.
- Compression plating (usually two plates) is the treatment of choice for foals with diaphyseal fractures when athletic soundness is desired.
- Intramedullary pinning using the stacked pin technique or interlocking nails have also been reported to treat diaphyseal fractures in young foals.
- Minimally displaced distal physeal fractures may heal with conservative therapy (Figure 4.51).
- Unstable distal physeal fractures can be treated with an angled blade plate, condylar

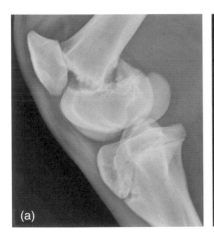
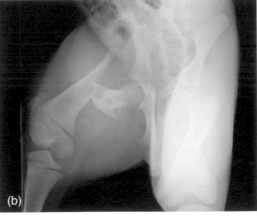

Figure 4.50 (a) Lateromedial oblique view of the stifle of a weanling taken standing, showing a Salter–Harris type II fracture of the distal physis of the femur. (b) Radiograph taken with the horse in a recumbent position under anesthesia demonstrating a closed, oblique, mid-diaphyseal fracture of the femur in a miniature foal. *Source*: Courtesy of Troy Trumble.

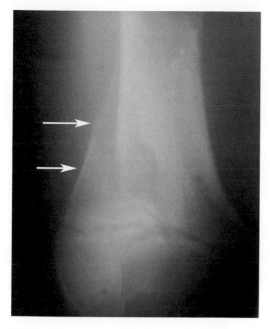

Figure 4.51 Lateral radiograph of a weanling with a Type II distal femoral fracture (arrows) that was successfully treated with confinement.

buttress plate, cobra-head and dynamic compression plate, and cross-pins or Rush pins.

Prognosis

- Femoral fractures in horses older than yearlings carry a very poor prognosis for a successful outcome.
- Approximately 50% of foals treated surgically were successful in one report. The mean age for successfully treated foals was two months vs. four months for unsuccessfully treated foals.
- Three of four foals with oblique mid-shaft femoral fractures treated by stall rest alone became sound for breeding but fracture disease associated with prolonged non-weight-bearing presented problems during the healing period.

Capital Physeal Fractures of the Femoral Head

Overview

- Fractures of the capital physis of the femoral neck occur commonly in foals less than one year of age.

- These fractures are usually a Type I Salter-Harris physeal fracture but Types II and III can also occur.
- Another term that has been used to describe these fractures is a "slipped capital physis" since the epiphysis is often displaced from the femoral neck (Figure 4.52).

Anatomy

- The femoral head and the acetabulum form a ball-and-socket articulation that makes up the coxofemoral joint (Figure 4.1).
- In young animals, the proximal femur contains a physis within the femoral neck called the capital physis that communicates directly with the acetabulum.
- The heavy musculature and extensive ligament network surrounding and within the joint make the hip joint inherently stable.
- Because of the inherent stability of the hip, excessive trauma to the hip region in young horses often results in displacement of the physis instead of luxation of the joint.

Imaging

- Radiography of the proximal femur is the ideal method to document fractures in this region and can be performed in both the standing and recumbent position.
- Better quality images are usually obtained in the recumbent animal.
- Rectal and transcutaneous ultrasound may be helpful to document capital physeal and acetabular fractures, and hip luxations.

Etiology

- Trauma such as violent falls, struggles, and kicks are the cause.
- Falling on the greater trochanter is thought to cause shearing forces across the physis, resulting in displacement between the epiphysis and metaphysis.

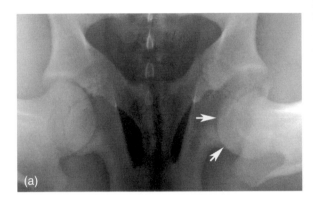

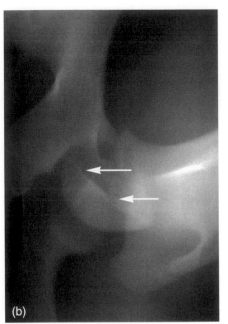

(a)

(b)

Figure 4.52 Recumbent radiographs of the pelvis of two different foals with capital physeal fractures (arrows) of the left proximal femur.

Clinical Signs
- Immediate severe lameness after a violent accident is usually present but the lameness can improve within a few days.
- Most foals are able to bear some weight and often stand with a toe-out, hock-in appearance.
- Swelling and pain over the hip, pelvic asymmetry, gluteal muscle atrophy, and crepitus with hip manipulation may be present but are not consistently seen.

Diagnosis
- Standing or recumbent radiography of the hip is usually necessary for an accurate diagnosis. Separation of the epiphysis and metaphysis of the femoral neck confirms the diagnosis (Figure 4.52).
- Ultrasound in the standing horse may also be used to document the fracture.
- Concurrent radiographic abnormalities may also be present, such as comminution of the epiphysis, greater trochanter or acetabular fracture, or coxofemoral joint luxation/subluxation that will preclude surgical repair.

Treatment
- Nonsurgical management of these fractures is not recommended because malunion, avascular necrosis, and secondary hip OA can lead to debilitating lameness.
- Surgical treatment is difficult and is not recommended in foals with concurrent radiographic abnormalities.
- Surgical options include the use of cancellous or cortical bone screws, IM or Knowles pins, and an interfragmentary compression system.
- Small foals with a Type I or II physeal fracture are the best candidates for surgery.

Prognosis
- The majority of foals with this condition are euthanized because of the poor prognosis with nonsurgical treatment and the questionable results with surgery.

- If the epiphysis can be reduced and maintained until healing, athletic soundness can be achieved.

Coxofemoral Joint Luxation/Subluxation (Dislocation of the HIP Joint)

Overview

- Luxation of the coxofemoral joint is an uncommon condition in horses because of the numerous ligaments and heavy musculature surrounding the joint.
- The ilium in adults or capital physis in young horses tends to fracture before the hip luxates.
- Foals, miniature horses, and ponies appear to be prone to hip luxation/subluxation, and it can occur in any age horse.
- Coxofemoral luxation is most often unilateral, and the head of the femur nearly always dislocates craniodorsal to the acetabulum.

Anatomy

- The femoral head and the acetabulum form a ball-and-socket articulation that makes up the coxofemoral joint (Figure 4.53).
- The lunate surface of the acetabulum, a cup-shaped cavity arcing around a deep nonarticular fossa, articulates with the head of the femur.
- The acetabulum is also surrounded by a fibrocartilaginous rim, the acetabular labrum, that increases the articular surface of the acetabulum.
- The heavy musculature and extensive ligament network surrounding and within the joint make the hip joint inherently stable.
- The transverse acetabular ligament, ligament of the head of the femur (round), and femoral accessory ligament help to stabilize the coxofemoral joint (Figure 4.53).
- Abduction of the thigh is restricted by the ligament of the head of the femur and the accessory femoral ligament.

Imaging

- Standing or recumbent radiography of the coxofemoral region is the ideal method to document abnormalities in the region.
- Better quality images are usually obtained in the recumbent animal.
- Rectal and transcutaneous ultrasound may be used to document capital physeal and acetabular fractures, and hip luxation.

Etiology

- Both the accessory and the ligament of the head of the femur (round) must rupture for a luxation to occur. Some type of violent trauma is nearly always the cause.
- Violent overextension and falling on the point of the stifle with the femur in a vertical position occasionally causes luxation of the coxofemoral joint.
- A tethered horse that catches its foot in a rope or a halter may dislocate the hip in the struggle to free itself.
- Partial tearing of the ligament of the head of the femur may predispose to subluxation and luxation with or without associated trauma.
- Luxation of the hip also may occur secondary to wearing a full limb hindlimb cast, especially in foals.

Clinical Signs

- A history of trauma resulting in a severe non-weight-bearing lameness is common.
- Some horses may toe-touch when walked because the affected limb is shorter than the opposite limb due to the craniodorsal position of the femur (Figure 4.54).
- The limb may "dangle" somewhat because of shortening, and the point of the hock on the affected side will be higher than that of the opposite limb. The toe and stifle turn outward, and the point of the hock turns inward.

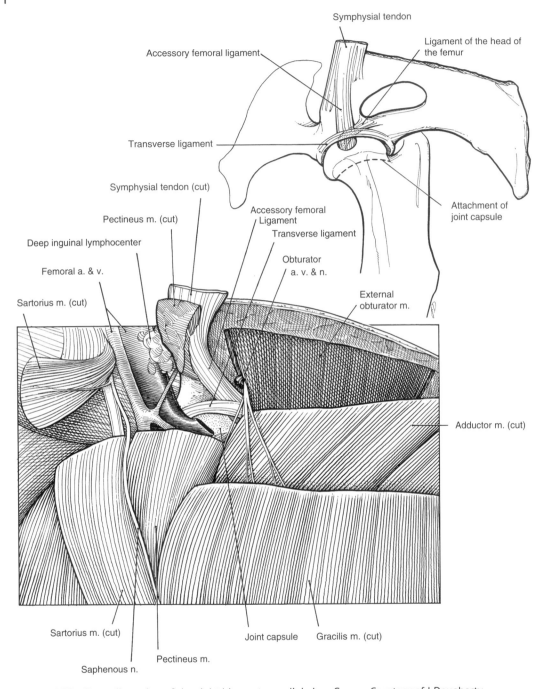

Symphysial tendon

Accessory femoral ligament

Ligament of the head of the femur

Transverse ligament

Symphysial tendon (cut)

Pectineus m. (cut)

Accessory femoral Ligament

Transverse ligament

Deep inguinal lymphocenter

Obturator a. v. & n.

Femoral a. & v.

External obturator m.

Attachment of joint capsule

Sartorius m. (cut)

Adductor m. (cut)

Sartorius m. (cut)

Joint capsule   Gracilis m. (cut)

Pectineus m.

Saphenous n.

Figure 4.53   Deep dissection of the right hip, ventromedial view. *Source*: Courtesy of J Daugherty.

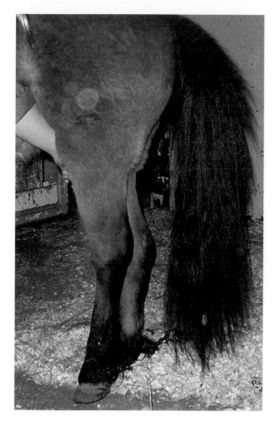

Figure 4.54 Image of the hind end of a pony demonstrating a shorter left hindlimb than the right hind. Notice that the point of the hock is higher, the heel does not completely contact the ground, and the limb is externally rotated. Horses with slipped capital epiphyses, femoral neck fractures, or coxofemoral luxations can all have this clinical appearance. *Source*: Courtesy of Troy Trumble.

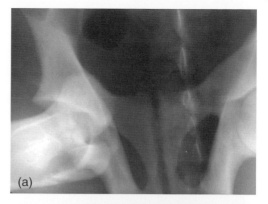

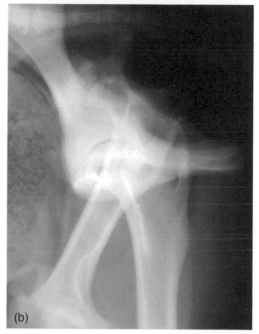

Figure 4.55 Ventrodorsal (a) and standing lateral (b) radiographs of the pelvis confirming luxation of the coxofemoral joint. The femoral head is outside the acetabulum in a craniodorsal location.

- Crepitus with limb manipulation may be present as a result of the femur rubbing on the shaft of the ilium.
- Luxation of the coxofemoral joint also may be complicated by UFP.

Diagnosis
- A presumptive diagnosis can often be made based on the history and clinical signs.
- Standing or recumbent radiography confirms the diagnosis and also rules out other possible causes of the lameness such as pel-

vic, acetabular, and capital physeal fractures (Figure 4.55).
- In suspected cases of subluxation, radiographs should be performed with the limb weight-bearing in order to identify the problem.
- Ultrasound of the hip region also may be used to confirm luxation/subluxation of the femoral head and should be performed with

the horse in both weight- and non-weight-bearing positions.

Treatment

- Many horses with this condition are euthanized because of the often, unsuccessful treatment options and the poor prognosis.
- Closed reduction of the luxation is usually the best treatment option but can be very difficult to perform in adult horses, and re-luxation is common.
- Horses with an acute luxation with no secondary fracture of the dorsal rim of the acetabulum are the best candidates for closed reduction.
- Several surgical approaches applicable for foals or small breed horses have been reported. They include open reduction alone, transposition of the greater trochanter, femoral head and neck resection, toggle pinning, or augmentation of the lateral joint capsule with synthetic sutures attached to screws.
- A combination of toggle pinning, synthetic capsular repair, and trochanteric transposition was used to successfully repair a hip luxation in an adult miniature horse.
- Some miniature horses may develop a pseudoarthrosis outside the coxofemoral joint without treatment and excision of the femoral head and neck and dorsal rim of the fractured acetabulum may aid in the development of a pseudoarthrosis.

Prognosis

- In cases where there is a combination of an acetabular fracture and subluxation, the prognosis is poor. The prognosis is improved with subluxation alone.
- The prognosis is typically guarded to poor because successful closed reduction is not always possible.
- There is usually a better chance of maintaining permanent reduction if the femur stays

in place for approximately three months after treatment.
- Most horses can become sound enough for breeding purposes if the reduction can be maintained or a pseudoarthrosis develops.

OA of the Coxofemoral Joint

Overview

- OA of the coxofemoral joint is a sequel to almost any orthopedic problem that occurs within the joint.
- It may occur from any type of soft tissue trauma to the hip region that does not necessarily result in intra-articular ligament damage or fracture.
- Hip OA is seen most frequently in older animals and should be considered in any horse with chronic hindlimb lameness.

Anatomy (See previous section on coxofemoral joint luxation/subluxation)

Imaging (See previous section on coxofemoral joint luxation/subluxation)

Etiology

- Any hip-related traumatic injury can lead to OA.
- Reported causes of coxofemoral joint OA include abnormal development of the coxofemoral joint (OC or hip dysplasia), infection in young foals, rupture or partial tearing of the round ligament, and trauma.

Clinical Signs

- No clinical signs are specific for coxofemoral joint OA, but it should be suspected in older horses with chronic hindlimb lameness that have a history of trauma.
- Many affected horses have a significant lameness (grade 3 to 4/5) and have a low arc of foot flight and a reduced cranial phase of the stride.
- Horses with hip pain tend to move with the limb rotated externally and carry the limb abducted during advancement.

- Firm swelling over the greater trochanter and hip area may be present in chronic cases and the characteristic toe-out, hock-in stance may or may not be observed (Figure 4.56).
- Swelling over the hip region and pain on direct palpation over the hip may be observed in some horses (Figure 4.57).

Diagnosis

- A presumptive diagnosis of severe hip OA often can be made based on the history and clinical exam.
- Milder cases of hip OA can be a diagnostic challenge. Intra-articular anesthetic of the coxofemoral joint is often the best method to localize the lameness to the hip.

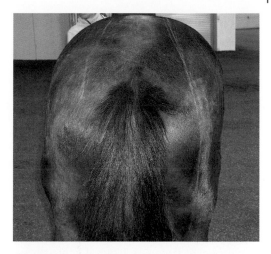

Figure 4.57 An older Quarter horse mare with grade 3/5 hindlimb lameness. Swelling over the left greater trochanter region could be seen when compared with the opposite side, and pain was elicited with firm palpation.

- Radiographs are often necessary for a definitive diagnosis and usually reveal evidence of bone remodeling and osteophytes production in chronic cases (Figure 4.58).

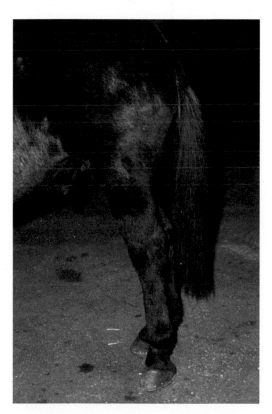

Figure 4.56 Lateral view of an aged pony with the typical toe-out, hock-in stance characteristic of a hip/pelvic problem. The left hindlimb is straighter than the contralateral limb and the horse is leaning to the right.

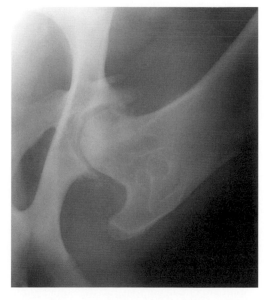

Figure 4.58 Ventrodorsal radiograph of the pelvis of the horse in Figure 4.57 (above), demonstrating severe OA of the coxofemoral joint. The OA was reportedly secondary to trauma to the area from a previous fall.

- Ultrasound can be helpful, but it can be challenging to determine whether the abnormalities are the result of the progression of OA or from the initial injury.

Treatment
- Treatment of hip OA is usually palliative because the lameness often progresses. Horses with mild OA usually respond well to oral NSAIDs and/or IA medication.
- Horses usually benefit from both systemic and IA medications directed at joint healing such PSGAGs, nutraceuticals, and biologics.
- Horses with unilateral mild or moderate OA may benefit from coxofemoral joint arthroscopy to debride cartilage lesions and determine the inciting cause.
- Confinement is usually not indicated because some type of controlled exercise often benefits horses with OA.

Prognosis
- The prognosis for athletic use in horses with severe OA is thought to be poor. However, many of these horses can be used for breeding or maintained as pets because they tend to do well at the walk.
- Horses with mild or moderate OA may respond well to treatment and may be used at a reduced performance level.

Infectious Arthritis and OC of the Coxofemoral Joint

Overview
- Infection of the coxofemoral joint and the capital physis of the femur are part of the joint ill complex in foals.
- Hematogenous infections around the hip occur less frequently than at other sites in foals and can be very difficult to diagnose.
- Developmental lesions of the coxofemoral joint are rare in comparison with other joints in the horse and can also be difficult to diagnose.

Anatomy (Please refer to previous sections on "Capital Physeal Fracture and Coxofemoral Joint Luxation")

Imaging (Please refer to previous sections on "Capital Physeal Fracture and Coxofemoral Joint Luxation")

Etiology
- Joint and physeal infections in foals are hematogenous in origin, and bacteria usually gain access to the circulation through the umbilicus, gastrointestinal tract, or respiratory tract.
- Affected foals usually have a history of failure of passive transfer and most infections are from Gram-negative bacteria.
- The cause of developmental lesions is assumed to be the same as for other OC-type lesions, but it is unknown why there is a low prevalence of OC in the hip compared with other locations.

Clinical Signs
- Infection of the coxofemoral joint can be a diagnostic challenge because joint effusion, heat, and pain are often not found on physical examination.
- Clinical signs of young horses with OC of the hip may be similar to those of any hindlimb lameness and physical abnormalities of the limb and palpable pain is often difficult to document.
- Typically, these foals are less than four months of age and often present with a unilateral hindlimb lameness of unknown cause. These foals may have a characteristic toe-out, stifle-out, hock-in appearance.
- Pain is often elicited with deep palpation over the greater trochanter and hip region.
- It can often be confused with trauma to the limb but the infection and therefore the lameness is often progressive, whereas a traumatic injury often improves with time.
- Young foals with severe hindlimb lameness without any definable lesions in the lower

limb should be suspected of having infection or OC of the hip joint.

Diagnosis

- A complete blood count is often very helpful in differentiating trauma and OC from a potential hip infection. High white blood cell count and fibrinogen concentrations help confirm the presence of an infection.
- Synovial fluid analysis should be performed when possible to document the infection.
- Infection can also be documented with radiographs - bone lysis around the capital physis, epiphysis, and occasionally the acetabulum may be seen (Figure 4.59b).
- Radiographic abnormalities consistent with OC of the hip are similar to those of other locations and include SCLs, osteochondral fragments, abnormal contour of the femoral head or acetabulum, and shallow and irregular acetabulum (Figure 4.59a).

Treatment

- Treatment of a hip infection is similar to other joint/physis with a hematogenous infection. Broad-spectrum systemic antimicrobials, IA antimicrobials, and joint lavage/drainage are all important.
- Arthroscopy can be performed in small horses and foals to help lavage and debride these lesions, but cannula lavage alone can be very helpful.
- Arthroscopic debridement of OC lesions is usually the treatment of choice, especially if a dissecans lesion is present, and is best performed in foals and weanlings.
- With severe unilateral hip malformation or dysplasia (Figure 4.59a), a femoral head ostectomy may provide a salvage procedure for breeding soundness.

Prognosis

- The prognosis is usually poor for infection because the diagnosis is seldom made before

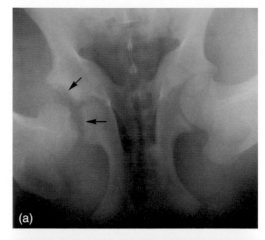
(a)

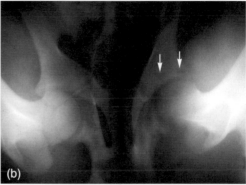
(b)

Figure 4.59 Ventrodorsal radiographs of the pelvis of two different three-month-old fillies with a history of increasing lameness. (a) Remodeling of the femoral head and acetabulum (arrows) consistent with a developmental abnormality. (b) Lysis of the left acetabulum (arrows) consistent with infectious arthritis and osteomyelitis.

significant joint abnormalities and osteomyelitis have occurred.

- Foals with coxofemoral infectious arthritis without radiographic abnormalities should respond well to aggressive treatment similar to infection in other locations.
- The coxofemoral joint is a major weight-bearing joint, and therefore the prognosis for most horses with hip OC is considered guarded to poor for future athletic use.

Bibliography

1 Adams WM, Thilsted JP: 1985. Radiographic appearance of the equine stifle from birth to 6 months. *Vet Radiol Ultrasound* 26:126–132.

2 Adkins AR, Yovich JV, Steel CM: 2001. Surgical arthrodesis of distal tarsal joints in 17 horses clinically affected with osteoarthritis. *Aust Vet J* 79:26–29.

3 Adrian AM, Barrett MF, Werpy NM, et al.: 2015. A comparison of arthroscopy to ultrasonography for identification of pathology of the equine stifle. *Equine Vet J* 49:314–321. doi:10.1111/evj.12541.

4 Arnold CE, Schaer TP, Baird DL, et al.: 2003. Conservative management of 17 horses with nonarticular fractures of the tibial tuberosity. *Equine Vet J* 35:202–206.

5 Auer JA, Watkins JP: 1999. Diseases of the Tibia. *In*: Colahan PT, Mayhew IG, Merritt AM, et al. (eds) *Equine Medicine and Surgery, Vol ii, Fifth Edition*. Santa Barbara, American Veterinary Publications, 1696–1701.

6 Axelsson M, Bjornsdottir S, Eksell P, et al.: 2001. Risk factors associated with hindlimb lameness and degenerative joint disease in the distal tarsus of Icelandic horses. *Equine Vet J* 33:84–90.

7 Baccarin RYA, Martins EAN, Hagen SCF, et al.: 2009. Patellar instability following experimental medial patellar desmotomy in horses. *Vet Comp Orth Traum* 22:27–31.

8 Baird DH, Pilsworth RC: 2001. Wedge-shaped conformation of the dorsolateral aspect of the third tarsal bone in the thoroughbred racehorse is associated with development of slab fractures in this site. *Equine Vet J* 33:617–620.

9 Barcelo Oliver F, Russell TM, Uprichard KL, et al.: 2017. Treatment of septic arthritis of the coxofemoral joint in 12 foals. *Vet Surg* 46:530–538.

10 Barker WHJ, Smith MRW, Minshall GI, et al.: 2013. Soft tissue injuries of the tarsocrural joint: A retrospective analysis of 30 cases evaluated arthroscopically. *Equine Vet J* 45:435–441.

11 Barr ED, Pinchbeck GL, Clegg PD, et al.: 2006. Accuracy of diagnostic techniques used in investigation of stifle lameness in horses—40 cases. *Equine Vet Educ* 18:326–331.

12 Barrett MF, McIlwraith CW, Contino EK, et al.: 2018. Relationship between repository radiographic findings and subsequent performance of Quarter Horses competing in cutting events. *J Am Vet Med Assoc* 252:108–115.

13 Bassage LH, Garcia-Lopez J, Currid EM: 2000. Osteolytic lesions of the tuber calcanei in two horses. *J Am Vet Med Assoc* 217:710–716.

14 Bathe AP, O'Hara LK: 2004. A retrospective study of the outcome of medial patellar desmotomy in 49 horses. *Proc Am Assoc Equine Pract* 50:476–478.

15 Baxter GM: 2005. Treatment of wounds involving synovial structures. *Clin Tech Equine Prac* 3: 204–210.

16 Beard WL, Bramlage LR, Schneider RK, et al.: 1994. Postoperative racing performance in standardbreds and thoroughbreds with osteochondrosis of the tarsocrural joint: 109 cases (1984–1990). *J Am Vet Med Assoc* 204:1655–1659.

17 Bergman EHJ, Puchalski SM, van der Veen H, et al.: 2007. Computed tomography and computed tomography arthrography of the equine stifle: Technique and preliminary results in 16 clinical cases. *Proc Am Assoc Equine Pract* 53:46–55.

18 Betsch JM, Albert N, Lienasson D: 2006. Retrospective study of 143 cases of osteochondritis of the distal tibia in French trotter horses. *Equine Vet J* 38:41–45.

19 Blaik MA, Hanson RR, Kincaid SA, et al.: 2000. Low-field magnetic resonance imaging of the equine tarsus: Normal anatomy. *Vet Rad Ultra* 41:131–141.

20 Bohanon TC: 1999. The Tarsus. *In*: Auer JA, Stick JA (eds) *Equine Surgery, Second Edition*. Philadelphia, W.B. Saunders, 848–862.

21 Bourzac C, Alexander K, Rossier Y, et al.: 2009. Comparison of radiography and ultrasonography for the diagnosis of osteochondritis dissecans in the equine femoropatellar joint. *Equine Vet J* 41:686–692.

22 Bramlage LR, Hanes GE: 1982. Internal fixation of a tibial fracture in an adult horse. *J Am Vet Med Assoc* 180:1090–1094.

23 Bramlage LR, Reed SM, Embertson RM: 1985. Semitendinosus tenotomy for treatment of fibrotic myopathy in the horse. *J Am Vet Med Assoc* 186:565–567.

24 Branch M, Murray RC, Dyson SJ, et al.: 2007. Magnetic resonance imaging of the equine tarsus. *Clin Tech Equine Pract* 6:96–102.

25 Branch MV, Murray RC, Dyson SJ, et al.: 2007. Alteration of distal tarsal subchondral bone thickness pattern in horses with tarsal pain. *Equine Vet J* 39:101–105.

26 Brenner S, Whitcomb MB: 2009. Ultrasonographic diagnosis of coxofemoral subluxation in horses. *Vet Radiol Ultrasound* 50:423–428.

27 Brunsting JY, Pille FJ, Oosterlinck M, et al.: 2018. Incidence and risk factors of surgical site infection and septic arthritis after elective arthroscopy in horses. *Vet Surg* 47:52–59.

28 Byam-Cook KL, Singer ER: 2009. Is there a relationship between clinical presentation, diagnostic and radiographic findings and outcome in horses with osteoarthritis of the small tarsal joints? *Equine Vet J* 41:118–123.

29 Cahill JI, Goulden BE: 1992. Stringhalt—Current thoughts on aetiology and pathogenesis. *Equine Vet J* 24:161–162.

30 Carmalt JL, Bell CD, Panizzi L, et al.: 2012. Alcohol-facilitated ankyloses of the distal intertarsal and tarsometatarsal joints in horses with osteoarthritis. *J Am Vet Med Assoc* 240:199–204.

31 Cauvin ER, Munroe GA, Boyd JS, et al.: 1996. Ultrasonographic examination of the femorotibial articulation in horses: Imaging of the cranial and caudal aspects. *Equine Vet J* 28:285–296.

32 Cauvin ER, Tapprest J, Munroe GA, et al.: 1999. Endoscopic examination of the tarsal sheath of the lateral digital flexor tendon in horses. *Equine Vet J* 31:219–227.

33 Cohen JM, Richardson DW, McKnight AL, et al.: 2009. Long-term outcome in 44 horses with stifle lameness after arthroscopic exploration and debridement. *Vet Surg* 38:543–551.

34 Contino EK, King MR, Valdés-Martínez A, et al.: 2015. In vivo diffusion characteristics following perineural injection of the deep branch of the lateral plantar nerve with mepivacaine or iohexol in horses. *Equine Vet J* 47:230–234.

35 Crabill MR, Honnas CM, Taylor DS, ct al.: 1994. Stringhalt secondary to trauma to the dorsoproximal region of the metatarsus in horses: 10 cases (1986–1991). *J Am Vet Med Assoc* 205:867–869.

36 Dabareiner RM, Sullins KE, White NA: 1993. Progression of femoropatellar osteochondrosis in nine young horses. Clinical, radiographic and arthroscopic findings. *Vet Surg* 22:515–523.

37 Daglish J, Frisbie DD, Selberg KT, et al.: 2018. High field magnetic resonance imaging is comparable with gross anatomy for description of the normal appearance of soft tissues in the equine stifle. *Vet Radiol Ultrasound* 59:721–736.

38 David F, Rougier M, Alexander K, et al.: 2007. Ultrasound-guided coxofemoral arthrocentesis in horses. *Equine Vet J* 39:79–83.

39 Davis W, Caniglia CJ, Lustgarten M, et al.: 2014. Clinical and diagnostic imaging characteristics of lateral digital flexor tendinitis within the tarsal sheath in four horses. *Vet Radiol Ultrasound* 55: 166–173.

40 De Busscher V, Verwilghen D, Bolen G, et al.: 2006. Meniscal damage diagnosed by ultrasonography in horses: A retrospective study of 74 femorotibial joint ultrasonographic examinations (2000–2005) *J Equine Vet Sci* 26:453–461.

41 Dechant JE, Southwood LL, Baxter GM, et al.: 2003. Use of a three-drill-tract technique for arthrodesis of the distal tarsal joints in horses with distal tarsal osteoarthritis: 54 cases (1990–1999). *J Am Vet Med Assoc* 223:1800–1805.

42 Derungs S, Fuerst A, Haas C, et al.: 2001. Fissure fractures of the radius and tibia in 23 horses: A retrospective study. *Equine Vet Educ* 13:313–318.

43 Dik KJ, Enzerink E, Weeren PR: 1999. Radiographic development of osteochondral abnormalities, in the hock and stifle of Dutch warmblood foals, from age 1 to 11 months. *Equine Vet J* 31: 9–15.

44 Dik KJ, Merkens HW: 1987. Unilateral distension of the tarsal sheath in the horse: A report of 11 cases. *Equine Vet J* 19:307–313.

45 Dubuc J, Girard C, Richard H, et al.: 2018. Equine meniscal degeneration is associated with medial femorotibial osteoarthritis. *Equine Vet J* 50:133–140. doi:10.1111/evj.12716.

46 Ducharme NG: 1996. Pelvic Fracture and Coxofemoral Luxation. *In*: Nixon AJ (ed) *Equine Fracture Repair*. Philadelphia, WB Saunders Co., 295–298.

47 Dumoulin M, Pille F, Desmet P, et al.: 2007. Upward fixation of the patella in the horse: A retrospective study. *Vet Comp Orth Traum* 20:119–125.

48 Dyson S, Wright I, Kold S, et al.: 1992. Clinical and radiographic features, treatment and outcome in 15 horses with fracture of the medial aspect of the patella. *Equine Vet J* 24:264–268.

49 Dyson SJ, Blunden A, Murray R: 2017. Magnetic resonance imaging, gross postmortem, and histological findings for soft tissues of the plantar aspect of the tarsus and proximal metatarsal region in non-lame horses. *Vet Radiol Ultrasound* 58:216–227.

50 Dyson SJ, Kidd L: 1992. Five cases of gastrocnemius tendinitis in the horse. *Equine Vet J* 24:351–356.

51 Dyson SJ: 1994. Stifle trauma in the event horse. *Equine Vet Educ* 6: 234–240.

52 Dyson SJ: 2002. Normal ultrasonographic anatomy and injury of the patellar ligaments in the horse. *Equine Vet J* 34:258–264.

53 Edwards RB, Nixon AJ: 1996. Avulsion of the cranial cruciate ligament insertion in a horse. *Equine Vet J* 28:334–336.

54 Ehrlich PJ, Seeherman HJ, MW O'Callaghan, et al.: 1998. Results of bone scintigraphy in horses used for show jumping, hunting, or eventing: 141 cases (1988–1994). *J Am Vet Med Assoc* 213:1460–1467.

55 Fleck SKV, Dyson SJ: 2012. Lameness associated with tarsocrural joint pathology in 17 mature horses (1997–2010). *Equine Vet Educ* 24:628–638.

56 Foland JW, McIlwraith CW, Trotter GW: 1992. Arthroscopic surgery for osteochondritis dissecans of the femoropatellar joint of the horse. *Equine Vet J* 24:419–423.

57 Fowlie JG, Stick JA, Nickels FA: 2012. The stifle. *In*: Auer JA, Stick JA (eds) *Equine Surgery, Fourth Edition*. St. Louis, MO, Elsevier, 1419–1442.

58 Frisbie DD, Barrett MF, McIlwraith CW, et al.: 2014. Diagnostic stifle joint arthroscopy using a needle arthroscope in standing horses. *Vet Surg* 43:12–18.

59 Fürst AE, Oswald S, Jäggin S, et al.: 2008. Fracture configurations of the equine radius and tibia after a simulated kick. *Vet Comp Orth Traum* 21:49–58.

60 Garcia-Lopez JM, Boudrieau RJ, Provost PJ: 2001. Surgical repair of a coxofemoral joint luxation in a horse. *J Am Vet Med Assoc* 219:1254–1258.

61 Geburek F, Rötting AK, Stadler PM: 2009. Comparison of the diagnostic value of ultrasonography and standing radiography for pelvic femoral disorders in horses. *Vet Surg* 38:310–317.

62 Gibson KT, McIlwraith CW, Park RD, et al.: 1989. Production of patellar lesions by medial patellar desmotomy in normal horses. *Vet Surg* 18:466–471.

63 Gomez-Villamandos R, Santisteban J, Ruiz I, et al.: 1995. Tenotomy of the tibial insertion of the semitendinosus muscle of two horses with fibrotic myopathy. *Vet Rec* 136:67–68.

64 Gough MR, Thibaud D, Smith RK: 2010. Tiludronate infusion in the treatment of bone spavin: A double-blind placebo-controlled trial. *Equine Vet J* 42:381–387.

65 Graham S, Solano M, Sutherland-Smith J, et al.: 2015. Diagnostic sensitivity of bone scintigraphy for equine stifle disorders. *Vet Radiol Ultrasound* 56:96–102. doi:10.1111/vru.12184.

66 Greet G, Greet TRC: 1996. The use of specific radiographic projections to demonstrate three intra-articular fractures. *Equine Vet Educ* 8:208–211.

67 Hague BA, Guccione A: 2002. Laser-facilitated arthrodesis of the distal tarsal joints. *Tech Equine Pract* 1:32–35.

68 Hance SR, Bramlage LR, Schneider RK, et al.: 1992. Retrospective study of 38 cases of femur fractures in horses less than one year of age. *Equine Vet J* 24: 357–363.

69 Hance SR, Bramlage LR: 1996. Fractures of the Femur and Patella. *In*: Nixon AJ (ed) *Equine Fracture Repair*. Philadelphia, W.B. Saunders Co., 284–293.

70 Hand R, Watkins JP, Honnas CM, et al.: 1999. Treatment of osteomyelitis of the sustentaculum tali and associated tenosynovitis in horses: 10 cases (1992–1998). *Proc Am Assoc Pract* 45:158–159.

71 Harrison LJ, May SA, Richardson JD, et al.: 1991. Conservative treatment of an incomplete long bone fracture of a hindlimb of four horses. *Vet Rec* 129:133–136.

72 Hoegaerts M, Nicaise M, Van Bree H, et al.: 2005. Cross-sectional anatomy and comparative ultrasonography of the equine medial femorotibial joint and its related structures. *Equine Vet J* 37:520–529.

73 Howard RD, McIlwraith CW, Trotter GW: 1995. Arthroscopic surgery for subchondral cystic lesions of the medial femoral condyle in horses: 41 cases (1988–1991). *J Am Vet Med Assoc* 206:842–850.

74 Hunt DA, Snyder JR, Morgan JP: 1990. Femoral capital physeal fractures in 25 foals. *Vet Surg* 19: 41–49.

75 Hunt RJ, Baxter, GM, Zamos DT: 1992. Tension band wiring and lag screw fixation of a transverse, comminuted fracture of a patella in a horse. *J Am Vet Med Assoc* 200:819–820.

76 Huntington PJ, Jeffcott LB, Friend SCE, et al.: 1989. Australian stringhalt—Epidemiological, clinical and neurological. *Equine Vet J* 21:266–273.

77 Huntington PJ, Seneque S, Slocombe RF, et al.: 1991. Use of phenytoin to treat horses with Australian stringhalt. *Aust Vet J* 68:221–224.

78 Ingle-Fehr JE, Baxter GM: 1998. Endoscopy of the calcaneal bursa in horses. *Vet Surg* 27:561–567.

79 Jacquet S, Audigie F, Denoix JM: 2007. Ultrasonographic diagnosis of subchondral bone cysts in the medial femoral condyle in horses. Tutorial article. *Equine Vet Educ* 19:47–50.

80 James SJ, Eastman TG, McCormick JD: 2014. Long-term outcome of standing medial patellar ligament splitting to manage horses exhibiting delayed patellar release: 64 horses. *J Equine Vet Sci* 34:479–483.

81 Janicek J, Lopes MA, Wilson DA, et al.: 2012. Hindlimb kinematics before and after laser fibrotomy in horses with fibrotic myopathy. *Equine Vet J Suppl* 43:126–131.

82 Jansson N: 1996. Treatment for upward fixation of the patella in the horse by medial patellar desmotomy: Indications and complications. *Equine Pract* 18:24–29.

83 Jesty SA, Palmer JE, Parente EJ, et al.: 2005. Rupture of the gastrocnemius muscle in six foals. *J Am Vet Med Assoc* 227:1965–1968.

84 Kelmer G, Wilson DA, Essman SC: 2008. Computed tomography assisted repair of a central tarsal bone slab fracture in a horse. *Equine Vet Educ* 20:284–287.

85 Koenig J, Cruz A, Genovese R, et al.: 2002. Rupture of the peroneus tertius tendon in 25 horses. *Proc Am Assoc Equine Pract* 48:326–328.

86 Labens R, Mellor DJ, Voute LC: 2007. Retrospective study of the effect of intra-articular treatment of osteoarthritis of the distal tarsal joints in 51 horses. *Vet Rec* 161:611–616.

87 Latorre R, Arencibia A, Gil F, et al.: 2006. Correlation of magnetic resonance images with anatomic features of the equine tarsus. *Am J Vet Res* 67:756–761.

88 Leveille R, Lindsay WA, Biller DS: 1993. Ultrasonographic appearance of ruptured peroneus tertius in a horse. *J Am Vet Med Assoc* 202: 1981–1982.

89 Levine DG, Aitken MR: 2017. Physeal fractures in foals. *Vet Clin North Am Equine Pract* 33:417–430.

90 Lugo J, Gaughan EM: 2006. Septic arthritis, tenosynovitis, and infections of hoof structures. *Vet Clin NA Equine Pract* 22:363–388.

91 MacDonald MH, Honnas CM, Meagher DM: 1989. Osteomyelitis of the calcaneus in horses: 28 cases (1972–1987). *J Am Vet Med Assoc* 194:1317–1323.

92 Magee AA, Vatistas N: 1998. Standing semitendinosus myotomy for the treatment of fibrotic myopathy in 39 horses (1989–1997). *Proc Am Assoc Equine Pract* 44:263–264.

93 Malark JA, Nixon AJ, Haughland MA, et al.: 1992. Equine coxofemoral luxations: 17 cases (1975–1990). *Cornell Vet* 82:79–90.

94 Marble GP, Sullins KE: 2000. Arthroscopic removal of patellar fracture fragments in horses: Five cases (1989– 1998). *J Am Vet Med Assoc* 216:1799–1801.

95 Martinelli MJ, Rantanen NW: 2009. Lameness originating from the equine stifle joint: A diagnostic challenge. *Equine Vet Educ* 21:648–651.

96 Martins EAN, Silva LC, Baccarin RYA: 2006. Ultrasonographic changes of the equine stifle following experimental medial patellar desmotomy. *Can Vet J* 47:471–474.

97 McCann ME, Hunt RJ: 1993. Conservative management of femoral diaphyseal fractures in four foals. *Cornell Vet* 83:125–132.

98 McCoy AM, Smith R, Herrera S, et al.: 2019. Long-term outcome after stifle arthroscopy in 82 Western performance horses (2003–2010). *Vet Surg* 48:956–965.

99 McIlwraith CW, Frisbie DD: 2014. Diagnostic and Surgical Arthroscopy of the Femoropatellar and Femorotibial Joints. *In*: McIlwraith CW, Nixon AJ, Wright IM (eds) *Diagnostic and Surgical Arthroscopy in the Horse, Fourth Edition*. London, Elsevier, 175–242.

100 McIlwraith CW, Nixon AJ, Wright IM, et al.: 2005. Arthroscopic Surgery of the Tarsocrural Joint. *In*: McIlwraith CW, Nixon AJ, Wright IM (eds) *Diagnostic and Surgical Arthroscopy in the Horse, Third Edition*. Philadelphia, Elsevier, 280–294.

101 McIlwraith CW, Nixon AJ, Wright IM, et al.: 2005. Diagnostic and Surgical Arthroscopy of the Coxofemoral (Hip) Joint. *In*: *Diagnostic and Surgical Arthroscopy in the Horse*. Philadelphia, Elsevier, 337–246.

102 McIlwraith CW: 2016. Osteochondrosis dissecans. *In*: McIlwraith CW, et al. (eds) *Joint Disease in the Horse, Second Edition*. St. Louis, MO, Elsevier, 57–84.

103 McIlwraith CW: 2010. The use of intra-articular corticosteroids in the horse: What is known on a scientific basis? *Equine Vet J* 42:563–571.

104 McIlwraith CW: 1990. Osteochondral fragmentation of the distal aspect of the patella in horses. *Equine Vet J* 22:157–163.

105 McLellan J, Plevin S, Hammock PD, et al.: 2009. Comparison of radiography, scintigraphy and ultrasonography in the diagnosis of patellar chondromalacia in a horse, confirmed by arthroscopy. *Equine Vet Educ* 21:642–647.

106 Meagher DM, Aldrete AV: 1989. Lateral luxation of the superficial digital flexor tendon from the calcaneal tuber in two horses. *J Am Vet Med Assoc* 195: 495–498.

107 Moll HD, Slone DE, Humburg JM, et al.: 1987. Traumatic tarsal luxation repaired without internal fixation in three horses and three ponies. *J Am Vet Med Assoc* 190:297–300.

108 Mueller PO, Allen D, Watson E, et al.: 1994. Arthroscopic removal of a fragment from an intercondylar eminence fracture of the tibia in a two-year-old horse. *J Am Vet Med Assoc* 204:1793–1795.

109 Murphey ED, Schneider RK, Adams SB, et al.: 2000. Long-term outcome of horses with a slab fracture of the central or third tarsal bone treated conservatively: 25 cases (1976–1993). *J Am Vet Med Assoc* 216: 1949–1954.

110 Murray RC, Dyson SJ, Weekes JS, et al.: 2005. Scintigraphic evaluation of the distal tarsal region in horses with distal tarsal pain. *Vet Rad Ultra* 46: 171–178.

111 Nelson BB, Kawcak CE, Goodrich LR, et al.: 2016. Comparison between computed tomographic arthrography, radiology, ultrasonography, and arthroscopy for the diagnosis of femorotibial joint disease in Western performance horses. *Vet Radiol Ultrasound* 57: 387–402.

112 Nixon A: 1996. Fractures of Specific Tarsal Bones. *In*: Nixon A (ed) *Equine Fracture Repair*. Philadelphia, WB Saunders, 260–267.

113 Nixon A: 1996. Luxations of the Hock. *In*: Nixon A (ed) *Equine Fracture Repair*. Philadelphia, WB Saunders, 270–271.

114 O'Brien T, Koch C, Livesey MA: 2012. What is your diagnosis? Avulsion fracture of the insertion of the round ligament of the head of the femur. *J Am Vet Med Assoc* 240:1059–1060.

115 O'Neill HDO, Bladon BM: 2010. Arthroscopic removal of fractures of the lateral malleolus of the tibia in the tarsocrural joint: A retrospective study of 13 cases. *Equine Vet J* 42:558–562.

116 O'Sullivan CB, Lumsden JM: 2003. Stress fractures of the tibia and humerus in thoroughbred racehorses: 99 cases (1992–2000). *J Am Vet Med Assoc* 222:491–498.

117 Ortved KF: 2017. Surgical management of osteochondrosis in foals. *Vet Clin North Am Equine Pract* 33:379–396.

118 Parks AH, Wyn-Jones G: 1988. Traumatic injuries of the patella in five horses. *Equine Vet J* 20:25–28.

119 Pease T, Redding WR: 2011. Computed Tomography of the Musculoskeletal System in Horses. *In*: Baxter GM (ed) *Adams Lameness in the Horse*. Hoboken, NJ, Wiley-Blackwell, 451–459.

120 Peloso JG, Watkins JP, Keele SR, et al.: 1993. Bilateral stress fractures of the tibia in a racing American Quarter horse. *J Am Vet Med Assoc* 203:801–803.

121 Peroni JF, Stick JA: 2002. Evaluation of a cranial arthroscopic approach to the stifle joint for the treatment of femorotibial joint disease in horses: 23 cases (1998–1999). *J Am Vet Med Assoc* 220:1046–1052.

122 Post EM, Singer ER, Clegg PD, et al.: 2003. Retrospective study of 24 cases of septic calcaneal bursitis in the horse. *Equine Vet J* 35: 662–668.

123 Post EM, Singer ER, Clegg PD: 2007. An anatomic study of the calcaneal bursae in the horse. *Vet Surg* 36: 3–9.

124 Prades M, Grant BD, Turner TA, et al.: 1989. Injuries to the cranial cruciate ligament and associated structures: Summary of clinical, radiographic, arthroscopic and pathological findings from 10 horses. *Equine Vet J* 21:354–357.

125 Ramzan PHL, Newton JR, Shepherd MC, et al.: 2003. The application of a scintigraphic grading system to equine tibial stress fractures: 42 cases. *Equine Vet J* 35:382–388.

126 Ray CS, Baxter GM, McIlwraith CW: 1996. Development of subchondral cystic lesions after articular cartilage and subchondral bone damage in young horses. *Equine Vet J* 28:225–232.

127 Redding WR, Tomlinson J, Berry C, et al.: 2003. Computed tomographic anatomy of the equine tarsus. *Vet Radiol Ultrasound* 44:174–178.

128 Reef VB: 1998. *Equine Diagnostic Ultrasound*. Philadelphia, WB Saunders Co., 74–75, 160–164.

129 Reiners S, Jann HW, Gillis E: 2000. Repair of medial luxation of the superficial digital flexor tendon in the pelvic limb of a filly. *Equine Pract* 22:18–19, 21.

130 Reiners SR, May K, DiGrassie W, et al.: 2005. How to perform a standing medial patellar ligament splitting. *Proc Am Assoc Equine Pract* 51:481–483.

131 Richard E, Alexander K: 2007. Nonconventional radiographic projections in the equine orthopaedic examination. *Equine Vet Educ* 19:551–559.

132 Rose PL, Graham JP, Moore I, et al.: 2001. Imaging diagnosis—Caudal cruciate ligament avulsion in a horse. *Vet Radiol Ultrasound* 42:414–416.

133 Rottensteiner U, Palm F, Kofler J: 2012. Ultrasonographic evaluation of the coxofemoral joint region in young foals. *Vet J* 191:193–198.

134 Rubio-Martínez LM, Redding WR, Bladon B, et al.: 2018. Fracture of the medial intercondylar eminence of the tibia in horses treated by arthroscopic fragment removal (21 horses). *Equine Vet J* 50:60–64.

135 Ruggles AJ, Moore RM, Bertone AL, et al.: 1996. Tibial stress fractures in racing standardbreds: 13 cases (1989–1993). *J Am Vet Med Assoc* 209:634–637.

136 Santschi EM, Williams JM, Morgan JW, et al.: 2015. Preliminary investigation of the treatment of equine medial femoral condylar subchondral cystic lesions with a transcondylar screw. *Vet Surg* 44:281–288. doi:10.1111/j.1532-950X.2014.12199.x.

137 Schneider RK, Jenson P, Moore RM: 1997. Evaluation of cartilage lesions on the medial femoral condyle as a cause of lameness in horses: 11 cases (1988–1994). *J Am Vet Med Assoc* 210:1649–1652.

138 Scott EA: 1983. Surgical repair of a dislocated superficial digital flexor tendon and fractured fibular tarsal bone in a horse. *J Am Vet Med Assoc* 183: 332–333.

139 Scott GS, Crawford WH, Colahan PT: 2004. Arthroscopic findings in horses with subtle radiographic evidence of osteochondral lesions of the medial femoral condyle: 15 cases (1995–2002). *J Am Vet Med Assoc* 224:1821–1826.

140 Scruton C, Baxter GM, Cross MW, et al.: 2005. Comparison of intra-articular drilling and diode laser treatment for arthrodesis of the distal tarsal joints in normal horses. *Equine Vet J* 37:81–86.

141 Serena A, Schumacher J, Schramme M, et al.: 2005. Concentration of methylprednisolone in the distal intertarsal joint after administration of methylprednisolone acetate into the tarsometatarsal joint. *Equine Vet J* 37:172–174.

142 Sherlock CE, Eggleston RB, Peroni JF, et al.: 2012. Desmitis of the medial tarsal collateral ligament in 7 horses. *Equine Vet Educ* 24:72–80.

143 Shoemaker RW, Allen AL, Richardson CE, et al.: 2006. Use of intra-articular administration of ethyl alcohol for arthrodesis of the tarsometatarsal joint in healthy horses. *Am J Vet Res* 67:850–857.

144 Smith BL, Auer JA, Watkins JP: 1990. Surgical repair of tibial tuberosity avulsion fractures in four horses. *Vet Surg* 19:117–121.

145 Smith MA, Walmsley JP, Phillips TJ, et al.: 2005. Effect of age at presentation on outcome following arthroscopic debridement of subchondral cystic lesions of the medial femoral condyle: 85 horses (1993–2003). *Equine Vet J* 37:175–180.

146 Smith RKW, Dyson SJ, Schramme MC, et al.: 2005. Osteoarthritis of the talocalcaneal joint in 18 horses. *Equine Vet J* 37:166–171.

147 Sparks HD, Nixon AJ, Fortier LA, et al.: 2011. Arthroscopic reattachment of osteochondritis dissecans cartilage flaps of the femoropatellar joint: long-term results. *Equine Vet J* 43:650–659.

148 Squire KRE, Blevins WE, Frederick M, et al.: 1990. Radiographic changes in an equine patella following medial patellar desmotomy. *Vet Rad* 31:208–209.

149 Steel CM, Hunt AR, Adams PL, et al.: 1999. Factors associated with prognosis for survival and athletic use in foals with septic arthritis: 93 cases (1987–1994). *J Am Vet Med Assoc* 215:973–977.

150 Stock KF, Hamann H, Distl O: 2005. Prevalence of osseous fragments in distal and proximal interphalangeal-geal, metacarpo- and metatarsophalangeal and tarsocrural joints of Hanoverian warmblood horses. *J Vet Med Ser A* 52:388–394.

151 Suarez-Fuentes DG, Tatarniuk DM, Caston SS, et al.: 2018. Tenotomy of the semitendinosus muscle under standing sedation versus general anesthesia: Outcomes in 20 horses with fibrotic myopathy. *Vet Surg* 47:350–356.

152 Sullins KE, Baxter GM: 2011. *The Femur and Coxofemoral Joint, Sixth Edition*. Hoboken, NJ, Blackwell Publishing, Ltd., 814–832.

153 Swor TM, Schneider RK, Ross MW, et al.: 2001. Injury to the origin of the gastrocnemius muscle as a possible cause of lameness in four horses. *J Am Assoc Vet Med* 219:215–219.

154 Talbot AM, Barrett EL, Driver AJ, et al.: 2006. How to perform standing lateral oblique radiographs of the equine pelvis. *Proc Am Assoc Equine Pract* 52:613–614.

155 Textor JA, Nixon AJ, Lumsden J, et al.: 2001. Subchondral cystic lesions of the proximal extremity of the tibia in horses: 12 cases (1983–2000). *J Am Vet Med Assoc* 218:408–413.

156 Tnibar MA: 2002. Medial patellar ligament splitting for the treatment of upward fixation of the patella in 7 equids. *Vet Surg* 31:462–467.

157 Tomlinson J, Redding WR, Sage A: 2000. Ultrasonographic evaluation of tarsocrural joint cartilage in normal adult horses. *Vet Radiol Ultrasound* 41:457–460.

158 Tomlinson JE, Redding WR, Berry C, et al.: 2003. Computed tomographic anatomy of the equine tarsus. *Vet Rad Ultrasound* 44:174–178.

159 Toth F, Schumacher J, Schramme HS: 2011. Evaluation of four techniques for injecting the trochanteric bursa of horses. *Vet Surg* 40:489–493.

160 Trump M, Kircher PR, Fürst A: 2011. The use of computed tomography in the diagnosis of pelvic fractures involving the acetabulum in two fillies. *Vet Comp Orthop Traumatol* 24:68–71.

161 Tull TM, Woodie JB, Ruggles AJ, et al.: 2009. Management and assessment of prognosis after gastrocnemius disruption in thoroughbred foals: 28 cases (1993–2007). *Equine Vet J* 41:541–546.

162 Updike SJ: 1984. Anatomy of the tarsal tendons of the equine tibialis cranialis and peroneus tertius muscles. *Am J Vet Res* 45:1379–1382.

163 Valdés-Martínez A, Seiler G, Mai W, et al.: 2008. Quantitative analysis of scintigraphic findings in tibial stress fractures in thoroughbred racehorses. *Am J Vet Res* 69:886–890.

164 Valentine BA, Rousselle SD, Sams AE, et al.: 1994. Denervation atrophy in three horses with fibrotic myopathy. *J Am Vet Med Assoc* 205:332–336.

165 Van Hoogmoed LM, Agnew DW, Whitcomb M, et al.: 2002. Ultrasonographic and histologic evaluation of medial and middle patellar ligaments in exercised horses following injection with ethanolamine oleate and 2% iodine in almond oil. *Am J Vet Res* 63:738–743.

166 Von Rechenberg B, Guenther H, McIlwraith CW, et al.: 2000. Fibrous tissue of subchondral cystic lesions in horses produce local mediators and neutral metalloproteinases and cause bone resorption in vitro. *Vet Surg* 29:420–429.

167 Wallis TW, Goodrich LR, McIlwraith CW, et al.: 2008. Arthroscopic injection of corticosteroids into the fibrous tissue of subchondral cystic lesions of the medial femoral condyle in horses: A retrospective study of 52 cases (2001–2006). *Equine Vet J* 40:461–467.

168 Walmsley JP: 2005. Diagnosis and treatment of ligamentous and meniscal injuries in the equine stifle. *Vet Clin North Am Equine Pract* 21:651–672.

169 Walmsley JP: 1994. Medial patellar desmotomy for upward fixation of the patella. *Equine Vet Educ* 6: 148–150.

170 Walmsley JP: 1997. Fracture of the intercondylar eminence of the tibia treated by arthroscopic internal fixation. *Equine Vet J* 29:148–150.

171 Walmsley JR, Phillips TJ, Townsend HG: 2003. Meniscal tears in horses: An evaluation of clinical signs and arthroscopic treatment of 80 cases. *Equine Vet J* 35:402–406.

172 Watkins JP: 1996. Fractures of the Tibia. *In:* Nixon AJ (ed) *Equine Fracture Repair.* Philadelphia, WB Saunders, 273–283.

173 Watkins JP: 2004. Intramedullary interlocking nail fixation in equine fracture management. *Euro Soc of Vet Orthopaed and Traumat* 12:195–196.

174 Welch RD, Auer JA, Watkins JP, et al.: 1990. Surgical treatment of tarsal sheath effusion associated with an exostosis on the calcaneus of a horse. *J Am Vet Med Assoc* 196:1992–1994.

175 Whitcomb MB, Vaughan B: 2015. Ultrasonographic evaluation of the coxofemoral joint. *Proc Am Assoc Equine Pract* 61:346–354.

176 Whitcomb MR: 2006. Ultrasonography of the equine tarsus. *Proc Am Assoc Equine Pract* 52:13–30.

177 Winberg FG, Pettersson H: 1999. Outcome and racing performance after internal fixation of third and central tarsal bone slab fractures in horses. A review of 20 cases. *Acta Vet Scand* 40:173–180.

178 Wright IM, Minshall GJ: 2012. Injuries of the calcaneal insertions of the superficial digital flexor tendon in 19 horses. *Equine Vet J* 44:136–142.

179 Wright IM, Montesso F, Kidd LJ: 1995. Surgical treatment of fractures of the tibial tuberosity in 6 adult horses. *Equine Vet J* 27:96–102.

180 Wright IM: 1992. Fractures of the lateral malleolus of the tibia in 16 horses. *Equine Vet J* 24:424–429.

181 Zamos DT, Honnas CM, Hoffman AG: 1994. Arthroscopic and intra-articular anatomy of the plantar pouch of the equine tarsocrural joint. *Vet Surg* 23:161–166.

182 Zubrod CJ, Schneider RK, Hague BA, et al.: 2005. Comparison of three methods for arthrodesis of the distal intertarsal and tarsometatarsal joints in horses. *Vet Surg* 34:372–382.

Revised from "Lameness of the Proximal Limb" in *Adams and Stashak's Lameness in Horses, 7th Edition,* **by W. Rich Redding, Chris Kawcak, Troy N. Trumble, Nicolas S. Ernst, Ken E. Sullins, and Gary M. Baxter.**

5

Common Conditions of the Axial Skeleton

The Pelvis

Pelvic Fractures

Overview
- Pelvic fractures are more common in young horses and are usually due to trauma.
- Ileal stress fractures are seen in racehorses.
- Pelvic fractures are nearly always unilateral but may involve multiple bones of the pelvis such as the ilium and pubis.
- Non-displaced fractures may be difficult to diagnose.
- Severe pelvic fractures in adult horses that involve the ilium can lacerate the iliac arteries and contribute to acute death.

Anatomy

- The pelvis is comprised of the ilium, ischium, and pubis, and the acetabulum is formed through contributions from all three of these bones.
- The lunate surface of the acetabulum, a cup-shaped cavity arcing around a deep nonarticular fossa, articulates with the head of the femur.
- The wing-shaped ilium forms a prominence on each side of the pelvis known as the tuber coxae or point of the hip (Figure 5.1).
- The dorsally directed tuber sacrale inclines medially toward the opposite side so that

the two sacral tubers come within 2–3 cm over the first sacral spinous process (Figure 5.1).
- The ischial tuberosity is the caudal and lateral ridge of the ilium to which muscles of the thigh attach.
- The pelvis is surrounded by a complicated network of ligaments and musculature that serves to both stabilize and protect the pelvis from injury.

Imaging
- The pelvis can be difficult to image, especially in the standing horse.
- Both standing and recumbent radiography can be used to identify pelvic fractures depending on their location, the amount of displacement, and the size of the horse.
- Ultrasonography can be used to identify fractures of the ilium and acetabulum.
- Nuclear scintigraphy can be useful to identify more subtle lesions within the pelvis such as non-displaced or stress fractures and lesions in the sacroiliac region.
- CT has been used to document select fractures within the coxofemoral joint.

Etiology
- Most are single-event traumatic fractures from falling, slipping, fighting, and other types of accidents.

Manual of Equine Lameness, Second Edition. Gary M. Baxter.
© 2022 John Wiley & Sons, Inc. Published 2022 by John Wiley & Sons, Inc.
Companion website: www.wiley.com/go/baxter/manual

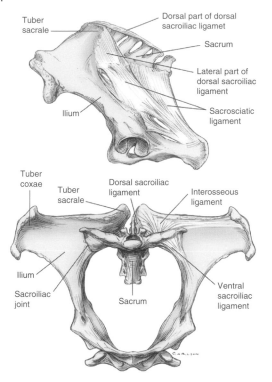

Figure 5.1 Pelvis and sacroiliac joint, lateral (top) and cranial (bottom) views. *Source:* Courtesy of Dave Carlson.

- Ilial fractures in racehorses are common stress-type fractures caused by repetitive overloading.

Clinical Signs
- There is acute onset of lameness, which is usually severe (4 to 5/5).
- The horse may have a toe-out, hock-in limb conformation (Figure 5.2).
- There is often pain on deep palpation of the gluteal muscles and/or manipulation of the pelvis.
- Crepitus may be audible with manipulation of the pelvis or pelvic limb.
- An alteration in height of the tuber coxae or tuber ischii may be visible.
- Palpable hematoma, fracture, or asymmetry of the pelvic canal may be found on a rectal exam.

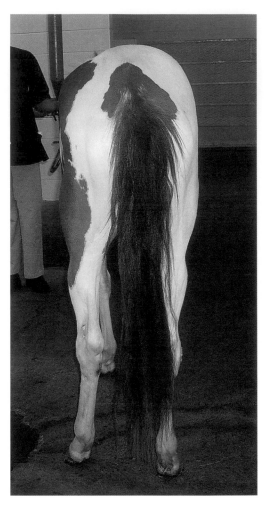

Figure 5.2 Young horse with asymmetry of the pelvis, muscle atrophy over the left hip, and a toe-out stance. The horse was lame at the walk and an acetabular fracture was present on radiographs.

- There may be differences in limb length; this is mostly seen with hip luxations.
- Gluteal muscle atrophy can occur quickly on the affected side with pelvic fractures.
- Chronic fractures are nearly always associated with gluteal muscle atrophy and outward rotation of the limb (Figure 1.50).

Diagnosis
- The diagnosis may be made strictly based on history and clinical findings.

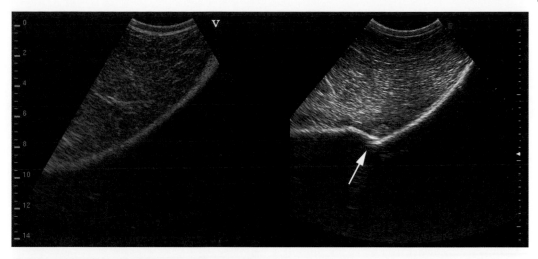

Figure 5.3 Ultrasonographic image of mildly displaced ilial wing fracture. At the left is the sonogram of a normal ilial wing; at the right is an ilial wing fracture (arrow). *Source:* Courtesy of Mary Beth Withcomb.

- Standing or recumbent radiography can be used to make the diagnosis.
- Percutaneous or transrectal ultrasonography is also useful to confirm the diagnosis (Figure 5.3).
- Scintigraphy is best used to identify ilial stress fractures in racehorses.

Treatment
- The treatment is usually confinement combined with variable periods of NSAIDs. Strict stall confinement for at least 30 days is considered important.
- The length of confinement and prognosis depend on the type of fracture.
- Euthanasia is recommended in horses with severely comminuted and displaced fractures, especially if they fail to improve with confinement.

Prognosis
- The prognosis varies, depending on the type of fracture.
- Most minimally displaced fractures should heal with a good prognosis.
- Horses with acetabular fractures have a reduced prognosis for future performance.

Ilial Wing Fractures

Anatomy (Please refer to previous section on "Pelvic Fractures")

Imaging (Please refer to previous section on "Pelvic Fractures")
Etiology
- Ilial wing fractures are incomplete, stress, or "fatigue" fractures associated with training and racing in young racehorses.
- They are usually unilateral but can occur bilaterally.

Clinical Signs and Diagnosis
- Young racehorse that presents with an acute onset of lameness.
- The severity of lameness varies from grade 2 to 5/5 and usually improves quickly with confinement.
- The horse may tend to plait with the hind limbs or cross over the hind limbs at the trot.
- Gluteal muscle atrophy may occur within two weeks.
- Scintigraphy is usually necessary to make the diagnosis.

- Ultrasonography may be used to detect the fracture if it is displaced (Figure 5.3).
- Radiography of pelvis under general anesthesia is contraindicated because of the risk of fracture displacement.

Treatment and Prognosis

- Treatment consists of discontinuing training/racing and rest.
- Usually confinement is combined with NSAIDs, depending on severity of the lameness.
- The prognosis usually is very good for returning to racing.
- Complete, displaced fracture of the ilium is always a risk if the horse returns to training too soon.

Tuber Coxae Fractures

Anatomy (Please refer to previous section on "Pelvic Fractures")

Imaging (Please refer to previous section on "Pelvic Fractures")

Etiology

- The cause of tuber coxae fractures is single-event trauma such as running into a door, post, wood fence, side of a building, etc.
- It may be associated with a wound at the point of the hip and drainage if infection is present.

Clinical Signs and Diagnosis

- Moderate-to-severe lameness is usually present initially, which decreases to mild lameness within 48 hours.
- In an abnormally contoured tuber coxae, the fractured portion will move cranioventrally due to traction of the internal abdominal oblique muscle.
- The horse may have an associated wound with a draining tract with or without sequestration in chronic cases (Figure 5.4).

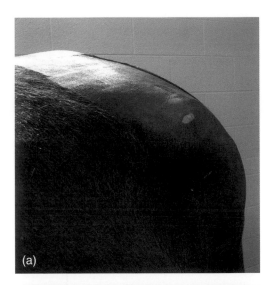

(a)

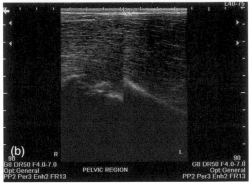

(b)

Figure 5.4 (a) Cranial view of the pelvis demonstrating swelling and a wound associated with the left tuber coxae. (b) Ultrasound image of the tuber coxae showing a disrupted contour of the ilial wing. *Source:* Courtesy of Rob van Wessum.

- The diagnosis is often based on clinical signs alone, but ultrasonography usually aids in making the diagnosis (Figure 5.4).
- A dorsomedial–centrolateral 50° oblique radiograph of the tuber coxae in the standing horse may also be used to confirm the fracture.

Treatment and Prognosis

- The best treatment is confinement if the fracture is closed.
- Appropriate wound management is necessary if the fracture is open.

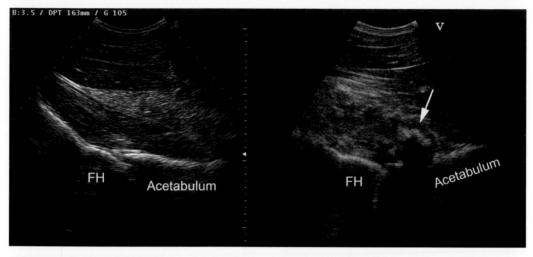

Figure 5.5 Ultrasonographic image of an acetabular fracture. At the left is a normal image; a fracture of the acetabulum (arrow) can be seen on the right. FH = femoral head. *Source:* Courtesy of Mary Beth Whitcomb.

- There is no need to remove the fracture fragment unless the wound fails to heal and a sequestrum develops. Surgery is usually necessary if this occurs.
- The prognosis is usually very good – 93% of the horses returned to athletic performance in one study.

Acetabular Fractures

Anatomy (Please refer to previous section on "Pelvic Fractures")

Imaging (Please refer to previous section on "Pelvic Fractures")

Etiology
- The cause is usually single-event trauma, such as a fall and are most common in young horses.

Clinical Signs and Diagnosis
- The horse is often very lame and reluctant to move, but this depends on the duration and degree of displacement.
- Crepitation can often be heard or ausculted when the horse is rocked back and forth.
- Swelling adjacent to the acetabulum may be palpable on rectal examination.

- Tentative diagnosis can usually be made based on history and clinical findings.
- Ultrasonography (transcutaneous or transrectal) is often diagnostic if the fracture is complete (Figure 5.5).
- Radiography can be performed under anesthesia but may cause further fracture displacement (Figure 5.6).

Treatment and Prognosis
- The treatment is similar to other types of pelvic fractures: conservative or euthanasia.
- The prognosis is unfavorable for return to performance if the fracture is significantly displaced due to development of OA of the coxofemoral joint.
- The prognosis is good if the fracture is minimally displaced.

Fractures of the Sacrum and Coccygeal Vertebrae

Anatomy

- The equine sacrum is a single bone formed through fusion of embryologically distinct sacral vertebrae, generally five of these, with

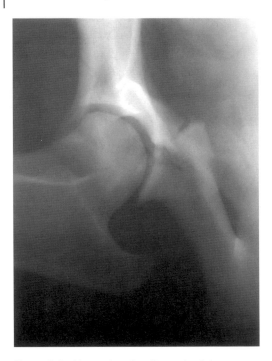

Figure 5.6 Ventrodorsal radiograph of the coxofemoral joint demonstrating a minimally displaced acetabular fracture. Intra-articular fragmentation was not identified, and the horse was treated with stall confinement.

four, six, and seven sacral vertebrae also being reported.
- The sacrum is triangular and gently curving so as to present a slightly concave ventral aspect.
- Although there is considerable individual variation, the average horse has 18 caudal vertebrae, and the first caudal vertebra is not uncommonly fused with the sacrum.

Imaging
- Radiography can usually document the fracture depending on the location.
- Both ultrasonography and scintigraphy may also be used aid the diagnosis depending on the location and duration of injury.

Etiology
- The cause is usually trauma such as a fall.
- Often no cause is known.

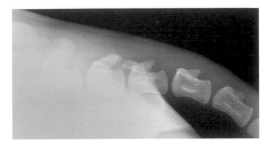

Figure 5.7 Radiograph of a horse with bone proliferation between the coccygeal vertebrae 1 and 2 at the dorsal aspect as the result of an avulsion fracture of the intervertebral ligament. *Source:* Courtesy of Rob van Wessum.

Clinical Signs
- The clinical signs are variable; one indication is the horse's reluctance to back up.
- The normal "snake-like" locomotion pattern to the spine at the walk and canter is altered due to pain.
- Focal swelling and palpable pain are often present, with reduced mobility of the sacrum or tail.

Diagnosis
- Radiography is best used to diagnose coccygeal fractures (Figure 5.7).
- Ultrasound may also be able to identify the fracture depending on its location.

Treatment
- Treatment consists of a reduced workload or complete rest if a displaced fracture is present.
- Caudal epidural may be administered using corticosteroids if the problem is chronic.
- Topical NSAIDs, ESWT, PRP or other types of biological therapies may be used for concurrent soft-tissue injuries of the sacrum.

Prognosis
- The prognosis is usually very good.

The Sacroiliac (SI) Region

Overview

- Conditions of the sacroiliac region are recognized as a cause for (low-grade) lameness or lack of performance in many types of horses.
- The sacroiliac (SI) joint itself and/or the soft-tissue structures adjacent to the joint can cause SI problems.
- Differentiating true SI joint problems from other soft-tissue injuries in the area is difficult, and therefore, lameness issues in the SI region are often treated collectively.

Anatomy

- The axial skeleton and appendicular skeleton of the hind limb are united at the sacroiliac joint (Figure 5.1). This joint is capable of only extremely limited gliding movement; its principal purpose is most likely absorption of concussive forces transmitted through the appendicular skeleton to the vertebral column.
- The SI joint is located where the ventral aspect of the ilium comes into close contact with the sacrum.
- The joint is substantially reinforced by a series of sacroiliac ligaments (ventral sacroiliac ligament, the dorsal sacroiliac ligament, and the interosseous ligament) that contribute markedly to the overall stability of the joint and probably act to transfer most of the weight of the trunk to the pelvic limbs.
- The ventral sacroiliac ligament surrounds the joint and fills the space between the ilium and the wing of the sacrum and provides support to the ventral SI joint.
- The dorsal sacroiliac ligament has two distinct portions – one that arises from the tuber sacrale and inserts on the spinous processes of the sacral vertebrae and the other arises from the tuber sacrale and the caudal edge of the ilial wing and inserts along the

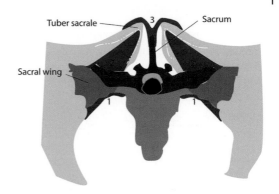

Figure 5.8 Schematic drawing of the sacroiliac joint region and the adjacent ligamentous structures (cranial aspect). (1) Ventral sacral ligaments. (2) Interosseus sacroiliac ligaments. (3) Dorsal sacral ligaments. *Source:* Drawing by Maggie Hofmann.

lateral aspect of the sacrum (Figures 5.1 and 5.8)
- The interosseous ligament consists of strong, vertically oriented fibers between the ventral part of the wing of the ilium and the dorsal aspect of the wing of the sacrum.

Imaging

- Scintigraphy and ultrasound are the two preferred imaging techniques with scintigraphy considered the best diagnostic method.
- Percutaneous ultrasound can be used to detect lesions in the dorsal sacral ligaments.
- Transrectal examination can be performed to evaluate the bony edges of the SI joint.

Etiology

- The pelvic musculature is important in providing stability and mobility to the SI region, and weakness in these muscles may contribute to injuries.
- SI conditions may involve damage to the dorsal sacral ligaments, the interosseus and ventral sacral ligaments (i.e. subluxation), or the SI joint itself (OA).
- Injuries can range from single-event trauma such as getting "cast" or repetitive injury to the area associated with performance.

Clinical Signs

- Variable presenting complaints including reduced stride length in one or both hind limbs, reduced propulsion and engagement, refusal to jump, and unwillingness to go downhill.
- Lameness or gait abnormalities may be most noticeable at the canter—a "bunny hop" in which there is less separation of footfalls of the hind limbs.
- The horse may change leads or cross canter frequently.
- The horse may appear stiff and rigid with a lack of lateroflexion in the lumbosacral region.
- The performance of racehorses may be reduced.
- Horses display behavioral issues such as kicking, rearing, striking, and bucking, especially when asked to canter.
- Asymmetry of the tuber sacrales can be observed but is not a consistent finding (Figure 5.9).
- Gluteal muscle atrophy is often present.
- During flexion tests, the horse may show reluctance to stand on the affected limb or lean over to the affected side, so the stance limb is in midposition, reducing rotational forces to the pelvic structures.

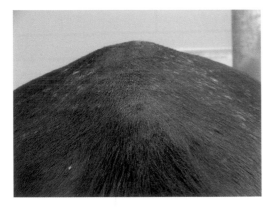

Figure 5.9 Caudal view of a horse with asymmetric tuber sacrales. Due to ligament damage, the right tuber sacrale is much higher than the left. *Source:* Courtesy of Rob van Wessum.

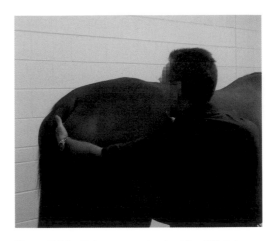

Figure 5.10 Pain provocation test for SI joint pain. The left hand of the examiner is on the right tuber ischium and the right hand is on the tuber coxae, creating a rocking motion in the cranial direction. *Source:* Courtesy of Rob van Wessum.

- There may be palpable pain on deep palpation over the tuber sacrale or with pelvic manipulation (Figure 5.10).
- Severe hind limb lameness is associated with severe SI injury such as acute subluxation, dislocation, or rupture of the sacral ligaments.

Diagnosis

- Scintigraphy is the best diagnostic method.
- Percutaneous ultrasound can be used to detect damage to the dorsal sacral ligaments.
- Transrectal examination can be performed to evaluate the bony edges of the SI joint.

Treatment

- Confinement and rest are indicated if an acute injury is suspected.
- A complete and intensive rehabilitation program is important in chronic injuries, with the goal of developing better muscle support of the SI region.
- Injection of the SI joint/area with corticosteroids is most useful if OA or chronic trauma to the joint is suspected.
- PRP or other biological therapies are most useful for injuries to the dorsal sacral

ligament and/or damage to other soft-tissue structures.

Prognosis

- The prognosis is variable and is difficult to predict.
- Most reports suggest a guarded prognosis for return to the previous level of performance.
- The prognosis may be improved with a structured rehabilitation program with frequent reevaluations.

Thoracolumbar Region/Back

Overriding/Impingement of Dorsal Spinous Processes

Overview

- Overriding/impingement of the dorsal spinous processes is known as "kissing spines."
- It is a common diagnosis in horses with back pain but is not always a contributing problem.
- The most common location for these lesions is in the thoracic spine (between T5 and T18), but impingement of the lumbar dorsal processes also has been reported.

Anatomy

- There are usually 18 thoracic vertebrae and 6 lumbar vertebrae in the horse, although there may be on occasion one more or one less than typical (Figure 5.11).
- The bodies of the thoracic vertebrae tend to be short with a small vertebral arch dorsally and the spinous processes are relatively tall (Figure 5.11).
- The tall spinous processes of the first 12 vertebrae constitute the withers and the anticlinal vertebra is usually the 16th, and occasionally the 14th.
- The vertebral arches of the lumbar vertebrae tend to overlap dorsally, except at the L5–L6

and L6-S1 interspaces, where the larger interarcuate spaces are much larger and clinically accessible.

- The joints of the vertebral column all permit flexion, extension, lateral flexion, and limited rotation, but these movements are fairly limited throughout the thoracic and lumbar regions. Intervertebral discs of fibrocartilage are interposed between adjacent vertebral bodies.
- Stabilization of the thoracolumbar vertebral column is provided by (i) the continuous dorsal and ventral longitudinal ligaments on their respective surfaces of the vertebral bodies; (ii) a supraspinous ligament that passes along the dorsal aspect of the spinous processes of the thoracic, lumbar, and sacral vertebrae; and (iii) interspinal ligaments that pass between adjacent spinous processes.
- The epaxial muscles are extensors of the vertebral column and are roughly divided into three parallel bundles of fascicles: from lateral to medial, these are the iliocostalis system, the longissimus system, and the transversospinalis system.

Imaging

- Radiography, scintigraphy, and ultrasonography are all potential imaging techniques that can be used in the thoracolumbar region and multiple imaging approaches are often necessary to confirm the diagnosis.
- Radiography alone can result in over diagnosis of boney abnormalities of the spinous processes.
- Scintigraphy is the best imaging technique to determine active bone remodeling and evidence of active inflammation within the spine.

Etiology

- Repetitive (traumatic) contact between the dorsal processes is thought to be the cause.
- Damage to the supraspinous or interspinous ligaments may also lead to impingement.

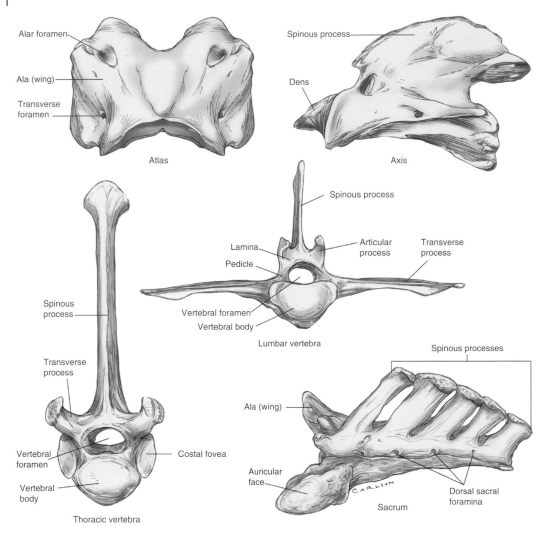

Figure 5.11 Vertebrae of the horse illustrating the varied size and shape of the dorsal spinous processes. *Source:* Courtesy of Dave Carlson.

- A primary injury to the ventral and ventrolateral support structures of the annulus fibrosis of the intervertebral disk may cause (asymmetrical) narrowing or collapse of the intervertebral joint.

Clinical Signs
- The horse may have a variety of signs, often related to the discipline in which they perform. Show jumpers and hunters seem to be more affected than others.
- Impingement reduces the ventrodorsal mobility of the spine most often, but when pain is present, the lateral mobility may be limited due to muscle spasm.
- There are often irregularities in the size of the summits of the spinous processes of the affected thoracic or lumbar vertebrae.
- Pain with localized digital pressure of the dorsal spinous processes or the supraspinous ligament is present at the affected site(s).
- When impingement is present in the cranial part of the thoracic spine (T5-T12-T13), the horse may have a painful or violent response when putting the saddle on or when the rider mounts.

Diagnosis

- The diagnosis is based on physical findings of irregularities and pain along the dorsal spinous processes of the affected vertebrae. It is important to differentiate between the resentment shown by some horses and distress resulting from other back conditions.
- Radiography can identify bony changes such as sclerosis, exostoses, and osteolysis.
- Ultrasonography can evaluate the contact and remodeling between adjacent spinous processes, transverse thickening of the processes, and abnormal alignment. Concomitant lesions in the supraspinous ligament and enthesiopathy on the summits of the spinous processes also can be imaged.
- Scintigraphy can identify evidence of active bone metabolism and remodeling of the spinous processes, as well as adjacent structures of the spine that may be involved (intervertebral disk, facet joint, vertebral body; Figure 5.12).

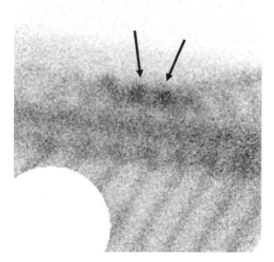

Figure 5.12 Delayed phase LDO view of the mid-thoracic vertebrae of a horse, showing focal and intense abnormal radiotracer uptake at two adjacent dorsal spinous processes (arrows) suggestive of impingement. *Source:* Courtesy of Kurt Selberg.

- Infiltration with a local anesthetic at suspected site(s) can provide information about the likelihood that the observed impingement is the cause of pain.

Treatment

- Conservative therapies include rest, NSAIDs, local injections of anti-inflammatory agents, acupuncture, and physiotherapy.
- Injections of corticosteroids between affected spinous processes, combined with NSAID therapy, can be very helpful in reducing or removing pain.
- Surgical removal of the affected spinous process(es) or transection of the interspinous ligaments can be performed if the area is determined to be contributing to the pain.
- Endoscopic resection of the spinous process and the interspinous ligament has also been reported.

Prognosis

- The prognosis is considered guarded in most reports.
- When ligamentous structures are involved (supraspinous ligament, intraspinous ligament, ventral longitudinal ligament), the prognosis is less favorable than when just osseous changes are seen on radiographs.
- The prognosis is also less favorable when there are adjacent pathologic conditions in the intervertebral disk or the facet joints.
- The prognosis in horses with severe lesions seems to be better with surgery than without surgery.

Supraspinous Ligament Injuries

Anatomy (Please refer to previous section on "Overriding Dorsal Spinous Processes")

Imaging (Please refer to previous section on "Overriding Dorsal Spinous Processes")
Etiology

- Supraspinous ligament injuries are most commonly found between T15 and L3.

- The specific cause is often unknown, but these injuries are often associated with repetitive-use trauma related to performance.
- Overriding dorsal spinous processes and supraspinous ligament injuries can occur concurrently along with other soft-tissue injuries in the thoracolumbar region.

Clinical Signs

- The clinical signs are similar to those of impingement of the dorsal spinous processes; when only ligament pathology is present, the signs can be mild and very difficult to detect.
- The signs are often associated with localized thickening of the ligament and palpable pain.
- The appearance of the contour of the spine can resemble kyphosis (roaching of the back) due to swelling at the site.

Diagnosis

- Ultrasonography is the imaging method of choice. It can usually document ligament pathology and surrounding swelling and edema.
- Radiography may show irregular bone margins of the summits of the dorsal spinal processes, avulsion fragments, and sclerosis.
- Scintigraphy can provide additional information about the involvement of the spinous processes (Figure 5.13).
- Local infiltration of anesthetic can be used to confirm that the supraspinous ligament is the cause of pain.

Treatment

- Conservative treatment focuses on rest, oral NSAIDs, and rehabilitation.
- Controlled stretching of the ligament with a lower position of the head (pasture, hay on the ground, ridden with a lower head and a longer neck) and a gradual increase in the workload are recommended.
- Local injection of anti-inflammatories (corticosteroids) can be used as treatment, as well as ESWT.

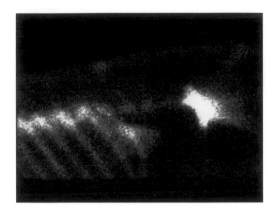

Figure 5.13 Scintigraphic image showing mild focal IRU at the summit of T18; it is indicative of desmitis of the supraspinous ligament. Radiography did not show any change, and ultrasonography showed mild desmitis with a roughened bone margin of the summit of the spinous process of T18. *Source:* Courtesy of Rob van Wessum.

- Local injection of PRP, stem cells, or other types of biological therapies can be used.

Prognosis

- The prognosis is favorable when only the supraspinous ligament is involved.
- The prognosis is reduced when concurrent structures are affected (dorsal spinous processes, facet joints, or intervertebral disk).

Fractures of the Spinous Processes

Anatomy (Please refer to previous section on "Overriding Dorsal Spinous Processes")

Imaging (Please refer to previous section on "Overriding Dorsal Spinous Processes")

Etiology

- Fractures of the spinous processes occur primarily in the cranial thoracic spine (withers region) when horses flip over, fall backward, or run into objects with their withers.
- Sporadic fractures in the lumbar spine can be caused by excessive trauma such as falling and turning (rotational force on the spine) and at high speed (cross country, jumping, barrel racing, hunting, etc.)

Clinical Signs

- The clinical signs include swelling and palpable pain in the affected region with deformation of the normal contour of the withers.
- An indentation may be observed in the withers, and the withers may appear wider than normal.
- Abnormal alignment of the spinous processes may be the only abnormality found in chronic cases.

Diagnosis

- Radiography of the withers usually reveals dislocated and fractures of the thoracic spines. The spinous processes of the withers region (T3–T12) can vary in shape and have accessory centers of ossification that can be misinterpreted as a fracture.
- Radiography of the lumbar spine can be difficult to perform depending on the size of the horse.
- Ultrasonography is most helpful to identify fractures of the spinous processes in the lumbar spine.
- Scintigraphy will often show increased radiopharmaceutical uptake at the affected site but cannot necessarily document a fracture (Figure 5.14).

Treatment

- Conservative treatment is used to manage the pain and swelling associated with the fracture.
- Surgery is not required in most cases unless the fractured spinous process of the withers becomes infected.

Prognosis

- The prognosis is usually very good for spinous process fractures of the withers, but an abnormal contour to the withers often remains.
- It may be difficult to make the saddle fit properly due to the changed shape of the withers.

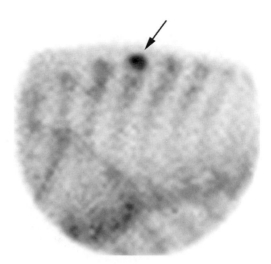

Figure 5.14 Delayed phase LDO view of the withers of a horse, showing a focal and intense abnormal radiotracer involving only the most proximal aspect of one of the spinous processes (arrow), suggestive of a fracture. *Source:* Courtesy of Dr. Erik Bergman.

Vertebral Fractures

Anatomy (Please refer to previous section on "Overriding Dorsal Spinous Processes")

Imaging (Please refer to previous section on "Overriding Dorsal Spinous Processes")

Etiology

- Vertebral fractures are usually traumatic in origin.
- Pathologic fractures can occur secondary to neoplasia or osteomyelitis, but this is uncommon.
- Stress fractures of the vertebrae can occur in racehorses, most often at the thoracolumbar junction and in the lumbar vertebrae.

Clinical Signs

- Horses with acute fractures often have severe pain. The horse may be reluctant to move the affected part of the spine and often demonstrates increased muscle tension in the region of the fracture.
- Neurological signs may be present secondary to soft-tissue swelling, hemorrhage, or

fragments compressing the spinal cord or nerve roots depending on the location.

- Most stress fractures cause lack of performance without well-defined signs.

Diagnosis

- Scintigraphy is usually the imaging modality of choice because radiography of the spine in adult horses is difficult.
- Scintigraphy is nearly the only modality that can determine an active stress fracture of a vertebrae.
- Computed tomography (CT) can be used to document vertebral fractures in the very caudal lumbar area (Figure 5.15).

Treatment

- Conservative treatment is indicated in horses with vertebral fractures without neurological signs.

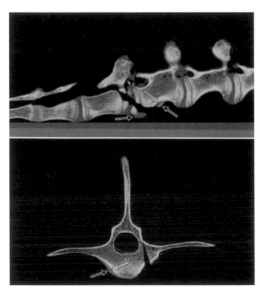

Figure 5.15 Parasagittal (a) and transverse (b) CT images illustrating a cranioventral to caudodorsal-oriented fracture and abnormal bone proliferation (arrows) on the ventral aspect of L5. *Source:* Reprinted with permission from Collar EM, Zavodovskaya R, Spreit M, et al.: 2015. Caudal lumbar vertebral fractures in California Quarter horse and Thoroughbred racehorses. *Equine Vet J* 47:573–579. Reproduced with permission of Equine Veterinary Journal. https://doi.org/10.1111/evj.12334.

- When neurological symptoms are present, treatment should be more focused on the reduction of swelling around the spinal structures; this includes systemic corticosteroids or NSAIDs, DMSO, and strict confinement.

Prognosis

- The prognosis is very good for stress fractures and non-displaced vertebral fractures without neurological signs.
- The prognosis is much reduced if neurological signs are present. In general, the longer the neurological signs persist, the worse the prognosis.

Discospondylitis

Overview

- Discospondylitis is an inflammatory condition involving the vertebral bodies adjacent to the symphysis between two vertebrae and includes the intervertebral disc.
- It is usually an infectious process but traumatic discospondylitis has been described at the lumbosacral junction and the cervical spine.
- Focal and generalized neurological signs may occur when there is compression of the spinal cord or nerve roots.

Anatomy (Please refer to previous section on "Overriding Dorsal Spinous Processes")

Imaging (Please refer to previous section on "Overriding Dorsal Spinous Processes")

Etiology

- Discospondylitis is usually a septic process from hematogenous spread. Bacteria isolated from adult horses include *Brucella abortus*, alpha-hemolytic *Streptococcus*, coagulase negative *Staphylococcus,* and *Staphylococcus aureus*. Rhodococcus equi has been implicated in foals.

- Traumatic discospondylitis has been described ultrasonographically and at post-mortem examination. Lesions include fissuration, calcification, and herniation of the intervertebral disk.

Clinical Signs

- Clinical signs include weight loss, back or neck pain, fever, stiffness, and ataxia
- Atrophy of the epaxial muscles in the thoracolumbar region may be evident in some horses suffering from chronic discospondylitis in this region.
- Some horses are so painful that they are reluctant to eat off the ground.

Diagnosis

- Leucocytosis and increased fibrinogen on a complete blood count support an infectious process.
- Radiography may reveal lysis and/or proliferation of the vertebral bodies adjacent to the affected disc. The intervertebral disk space may narrow and collapse, and a smooth bony bridge may unite the affected vertebrae.
- Scintigraphy, CT, and ultrasonography have all been used to facilitate the diagnosis of discospondylitis and vertebral osteomyelitis.
- Scintigraphy is especially helpful to determine if multiple sites of bone involvement are present.

Treatment

- Long-term (four to six months) antimicrobial therapy based on culture and sensitivity is used to treat septic discospondylitis.
- Broad-spectrum antimicrobials should be used if no causative organism is identified.
- Surgical curettage of the lesion is an option when access to the lesion is possible.

Prognosis

- The prognosis is guarded in cases of septic discospondylitis.

- Favorable outcomes have been associated with early detection, non-septic lesions, the absence of spinal cord compression, administration of long-term antimicrobial therapy, and surgical curettage.

Spondylosis

Overview

- Spondylosis (deformans) is a degenerative condition affecting the vertebral body that results in osteophyte/enthesiophyte formation on the ventrolateral aspects of the vertebral segment between T10 and T14 (Figure 5.16).
- The disease appears to be more common in event horses, show jumpers, hunters, and working draft horses.
- Reduced mobility of the spine at the site of the bone formation with complete ankylosis is seen as the end stage of the disease.

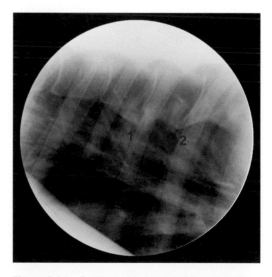

Figure 5.16 Radiographic image of the thoracic spine of a horse with severe spondylosis. There is proliferation of bone at the ventral aspect of the vertebral bodies. At (1), there is no complete contact between the proliferations. At (2), there seems to be complete bridging of the intervertebral disk space. *Source:* Courtesy of Rob van Wessum.

Anatomy (Please refer to previous section on "Overriding Dorsal Spinous Processes")

Imaging (Please refer to previous section on "Overriding Dorsal Spinous Processes")
Etiology

- Osteophyte and enthesiophyte formation are thought to occur from mechanical stress at the attachments of the most peripheral fibers of the intervertebral disk and the ventral longitudinal ligament.
- Postmortem results of acute cases have demonstrated damage to the intervertebral disk and erosion of cartilage and hemarthrosis of the facet joints.
- Thoracolumbar conformation and specific types of repetitive exercise may both contribute to the condition.

Clinical Signs

- In the acute stage, severe back pain with generalized stiffness and reluctance to work is often present. These cases seem to relate to the lay term of "cold-back," in which saddling, mounting, or starting to ride initiates a violent reaction of the horse (bucking, running away, and laying down).
- The chronic stage is less painful but limits the motion of the spine, giving the horse a "stiff" appearance.
- The horse may have the appearance of a "hollow back" or (acquired) lordosis that may contribute to chronic back problems.

Diagnosis

- Radiography and scintigraphy are the main diagnostic tools to confirm spondylosis (Figure 5.16).
- Scintigraphy can be used to demonstrate the amount of bone activity at the site(s) as an indicator for acuteness and bone activity.

Treatment

- Treatment in the acute stage includes rest and systemic NSAIDs.

- Horses with chronic disease are often treated with NSAIDs and other symptomatic treatments for chronic back pain.
- No surgical techniques have been described.

Prognosis

- In most cases, the prognosis is guarded to return to an athletic career.

Facet Joint OA and Vertebral Facet Joint Syndrome

Overview

- The development of OA in the thoracolumbar spine is often combined with a complex of processes in and around the vertebral facet joints known as facet joint syndrome.
- OA of the facet joints in the cervical spine is usually more isolated to the joint itself, but compression of the cervical nerve roots is more common than in the thoracolumbar region.

Anatomy (Please refer to previous section on "Overriding Dorsal Spinous Processes")

Imaging (Please refer to previous section on "Overriding Dorsal Spinous Processes")
Etiology

- The initiating incident in facet joint syndrome is damage to the facet joint, usually from trauma such as slipping, falling, flipping over backward, getting cast, and so on.
- Secondary muscle spasm often occurs in an attempt to stabilize the injured vertebral facet joints. This muscle contraction can be short, lasting from hours to days, or it can last weeks or even months.
- Due to the muscle spasm, no normal sequence of contraction–relaxation occurs in the muscle, and the normal supportive function is less effective.
- Repetitive injury to the facet joint related to exercise can also occur.

Clinical Signs

- In acute injuries, the horse may be reluctant to move and may stand with the hind feet parked out and the back lowered. Spasm and contraction of the muscles of the back and hind end is common.
- With severe pain in the thoracic or lumbar spine, signs of restlessness, pawing, looking at its back, etc. may be present.
- In chronic injuries, the locomotion of the horse can be altered, and a stiff back can be noticed. At the trot, the propulsion of the hind limbs can be reduced unilaterally or bilaterally.
- When the thoracic facet joints are involved, signs can include stiffness, reluctance to go downhill or jump, and refusal or difficulty in doing the extended trot. Lateral bending of the horse may be reduced, and pain may be initiated by tightening the girth or putting the saddle on because these actions can load the thoracic facet joints.
- When lumbar facet joints are involved, the most affected gait is the canter, because at the canter the dorsoventral flexion of the lumbar spine is most prominent.
- In racing, dorsoventral flexion of the lumbar spine is a prominent contribution to the propulsion phase of the hind limbs, so loss of performance may occur.

Diagnosis

- Scintigraphy is the best modality for imaging the vertebral column. One study showed 60% of horses with the complaint of back pain had increased uptake of radiopharmaceutical in one or more facet joints.
- There is a high predictive value for scintigraphy in the detection of radiographic lesions and a high sensitivity for scintigraphy in the detection of back pain.
- Ultrasonography can give information about ligamentous structures (supraspinous, interspinous, and dorsal sacral ligaments) and muscle conditions. Paramedian longitudinal views of the facet joints can be used to determine possible effusion, bony proliferations

at the joint margins, fractures and avulsion fragments, and ankylosis of the facet joints (Figure 5.17).
- With radiography, the thoracic vertebrae can be viewed through the lungs, facilitating radiographic imaging in the cranial part of the thorax (T1 through T15–T16). Oblique lateral views may be able to isolate the unilateral facet joints from T5–T7 to T18. Radiographic evidence of disease includes sclerosis of bone around the facet joint, narrowing of the joint space, irregular shape of the joint space and spur formation at the joint space, or complete ankylosis (Figure 5.18).

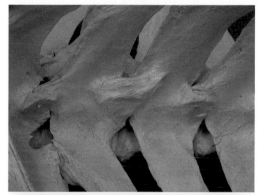
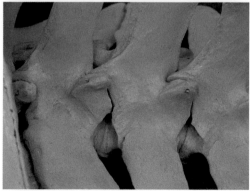

Figure 5.17 Anatomical specimen of the lumbar spine with the facet joints visible. In the lower image, the facet joints have smooth edges and appear to be normal. In the upper image, the facet joints have more irregular edges when compared to the facet joints in the lower image. Complete ankylosis is present in one of the facet joints. *Source:* Courtesy of Rob van Wessum.

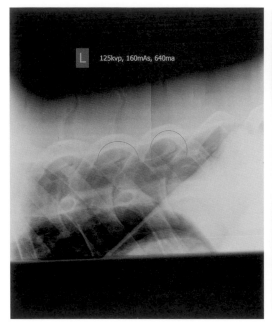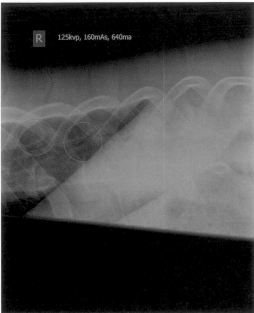

Figure 5.18 Radiographic image of the thoracic spine (oblique lateral view) to expose the left facet joints (circles) at the left and the right facet joints at the right. Note the more irregular joint space and some sclerosis in the right facet joints. This is indicative for OA of the right thoracic facet joints. *Source:* Courtesy of Rob van Wessum.

- Lumbar vertebrae are difficult to visualize with radiography. Oblique lateral views can sometimes facilitate imaging of the unilateral facet joints of the lumbar spine.
- The final diagnosis is often a summation of two or more imaging techniques.
- Local anesthesia as a tool to help confirm facet joint pain is not very reliable.

Treatment
- The initial goal of treatment is to break the inflammatory process triggering the nerves, which leads to muscle spasm, immobility of the spine, and repeated injury. Complex treatment plans that deal with several aspects of the vicious cycle are recommended.
- Treatments include local and systemic NSAIDs, muscle relaxants (methocarbamol), bisphosphonates, and ultrasound-guided injections of a corticosteroid into or close to the facet joint.
- A rehabilitation program is vital and should be aimed at gaining more mobility in the affected

part of the spine, as well as the development of better muscle support for that region.

Prognosis
- The prognosis varies, depending on the location of the facet joint pathology and the use of the horse.
- The prognosis appears better in racehorses with lumbar disease than thoracic disease.
- Three-day event horses and jumpers appear to have a more guarded prognosis than dressage horses.

Neck and Poll

Nuchal Ligament Desmopathy/Nuchal Bursitis

Overview
- The nuchal ligament connects the dorsal processes of the cervical vertebrae with the withers and has an important function in supporting the entire neck.

- The nuchal bursa, present at the proximal aspect at the first cervical vertebra (C1) in most horses and less frequently at the second cervical vertebra (C2) can be involved in pathology of the nuchal ligament.
- Both trauma and training methods may contribute to problems within the nuchal ligament and bursa.

Anatomy

- There are seven cervical vertebrae in the neck that serve to protect the spinal cord within the spinal canal.
- The first two cervical vertebrae (atlas and axis) are highly modified to meet the specialized function of permitting movement of the head with the third to seventh being similar to one another and follow the basic pattern of most vertebrae (Figure 5.11).
- The articulations between articular processes on vertebral arches are true synovial joints in the cervical vertebrae and are oriented in a nearly horizontal plane so as to permit significant lateral bending.
- The topline of the neck is in part determined by the presence of the ligamentum nuchae (nuchal ligament), which extends from its cranial attachments on the external occipital protuberance to the spinous process of the third or fourth thoracic vertebra.
- Bursae are consistently found between the funicular part of the nuchal ligament and the atlas (bursa subligamentosa nuchalis cranialis) and between the nuchal ligament and the second thoracic spine (bursa subligamentosa supraspinalis).
- The extensive neck musculature surrounds the cervical vertebral column and contributes to its stability, as well as its function.

Imaging

- Radiography is usually the initial diagnostic technique of choice to determine problems within the cervical region.
- Ultrasonography and scintigraphy may also be utilized depending on the clinical signs and suspected abnormalities.
- CT or MRI may be useful for suspected lesions within the proximal cervical region depending on the size of the horse and suspected lesion.

Etiology

- Desmopathy of the nuchal ligament is usually associated with trauma such as falling down, pulling backward when tied, head caught in fences, trailering accidents, etc.
- Training methods such as tying the horse's head to the side or between the front limbs or the "hyperflexion or Rollkur" as practiced by some dressage trainers can predispose to nuchal ligament pathology.
- The nuchal bursa is often secondarily involved with damage to the nuchal ligament, but infection of the nuchal bursa has also been reported.

Clinical Signs

- Signs can be diverse and very often more visible when the horse is worked. The horse may appear stiff with very little neck movement at the walk, with minimal to no flexion of the neck when worked in a circle.
- When ridden or driven, the contact with the bit through the reins or lines can feel different to the rider/driver, with one side feeling more rigid or as if the horse is pulling on one side.
- Dental issues can have similar signs, and particular head positions can cause the horse pain, making it behave defensively or reluctant to perform certain exercises.
- General lack of performance can be one of the more indistinctive signs.

Diagnosis

- With radiography, occasionally enthesophytes can be seen at the attachment of the ligament to the bone at the poll, which may suggest desmopathy or nuchal bursitis.

- Ultrasonography may be able to detect damage to the ligament itself and/or the nuchal bursa.
- Endoscopy of the nuchal bursa has been reported as both a diagnostic and treatment tool.

Treatment

- Therapy is similar to that of any desmopathy and may include rest, NSAIDs, ESWT, and injection of biological products such as PRP and stem cells.
- Ultrasound-guided injection of corticosteroids into the nuchal bursa can be performed if the bursa is thought to be involved.
- Endoscopy of the nuchal bursa has been reported as an effective treatment for nuchal bursitis.

Prognosis

- The prognosis is usually favorable if the horse is given time for complete recovery and rehabilitation of the nuchal ligament injury.
- Chronic injuries may lead to pain or defensive behavior (rearing, shaking the head, etc.) when the head is in a very high and upright position.
- Horses with nuchal bursitis appear to have a good prognosis for complete recovery.

Cervical Facet Joint OA

Overview

- Reduced neck mobility limiting athletic performance is often attributed to OA within the cervical facet joints.
- Cervical facet joint OA can be found radiographically in many older horses, even without clinical signs (Figure 5.19a).
- The condition may be associated with diverse clinical sign, ranging from performance-limiting lameness to severe neurological signs.

Anatomy (Please refer to previous section of "Nuchal Ligament Desmopathy")

Imaging (Please refer to previous section of "Nuchal Ligament Desmopathy")

Etiology

- Cervical facet joint OA can develop secondary to OC of the articular surfaces of the cervical joints similar to many other joints in the horse. Severe developmental lesions can lead to cervical instability and malformation, causing neurological signs (Wobbler syndrome).
- Trauma to the neck can damage the cervical joints, leading to secondary OA (Figure 5.19b).
- Major trauma to the neck region is often seen with trailering accidents, falling or hanging in cross ties, running into objects with the neck, falling during exercise, flipping over backward, etc.
- OA of the cervical facet joint can be found as an incidental finding radiographically in many asymptomatic older horses suggesting that it may occur as the result of normal aging and use.

Clinical Signs

- Clinical signs are often varied and may range from abnormal head carriage to severe neurological signs.
- Reduced neck mobility from the OA is thought to limit performance. The dressage horse may be reluctant to bend the neck in a lateral direction, bring the head vertical in the collection position, or stretch down. A jumping horse may lack balance during the jump due to neck stiffness, while a barrel racing horse may have difficulty turning around the barrels.
- Contraction of the muscles in the neck secondary to facet joint pain may alter the forelimb gait (shorter anterior stride, reduced protraction of the scapula) and mimic a forelimb lameness.

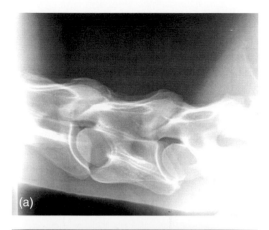

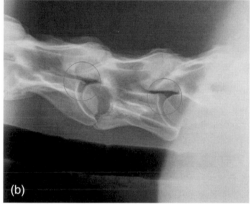

(a)

(b)

Figure 5.19 (a) Radiographic image of the cervical spine with C5, C6, and C7 in view. There is mild enlargement of the facet joints, indicative of OA, between C5 and C6 and between C6 and C7 with irregular joint spaces. This can be a common finding in horses without clinical signs. (b) Radiographic image of the cervical spine. Note the change at the caudal aspect of the endplate of C5 and the small fragment (circle 1) when compared to the clean appearance at C6 (circle 2). This is most likely caused by trauma to the intervertebral ligament at the ventral base of the spinal canal. *Source:* Courtesy of Rob van Wessum.

- Severe cervical malformation and cervical joint OA can cause compression of the spinal column and neurological deficits.
- Evidence of cervical pain and reduced range of motion may or may not be present.
- Asymmetrical enlargement of the left and right cervical vertebrae may be found on palpation but is not a consistent finding.

Diagnosis

- Cervical facet joint OA should be suspected when the range of motion in the neck is limited and palpable abnormalities are present.
- Radiography is the imaging technique of choice. Slight oblique views from the horizontal plane can be used to project the left or right facet joint without superimposing on top of the ipsilateral joint.
- Ultrasonography can be used to obtain information about joint space size and shape and bone proliferation at the edges of the joint.
- Scintigraphy can also be used to document active inflammation from older inactive lesions seen on radiographs, which is important in decision-making about whether to treat a facet joint(s) with medication (Figure 5.20).
- Ultrasound-guided intra-articular block of the facet joint(s) can be performed to verify it as the cause of the clinical signs but typically the joint is treated instead.
- Myelography documents spinal cord compression in horses with neurological signs or CT and MRI can be used if the suspected lesion is in the proximal cervical region.
- Electromyography may identify changes in muscle signals in the segmental muscles in

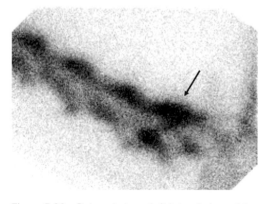

Figure 5.20 Delayed phase left lateral view of the caudal cervical region of a horse, showing marked, focal, and intense abnormal radiotracer at the articular facets of C6 to C7 (arrow), compatible with osteoarthritis. *Source:* Courtesy of Kurt Selberg.

the neck to demonstrate denervation of these muscles as a sign of nerve root compression.

Treatment

- Acute injuries are usually treated with topical and oral NSAIDs, muscle relaxants, and reduced activity.
- Chronic OA is often treated with ultrasound-guided injection of the facet joints usually with corticosteroids.
- Rehabilitation and physical therapy of the cervical region should also be performed.

- Surgical fusion of the vertebrae can be performed in horses with cervical vertebral malformation.

Prognosis

- The prognosis is variable, depending on the severity of the clinical signs.
- It is good for horses mild OA and minor clinical signs.
- The prognosis is poor for performance in horses with severe OA or cervical malformation together with neurological abnormalities.

Bibliography

1 Adams SB, Steckel R, Blevins W: 1985. Discospondylitis in five horses. *J Am Vet Med Assoc* 186:270–272.

2 Almanza A, Whitcomb MB: 2003. Ultrasonographic diagnosis of pelvic fractures in 28 horses. *Proc Am Assoc Equine Pract* 49:50–54.

3 Alward AA, Pease AP, Jones SL: 2007. Thoracic Discospondylitis with associated epaxial muscle atrophy in a quarter horse gelding. *Equine Vet Educ* 3:67–71.

4 Boswell J, Marr C, Cauvin E, et al.: 1999. The use of scintigraphy in the diagnosis or aorto-iliac thrombosis in a horse. *Equine Vet J* 31:537.

5 Brama PAJ, Rijkenhuizen ABM, van Swieten HA, et al.: 1996. Thrombosis of the aorta and the caudal arteries in the horse; additional diagnostics and a new surgical treatment. *Vet Quart* 18:S85–S89.

6 Bromiley MW: 1999. Physical therapy for the equine back. *Vet Clin NA Equine Pract* 15:223–246.

7 Brown K: 2008. Pelvic Fractures. *In*: Robinson E, Sprayberry KA (eds) *Current Therapy in Equine Medicine*, Sixth Edition. Philadelphia, Saunders, 488–491.

8 Butler J, Colles C, Dyson SJ, et al. 2000. The Spine. *In*: Butler J, Colles C, Dyson SJ, et al. (eds) *Clinical Radiology of the Horse*, Second Edition. Oxford, Blackwell Science.

9 Carrier TK, Estberg L, Stover SM, et al.: 1998. Association between long periods without high-speed workouts and risk of complete humeral or pelvic fracture in Thoroughbred racehorses: 54 cases (1991–1994). *J Am Vet Med Assoc* 212:1582–1587.

10 Chaffin MK, Honnas CM, Crabill MR, et al.: 1995. Cauda equina syndrome, Discospondylitis, and a para-vertebral abscess caused by Rhodococcus equi in a foal. *J Am Vet Med Assoc* 206: 215–220.

11 Chope K: 2008. How to perform sonographic examination and ultrasound-guided injection of the cervical vertebral facet joints in horses. *Proc Am Assoc Equine Pract* 54:186–189.

12 Collar EM, Zavodovskaya R, Spreit M, et al.: 2015. Caudal lumbar vertebral fractures in California Quarter horse and Thoroughbred racehorses. *Equine Vet J* 47:573–579.

13 Coomer RPC, McKane SA, Smith N, et al.: 2012. A controlled study evaluating a novel surgical treatment for kissing spines in standing sedated horses. *Vet Surg* 41:890–897.

14 Coudry V, Thibaud D, Riccio B, et al.: 2007. Efficacy of tiludronate in the treatment of horses with signs of pain associated with osteoarthritic lesions of the thoracolumbar vertebral column. *Am J Vet Res* 68:329–337.

15 Dabareiner RM, Cole CC: 2009. Fractures of the tuber coxae of the ilium in horses: 29 cases (996–2007). *J Am Vet Med Assoc* 243:1303–1307.

16 Denoix JM, Audigie F, Coudry V: 2005. Review of diagnosis and treatment of lumbosacral pain in sport and racehorses. *Proc Am Assoc Equine Pract* 51: 366–373.

17 Denoix JM, Audigie F: 2001. The Neck and Back. *In*: Back W, Clayton HM (eds) *Equine Locomotion*. London, W.B. Saunders, 167–191.

18 Denoix JM, Jacquet S: 2008. Ultrasound-guided injection of the sacroiliac area in horses. *Equine Vet Educ*;204:203–207.

19 Denoix JM: 1999. Ultrasonographic evaluation of back lesions. *Vet Clin North Am Equine Pract* 15:131–159.

20 Denoix JM: 2005. Thoracolumbar malformations or injuries and neurological manifestations. *Equine Vet Educ* 8:249–252.

21 Denoix JM: 2007. Discovertebral pathology in horses. *Equine Vet Educ* 3:72–73.

22 Desbrosse FG, Perrin R, Launois T, et al.: 2007. Endoscopic resection of dorsal spinous processes and interspinous ligament in ten horses. *Vet Surg* 36:149–155.

23 Dyson SJ, Murray RC. 2004. Clinical features of pain associated with the sacroiliac region: A European perspective. *Proc Am Assoc Equine Pract* 50:367–371.

24 Dyson SJ: 2004. Pain associated with the sacroiliac joint region: A diagnostic challenge. *Proc Am Assoc Equine Pract* 50:357–360.

25 Dyson, SJ: 2011. Lesions of the equine neck resulting in lameness or poor performance. *Vet Clin North Am Equine Pract*;27:417–437.

26 Engeli E, Haussler KK, Erb HN: 2004. Development and validation of a periarticular injection technique of the sacroiliac joint in horses. *Equine Vet J* 36:324–330.

27 Engeli E, Haussler KK: 2004. Review of sacroiliac injection techniques. *Proc Am Assoc Equine Pract* 50:372–378.

28 Engeli E, Yeager AE, Haussler KK: 2004. Use and limitations of ultrasonography in sacroiliac disease. *Proc Am Assoc Equine Pract* 50:385–391.

29 Erichsen C, Eksel P, Roethlisberger HK, et al.: 2004. Relationship between scintigraphic and radiographic evaluations of spinous processes in the thoracolumbar spine in riding horses without clinical signs of back problems. *Equine Vet J* 36:458–465.

30 Geburek F, Rotting AK, Stadler PM: 2009. Comparison of the diagnostic value of ultrasonography and standing radiography for pelvic–femoral disorders in horses. *Vet Surg* 38:307–310.

31 Gillen A, Dyson SJ, Murray R: 2009. Nuclear scintigraphic assessment of the thoracolumbar synovial intervertebral articulations. *Equine Vet J* 41:1–7.

32 Goff LM, Jeffcott LB, Jasiewicz, J, et al.: 2008. Structural and biomechanical aspects of equine sacroiliac joint function and their relationship to clinical disease. *Equine Vet J* 176;281–29.

33 Gorgas D, Kircher P, Doherr MG, et al.: 2007. Radiographic technique and anatomy of the equine sacroiliac region. *Vet Radiol Ultrasound* 48:501–506.

34 Haussler KK, Stover SM, Willits NH: 1999. Pathologic changes in the lumbosacral vertebrae and pelvis in Thoroughbred racehorses. *Am J Vet Res* 60:143–16.

35 Haussler KK, Stover SM: 1998. Stress fractures of the vertebral lamina and pelvis in Thoroughbred racehorses. *Equine Vet J* 30:374–381.

36 Haussler KK: 1999. Osseous spinal pathology. *Vet Clin North Am Equine Pract* 15:103–111.

37 Haussler KK: 2004. Functional anatomy and pathophysiology of sacroiliac joint disease. *Proc Am Assoc Equine Pract* 50:361–366.

38 Henson FMD, Lamas L, Knezevic S, et al.: 2007. Ultrasonographic evaluation of the supraspinous ligament in a series of ridden and unridden horses and horses with unrelated back pathology. *BMC Vet Res* 1:3.

39 Hudson NPH, Mayhew IG: 2005. Radiographic and myelographic assessment of the equine cervical vertebral column and spinal cord. *Equine Vet Educ* 2:43–48.

40 Hughes KJ: 2007. Spinal radiography of the horse. *Equine Vet Educ* 10:460–462.

41 Jeffcott LB: 1980. Disorders of the thoracolumbar spine of the horse—a survey of 443 cases. *Equine Vet J* 12:197–210

42 Jeffcott LB: 1999. Historical perspective and clinical indications. *Vet Clin NA Equine Pract* 15:1–12.

43 Johns S, Allen KA, Tyrrell LA: 2008. How to obtain digital radiographs of the thoracolumbar spine in the standing horse. *Proc Am Assoc Equine Pract* 54:455–458.

44 Kersten AA, Edinger J: 2004. Ultrasonographic examination of the equine sacroiliac region. *Equine Vet J* 36:602–608.

45 Marks D: 1999. Cervical nerve root compression in a horse, treated by epidural injection of corticosteroids. *J Equine Vet Sci* 19:399.

46 May SA, Patterson LJ, Peacock PJ, et al.: 1991. Radiographic technique for the pelvis in the standing horse. *Equine Vet J* 23:312–314.

47 Peters S, Ruggles AJ, Bramlage LR et al.: 2014. Short and long-term outcome of pelvic fractures in 136 thoroughbreds (2000–2010), *Proc Am Assoc Equine Pract* 60:249.

48 Pilsworth RC, Sheperd M, Herinckx BMB, et al.: 1994. Fracture of the wing of the ilium, adjacent to the sacroiliac joint, in Thoroughbred racehorses. *Equine Vet J* 26:94–99.

49 Prisk AJ, Garcia-Lopez JM: 2019. Long-term prognosis for return to athletic function after interspinous ligament desmotomy for treatment of impinging and overriding dorsal spinous processes in horses: 71 cases (2012–2017). *Vet Surg* 48:1278–1286.

50 Reef V, Roby K, Richardson DA, et al.: 1987. Use of ultrasonography for the detection of aortic-iliac thrombosis in horses. *J Am Vet Med Assoc* 190:286–289.

51 Ricardi G, Dyson SJ: 1993. Forelimb lameness associated with radiographic abnormalities of the cervical vertebrae. *Equine Vet J* 25:422.

52 Rutkowski JA, Richardson DW: 1989. A retrospective study of 100 pelvic fractures in horses. *Equine Vet J* 21:256–259.

53 Schulte TL, Pietilä TA, Heidenreich J, et al.: 2006. Injection therapy of lumbar facet syndrome: A prospective study. *Acta Neurochir* (Wien) 148:1165–72.

54 Shepherd MC, Pilsworth RC: 1994. The use of ultrasound in the diagnosis of pelvic fractures. *Equine Vet Educ* 6:223–225.

55 Ständer M, März U, Steude U, et al.: 2006. The facet syndrome: Frequent cause of chronic backaches. *Fortschr Med* 26;148:33–4.

56 Stewart AJ, Salazar P, Waldridge BM, et al.: 2007. Computed tomographic diagnosis of a pathological fracture due to rhodococcal osteomyelitis and spinal abscess in a foal. *Equine Vet Educ* 6:231–235.

57 Sweers L, Carsten A: 2006. Imaging features of Discospondylitis in two horses. *Vet Rad Ultrasound* 472:159–164.

58 Thomas WB: 2000. Discospondylitis and other vertebral infections. *Vet Clin N Am Small Anim Pract* 30; 169–182.

59 Tomlinson JE, Sage AM, Turner TA: 2003. Ultrasonographic abnormalities detected in the sacroiliac area in twenty cases of upper hindlimb lameness. *Equine Vet J* 35:48–54.

60 Tucker RL, Schneider RK, Sondhof AH, et al.: 1998. Bone scintigraphy in the diagnosis of sacroiliac injury in twelve horses. *Equine Vet J* 30:390–395.

61 van Wessum R, Nickels F, Pease AP, et al. Clinical data on 206 equine back pain cases. Unpublished data.

62 Van Wessum R, Sloet MM, Clayton HM: 1999. Electromyography in the horse; a review. *Vet Quart* 21:3–7.

63 Van Wessum R: 2009. Evaluation of Back Pain by Clinical Examination. *In*: Robinson NE, Sprayberry KA (eds) *Current Therapy in*

Equine Medicine, Sixth Edition. St. Louis, Elsevier, 469–473.

64 Van Wessum R: 2009. Sacroiliac Disease. *In*: Robinson NE, Sprayberry KA (eds) *Current Therapy in Equine Medicine, Sixth Edition.* St. Louis, Saunders Elsevier, 483–487.

65 Van Wessum, R: 2014. How to look for sacroiliac disease during lameness examination: some simple clinical indicators. *Proc Am Assoc Equine Pract* 60:244–246.

66 Zimmerman M, Dyson S and Murray R: 2012. Close, impinging and overriding spinous processes in the thoracolumbar spine: The relationship between radiological and scintigraphic findings and clinical signs. *Equine Vet J* 44;178–184.

Revised from "Lameness Associated with the Axial Skeleton" in *Adams and Stashak's Lameness in Horses, 7th Edition,* by Rob van Wessum.

6

Therapeutic Options

Systemic/Parenteral

Overview

- Systemic/parenteral medications used to treat musculoskeletal diseases in horses include IV or oral nonsteroidal anti-inflammatory drugs (NSAIDs), intramuscular (IM) polysulfated glycosaminoglycans (PSGAGs), pentosane polysulfate (PPS), IV hyaluronan (HA), IV bisphosphonates, and several other miscellaneous drugs.
- Excluding NSAIDs, the debate regarding many of these drugs in the horse revolves around whether they reach high enough concentrations at the intended area.
- Many (or most) of the drugs or nutraceuticals have been intended for systemic administration in humans, and levels high enough to be efficacious in the horse are often in question.

Parenteral NSAIDs

- The IV NSAIDs used most commonly are phenylbutazone and flunixin meglumine.
- Less commonly used IV NSAIDs are ketoprofen, carprofen, and firocoxib.
- Most of these NSAIDs can be delivered orally, but the IV route of delivery may be more effective and faster at yielding the desired pharmacological effect in the acute stages of disease.

- When NSAIDs are used consistently in horses, oral formulations are recommended. See "Oral/Nutritional" later in this chapter.

Polysulfated Glycosaminoglycans

- Adequan® (Luitpold Pharmaceuticals, Inc.) is produced from bovine trachea and lung and is in a class of drugs that exhibits chondroprotective properties in cartilage.
- PSGAG is a mixture of low-molecular-weight glycosaminoglycans (GAGs) that are very similar in structure to chondroitin sulfate, the major GAG in normal cartilage.
- PSGAG administration has been associated with reductions in the severity of clinical signs in both human and equine patients with OA.
- Modes of administration include IM and intra-articular (IA) routes. Elevated risks have been identified with IA administration; therefore, many practitioners still prefer to administer this drug IM.
- While there has been convincing evidence of the beneficial effects on cartilage, the exact mechanism of action of PSGAG remains unknown.
- It has been theorized that PSGAGs inhibit a plethora of degradative enzymes that contribute to the OA process, and an anti-inflammatory role based on the inhibitory effects on leukocyte migration and interleukin levels.

- Data is currently lacking in the benefit of IM PSGAG administration. However, in a survey of more than 400 equine practitioners, IM Adequan® was one of the most commonly administered medications (that was not in the steroid category). It is commonly administered as a prophylactic therapy for OA in horses.
- Currently, the dosing recommendations are 500 mg IM every three to five days for five to seven treatments. IA use is thought to provide greater benefit.

Pentosan Polysulfate (PPS; in a Sodium or Calcium Derivative)
- Within the same class of medications as PSGAGS, but produced from a plant source.
- Is not licensed in the United States, but widely used in Europe and Australia; compounded versions can be obtained for use in horses in the United States.
- PPS has been shown to reduce cartilage fibrillation experimentally suggesting that its benefit is likely through its disease-modifying effects.
- Current dosing recommendations are 3 mg/kg IM once a week for four weeks.
- PPS has been shown to provide greater benefit than Adequan® when administered IM.

Hyaluronan
- HA is a large, unbranched, nonsulfated GAG composed of repeating units of D-glucuronic acid and N-acetyl glucosamine.
- Intrasynovial injections are most likely the most efficacious route of administration; however, the desire to treat multiple joints simultaneously has resulted in its use IV.
- HA actions in the synovial joint include increasing viscosity of synovial fluid, lubricating unloaded joints, restoring the rheologic properties of synovial fluid, and most importantly, inhibiting inflammation.
- The clinical benefits of IV HA are debatable but are most likely due to its anti-inflammatory effects in the synovial membrane since the plasma half-life is less than an hour and the synovial membrane is highly vascularized.
- Currently, Legend® (Merial, Inc.) is the only licensed HA product for IV administration.
- Another product, Polyglycan® (Bimeda, Inc.) is licensed as a medical device and labeled for IA injection; however, it is used by practitioners off-label both IV and IM.
- Clinical indications for IV HA are similar to those for IM PSGAGs – IV HA may reduce inflammation in one or multiple joints and potentially prevent the inflammatory process within joints under heavy use.
- Although IA administration is the most effective way to deliver this drug to synovial cavities, often IA and IV administration are used concurrently.

Bisphosphonates
- Bisphosphonates have been used for decades to inhibit loss of bone mass in human patients with osteoporosis associated with age or steroid administration, and rheumatoid arthritis.
- Bisphosphonates inhibit osteoclast-mediated bone resorption, a property that may play a role in conditions such as OA and navicular bone edema/sclerosis.
- Three studies in horses report the effects of the bisphosphonate tiludronate (Tildren®) in clinical diseases such as navicular disease, vertebral pain related to OA of the thoracolumbar column, bone spavin, and bone loss due to cast immobilization. All three studies reported reduced lameness, back soreness, and loss of bone with administration of the drug.
- Clodronate (Osphos®, Dechra Veterinary Products) is an FDA-approved bisphosphonate licensed for treatment of navicular syndrome in horses. It has a similar mechanism of action as tiludronate but is hypothesized to also have analgesic properties through inhibition of glutamate transport.
- Dosage for Osphos® is 1.8 mg/kg by IM injection with a maximum dose of 900 mg per

horse (e.g. 900 mg dose standard for a 500 kg animal); recommended to divide the dose among three individual sites.

- More widespread use of bisphosphonates in horses has created concerns regarding their use in growing animals and in horses that have undergone therapy prior to sustaining a fracture.
- Off-label use or use of bisphosphonates in young, growing horses is not recommended at this time.

Tetracyclines

- The anti-inflammatory effect of tetracyclines, independent of their antimicrobial role, have been well documented for multiple disease processes.
- Both minocycline and doxycycline are considered to be disease-modifying osteoarthritic drugs (DMOADs) in horses.
- The mechanism of action, at least in part, is due to the ability of tetracyclines to reduce matrix metalloproteinase (MMP activity at dosages lower than what is required to inhibit bacterial growth.
- The recommended dose for doxycycline is 5 mg/kg once daily orally.

Estrogen

- Has been used to treat intermittent upward fixation of the patella in horses.
- It is hypothesized that estrogen affects muscle cell metabolism and muscle tone, particularly in the pelvic region, leading to the anecdotal benefit.
- Recommended dosage is 1 mg of estradiol cypionate IM for every 45 kg of body weight (i.e. 11 mg/500 kg) once weekly for three–five weeks. Concurrent anti-inflammatories along with exercise to strengthen the quadriceps muscles are usually recommended as well.

Robaxin (Methocarbamol)

- Methocarbamol is a centrally acting muscle relaxant commonly prescribed for various inflammatory and traumatic muscle disorders and to treat muscular spasms in the horse. Muscle relaxants are occasionally used in horses to treat various pathologies of muscle disease.
- Methocarbamol appears to produce variable results but may be most beneficial in horses that are prone to rhabdomyolysis or back soreness secondary to musculoskeletal disease of the axial skeleton or hind limbs.
- Can be used in conjunction with gabapentin in horses with suspected axial skeleton disease with associated secondary epaxial muscle sensitivity.
- The dose is variable ranging from 4.4 to 55 mg/kg but usually is 10 mg/kg orally twice daily for 5–10 days.

Gabapentin

- Gabapentin, an analog of γ-aminobutyric acid (GABA), has been shown to have analgesic effects through modulation of voltage-gated calcium ion channels.
- It is used as an antiepileptic medication and to treat neuropathic and chronic pain in humans, but very little data exists to support its analgesic properties in animals.
- Can be used in conjunction with methocarbamol in horses to combat chronic back soreness secondary to suspected axial skeleton disease.
- Dosages range from 5 to 20 mg/kg PO two to three times daily with dosages being titrated to effect.

Topical/Local

Overview

- Local and topical therapies are commonly used to treat equine musculoskeletal diseases both acutely, when inflammation is most pronounced, and chronically, when ongoing inflammation results in soreness and/or lameness.
- Local modes of therapy to control associated edema and release of inflammatory mediators

are often used concurrently with systemic NSAIDs.

- Effective use of topical therapy is thought to reduce the need for systemic NSAID therapy and secondary edema and tissue damage.

Topical NSAIDs

- A topical formulation of diclofenac liposomal cream (Surpass®, Boehringer Ingelheim Vetmedica, Inc.) is approved for treatment of horses with OA.
- Studies have reported that when applied locally the drug readily penetrates skin and significantly attenuates carrageenan-induced local production of PGE.
- Application of 7.3 g of Surpass® twice daily (label dose) to the skin showed significant improvement in lameness in a model of carpal OA.
- Surpass® can be used under a bandage and there are currently no reported adverse effects. However, proper bandage management is important.
- Although the dose is 7.3 g BID, some clinicians use this drug once daily or every other day for inflammation that is less acute.
- It can be used for a variety of musculoskeletal inflammatory conditions and concurrent use of this product with systemic NSAIDs is common.

Topical First Aid (Cold Therapy and Bandaging)

- Cold compression in the early stages of inflammation retards the inflammatory processes of exudation and diapedesis and reduces local circulation, tissue swelling, and pain.
- The application of cold therapy as a primary treatment for most acute joint or tendon injuries is commonly practiced and is extremely beneficial.
- Following an initial "cooling out" phase, usually 48–72 hours, warm hydrotherapy is often used to relieve pain and tension in tissues, as well as stimulate the vasodilatory effect to aid with fluid resorption and the stimulation of phagocytic cells.

- Cold therapy can be applied using ice boots, cold water hosing/hydrotherapy, or medical devices that provide cold therapy and compression (Game Ready®).
- Bandaging and pressure wraps are also commonly used to decrease edema formation and generalized swelling. Further benefits may include stimulation of mechanoreceptors that aid in reduction of pain sensation.
- The duration to use bandaging and pressure wraps is unknown, but the general practice is to apply them as long as ongoing inflammation is present. Any type of standard cotton compression bandage is usually effective and light elastic bandages over high motion areas like the carpus can be resistant to pressure changes with ambulation and helpful in reducing edema.

Dimethyl Sulfoxide (DMSO)

- The chemical solvent DMSO has been used alone or mixed with corticosteroids (CSs) to treat soft-tissue swelling and inflammation resulting from acute trauma. Its main benefit is considered to be the reduction of edema although analgesia through blockade of C-fiber transmission and/or blocking sensory neurons may also occur.
- DMSO has been shown to possess superoxide dismutase activity and inactivate superoxide radicals and enhance penetration of percutaneous steroids when it is mixed with DMSO.
- If applied under a bandage, it should be used with caution due to its predilection to cause skin irritation.

Extracorporeal Shock Wave Therapy (ESWT)

- Extracorporeal shock waves are acoustic waves generated outside the body, characterized by transient high peak pressures, followed by negative pressure and then return to zero pressure.
- Pressures reached by current equipment range from 10 to 100 MPa with a rapid rise time of 30–120 ns and a short pulse duration

(5 μs). Other variables include energy level, pulse frequency, and depth of penetration.

- Musculoskeletal conditions in horses that have been treated with ESWT include the bucked-shin complex, tibial stress fractures, proximal sesamoid bone fractures, incomplete proximal phalangeal fractures, subchondral bone pain, insertional desmopathies (most notably proximal ligament suspensory desmitis), impinging dorsal spinous processes, OA of the distal hock joints, navicular disease, and SDF tendinitis.
- The exact mechanism of action that ESWT has on specific tissues is not known. Suggested effects on bone include microfracture of the cortical bone, medullary hemorrhage, subperiosteal hemorrhage, and stimulation of osteogenesis.
- Analgesic properties attributed to ESWT are thought to be due to decreases in nerve conduction properties associated with disruption of the myelin sheath.
- Use of ESWT at racetracks has stimulated debate due to its abilities to reduce or eliminate pain from an injury that may become catastrophic if the horse continues to race.
- The most common clinical entity that is treated with ESWT is proximal suspensory ligament desmitis. Studies have reported variable success rates (55–80%) for horses returning to work six months following therapy.
- Clinical evidence for efficacy of ESWT in horses is sparse.

Regional Perfusion
- Intravenous regional limb perfusion (IVRLP) of the equine limb has become commonplace in equine veterinary practice over the last decade.
- Although it is used most commonly to deliver concentration-dependent antimicrobials, a variety of other medications can be substituted. These include local anesthetics, biologics such as mesenchymal stem cells, antifungal therapy such as amphotericin B, and anti-inflammatories such as DMSO.

- Efficacy of using IVRLP with antimicrobials in the presence of sepsis is well established. Documentation of using the other medications is lacking.

Therapeutic Ultrasound, Lasers, and Electromagnetics
- The empirical use of therapeutic ultrasound, lasers, and electromagnetics is common in the horse industry among owners and trainers.
- Therapeutic ultrasounds emit unfocused sound waves that may have the potential to penetrate underlying tissues, although the exact mechanism of action is unknown.
- Lasers used in a therapeutic setting are commonly referred to as low-level laser therapy (LLLT) or cold lasers. Cellular alterations from the laser may trigger mitosis and cellular proliferation that may have biomodulatory effects on circulation and analgesia.
- Electromagnetic devices are developed by passing an electric current through a coil of insulated wire creating an electromagnetic field.
- Electromagnetic therapy has been touted to improve both bone and soft-tissue healing, although clinical evidence in the horse remains sparse.

Counterirritation
- Topical blistering has long been part of veterinary medicine but is used rarely today.
- Topical blisters historically were made of iodine or mercuric iodide and were mainly used on splints, sore shins, or curbs. The technique involved application to the skin and light exercise.
- Firing typically involved the use of a pinpoint hot iron applied to the skin over the affected structure. Firing was used most commonly for bucked shins and plantar ligament desmitis (curb) when the condition had not responded favorably to other treatments. It is currently not a recommended therapy.

Intrasynovial

Overview

- Intrasynovial therapies are used to diminish the inflammatory response in synovium, cartilage, tendon (or tendon sheath), or meniscus.
- An effective therapy should halt progression of degradation of these structures, restore the normal intrasynovial environment, and alleviate pain.
- Intrasynovial therapies, specifically CSs, are used frequently to minimize or control pain and inflammation associated with synovitis and OA.
- New therapies such as disease-modifying agents of osteoarthritis drugs (DMOAD) are being used to prevent, retard, or reverse morphologic cartilaginous lesions of OA. While claims of these properties exist, evidence-based clinical studies about their true abilities to reverse OA are still in their infancy.

Corticosteroids

- CSs are the most potent anti-inflammatory drugs available that decrease the catabolic effects of joint disease.
- Clinical studies suggest judicious use of CSs may be beneficial and can result in long-lasting pain relief and control of inflammation.
- CSs have powerful inhibitory effects on inflammation through stabilization of cellular lysosomal membranes, reduction of vascular permeability and leukocyte adherence to vessel walls (margination), inhibition of platelet aggregation, and leukocyte diapedesis.
- CSs are also considered to be disease modifying by abrogation of important mediators of inflammation such as interleukin-1 (IL-1) and reducing degradative enzymes such as MMPs and other related proteinases.
- Detrimental effects of CSs include decreased chondrocyte size, loss of GAGs and decreased GAG synthesis, inhibition of proteoglycan synthesis, and chondrocyte necrosis.
- At high concentrations and prolonged exposure, CS inhibit production of important components of cartilage such as proteoglycans, collagen, and hyaluronic acid and result in chondrocyte necrosis.
- Detrimental effects are less noted, and more cartilage-sparing effects have been observed with low doses of CSs.
- Currently, the most commonly used formulations of CS are triamcinolone acetonide (TA), methylprednisolone acetate (MPA), and betamethasone acetate (BA) (Table 6.1).
- Doses vary depending on the volume of the joint, severity of inflammation, and the number of other joints that require treatment. However, lower dosages of CS are recommended compared to those used in the past (Table 6.1).
- In a survey of more than 400 equine practitioners, TA was found to be more commonly used in high-motion joints and MPA in low-motion joints.

Table 6.1 Commonly used intra-articular corticosteroids.

Corticosteroid	Trade name	Manufacturer	Drug conc. (mg/mL)	Dose (mg)	Duration of action
Triamcinolone acetonide	Kenalog-10	Bristol-Myers Squibb	10	6–18	Medium
	Vetalog	Boehringer Ingelheim	6		
Methylprednisolone acetate	Depo-Medrol	Zoetis US	40 or 20	40–100	Long
Betamethasone acetate/ sodium phosphate	Celestone Soluspan	Merck, Inc.	6	3–18	Medium to long
	BetaVet	Luitpold Pharmaceuticals			

- TA injected into one joint can affect other joints in the horse. This remote effect of TA has not been observed with other CS.
- Complications of using CS include postinjection flare and infection, and laminitis (all of which are rare). Recent studies have also suggested an association between the use of CS and subsequent musculoskeletal injuries in racehorses.

Hyaluronan

- HA is locally synthesized by chondrocytes, is the backbone of the proteoglycan aggregate in the extracellular matrix, and is secreted by the Type B synoviocytes of the synovial membrane.
- HA serves various important functions in the joint such as providing viscoelasticity to the joint fluid and boundary lubrication of the IA soft tissues.
- HA also may influence the composition of synovial fluid through steric hindrance of active plasma components and leukocytes from the joint cavity and modulates the chemotactic response within the synovial membrane by reducing cell migration and rates of diffusion.
- Although the exact mechanism of action is unclear, studies suggest that exogenously administered HA may replace the actions of depleted or depolymerized endogenous HA in the synovial fluid, which restores viscoelasticity, steric hindrance, and lubrication of the articular soft tissues.
- HA also may possess both anti-inflammatory and analgesic properties within the joint and increases synthesis of high-molecular-weight HA by the synoviocytes.
- Many clinical studies in horses and people have supported HA administration in joint disease as demonstrated by improvements in pain, activity level, and function.
- Although controversial, greater clinical efficacy is thought to occur with higher-molecular-weight products (Table 6.2). Efficacy is also often reduced in horses with advanced joint disease.

Corticosteroid and HA Combinations

- The combination of HA and CSs to treat inflammation intrasynovially is commonplace.
- Synergistic effects have been reported in human patients, and similar effects have been seen in vitro in horses.
- Clinically, the combination of CS and HA is thought to permit using a smaller dose of CS and provide a longer effect than either injection alone, especially in high motion joints.
- Based on a recent multicenter clinical trial, there is minimal clinical evidence to support combining HA and TA in horses.

Polysulfated Glycosaminoglycans

- PSGAG is principally composed of chondroitin sulfate and is a semisynthetic preparation from bovine trachea.
- PSGAG is reported to have chondroprotective and anti-inflammatory properties, as well as the ability to induce articular cartilage matrix synthesis and minimize matrix degradation.
- The exact mechanism of action of PSGAGs remains unclear but studies have revealed a significant ability of the drug to decrease lameness, modify OA through reducing bone remodeling, promote synthesis of endogenous HA, and inhibit mediators of inflammation, specifically PGE2 production.
- In one clinical study that compared PSGAGs to IA CS (Depo Medrol®, 40 mg), a regimen of weekly IA PSGAGs for three treatments had significantly improved clinical results (67%) compared to one treatment of CS (46%) in terms of returning horses back to athleticism.
- Currently, the recommended frequency of IA administration of PSGAG is three to five injections (250 mg) at weekly intervals.
- IA PSGAG may be most efficacious in joints with known or suspected articular cartilage pathology.
- IA administration is commonly combined with 125–250 mg of amikacin to reduce the risk of infection; this practice appears to be effective.

Table 6.2 Commonly used hyaluronan preparations.

Trade name	Concentration (mg/mL)	Manufacturer	Molecular weight (daltons)[a]	How packaged	Current recommended dose (mg) per joint
Hyvisc	11	Boehringer Ingelheim	2.1×10^6	2-mL syringe	22
HY-50	17	Dechra	7.5×10^5	3-mL syringe	51
Hyalovet	10	Boehringer Ingelheim	$5-7.3 \times 10^5$	2-mL syringe or vial	20
Legend[b]	10	Merial Inc.	3×10^5	2-mL vial	20
HyCoat (used IA)	5	Neogen	$>1.0 \times 10^6$	10-mL vial	30
MAP-5 (used IA at this dose)	10.3 (2 mL) 5 (10 mL)	Bioniche	7.5×10^5	2-mL or 10-mL vial	20

[a]Manufacturer's reported molecular weight
[b]Marketed for IV and IA use

Polyglycan®

- Polyglycan® is a patented formulation comprised of HA, chondroitin sulfate, and N-acetyl-D-glucosamine, but is not yet licensed for use as an IA medication.
- Currently, this product is used clinically in equine practice for viscosupplementation in horses with joint disease.
- In one controlled study in which Polyglycan® was administered IA at days 0, 7, 14, and 28, significant improvements were observed in lameness, bony proliferation, and the severity of full-thickness articular cartilage erosions seen grossly.
- Polyglycan is also thought to have anti-inflammatory properties.

Autologous Conditioned Serum (ACS)

- ACS (also called interleukin receptor antagonist protein; IRAP) has been used in practice to treat intrasynovial inflammation, especially in cases that are refractory to IA CSs.
- Due to cost, this treatment method is used less frequently; however, clinical impressions have been favorable.
- IRAP, a substance that inhibits IL-1 activity, decreases the progression of joint disease and is believed to be present in high amounts in ACS.
- Use of this medication requires incubation of equine serum with beads coated with chromium sulfate to obtain the ACS solution.
- ACS injected into the middle carpal joints on days 14, 21, 28, and 35 following induction of OA through a chip fragment model revealed clinical improvement in lameness and reduced gross cartilage fibrillation and synovial membrane pathology.
- The ACS is usually administered IA weekly for three to four treatments, depending on the quantity of ACS obtained.

Platelet rich Plasma (PRP)

- PRP is a platelet-concentrated, autologous blood product created through various centrifugation processes that delivers increased platelet-derived growth factors (PDGFs) to the site of injury.
- Various cytokines detected in PRP that can potentially promote healing include transforming growth factor-β (TGF-β), PDGF, insulin-like growth factor (IGF-I, IGF-II), fibroblast growth factor (FGF), epidermal growth factor (EGF), vascular endothelial growth factor (VEGF), and endothelial cell growth factor.
- PRP has been used primarily as an intralesional treatment but its use has recently emerged as a potential treatment of OA both in humans and horses.
- IA PRP is not yet a standard treatment for OA but has shown potential as a therapeutic option in refractory cases.
- Studies evaluating its use in healthy equine joints have found IA PRP to be safe without long-term detrimental effects. While largely positive, variable clinical results have been reported in both the equine and human literature.

Autologous Protein Solution (APS)

- APS (Pro-Stride®) is a newly developed, modified blood product generated from a dual-device system that concentrates plasma and WBC proteins and enriches platelet growth factors.
- APS is meant to achieve the goals of both autologous conditioned serum (IRAP) and PRP through a two-step centrifugation process – a small volume of plasma concentrated with platelets and WBCs, and is then filtered through polyacrylamide beads to desiccate and further concentrate growth factors and plasma proteins.
- APS can be drawn, processed, and injected stall-side without the need for incubation or processing.
- Current research on APS is limited, but one clinical trial that evaluated the efficacy of a single IA injection of APS in horses with OA in various high-motion joints found that treated horses had significant improvements

in lameness grade, asymmetry indices of vertical peak force, and range of joint motion by 14 days posttreatment.

Bone-Marrow- or Fat-Derived Mesenchymal Stem Cell Therapy

- The use of bone-marrow- or fat-derived mesenchymal stem cells (MSC) has grown in popularity in equine practice in the last decade.
- It is believed that these cells possess anti-inflammatory properties and also may contribute to healing of musculoskeletal tissues by becoming incorporated into the repair tissue.
- Although more is known regarding the efficacy of MSCs in tendon injuries, studies suggest these cells also may have a place as an intrasynovial therapy – IA administration of BMSCs postoperatively for stifle lesions has been reported in horses, with improved ability to return to work (75%).
- Concomitant IA use of CS or aminoglycoside antimicrobials with MSCs is not recommended because they contribute to MSC death.
- Concentrated bone marrow aspirate (BMAC) is another autologous source of MSCs being investigated for the treatment of OA and regeneration of cartilage in osteochondral defects.
- Although BMAC contains few MSCs, it provides a source of growth factors important for chondrogenesis and has the potential to be an effective, minimally invasive option to help repair cartilage defects and treat OA in the horse.

Polyacrylamide Hydrogel

- Polyacrylamide hydrogel (PAAG) is a non-toxic, non-immunogenic, nondegradable, biocompatible polymer gel consisting of 2.5% cross-linked polyacrylamide with a long-lasting viscous effect shown to support cellular growth and augment tissues.
- PAAG is a newly investigated therapeutic option to treat OA in horses and has just recently been approved for use in the United States.
- One multicenter study that evaluated the efficacy of IA PAAG in horses with OA showed a significant reduction in lameness and joint effusion. Another study demonstrated that horses with OA treated with PAAG had significantly improved clinical signs when compared to horses treated with TA and HA.
- Further studies are needed to determine the true efficacy of PAAG and the long-term effects of PAAG on the synovium and other articular structures.

Intralesional

Overview

- Therapies that are injected intralesionally are usually intended to augment the healing processes of tendons or ligaments by providing the necessary components of healing directly to the tissue.
- Alternatively, they may act locally to either reduce inflammation and/or signal the cellular and molecular components of the injured and surrounding tissue to begin the reparative processes.
- Intralesional approaches are directed at maximizing the chances for a more physiologically functioning tendon or ligament – rehabilitation and constant US monitoring must accompany any treatment.
- The ultimate goal of intralesional therapy is to maximize the chances for a tendon or ligament to repair with adequate strength and elasticity for a return to a similar level of performance with a reduced risk for reinjury.

Hyaluronan and Polysulfated Glycosaminoglycans

- The use of HA for tendon injuries is predicated on its abilities to decrease inflammation and prevent adhesion formation through its mechanical characteristics.

- The intralesional use of PSGAG is based on its known abilities to inhibit many of the enzymes associated with connective tissue degradation.
- Equivocal success has been reported in horses with tendinitis treated with intralesional HA or PSGAG – one clinical study reported no difference in outcome or reinjury rate in performance horses treated with intralesional HA, PSGAG, or nothing following diagnosis of SDF tendinitis.
- Intralesional HA or PSGAG is currently not the treatment of choice for tendon injuries in horses

Autologous Cell Therapies: Mesenchymal Stem Cell Therapy, Tendon-Derived Progenitor Cells

- MSCs have been used to treat a variety of musculoskeletal conditions but are mostly used in tendon injuries in performance horses.
- The mechanism of action of these cells is unknown, but the cells are thought to secrete bioactive molecules that:
  1) Inhibit apoptosis and limit the field of damage or injury
  2) Inhibit fibrosis or scarring at sites of injury
  3) Stimulate angiogenesis and bring in a new blood supply
  4) Stimulate the mitosis of tissue-specific and tissue-intrinsic progenitor cells
- Transplantation of MSCs into various injured skeletal tissues is thought to promote healing, and the use of autologous cells does not incite an immune response.
- Current theories on how transplanted MSCs act in tendon when injected intrathecally are that they either differentiate into cells capable of synthesizing tendon matrix or they secrete important factors that induce adjacent cells to synthesize tendon matrix.
- The two current techniques for MSC transplantation use cells derived from fat or cultured bone marrow aspirates.

- The fat-derived stem cells do not involve a culture step and have the advantage of lower cost and speed of preparation (cells are returned to the practitioner with 48 hours). However, the cell mixture is believed to be heterogeneous with regard to cell type.
- The bone-marrow-derived MSC technique involves aspirating bone marrow from the sternum or tuber coxae, transferring to a laboratory for culture and expansion, and then implanting the cell population (approximately $10–50 \times 106$) under US guidance.
- Most believe that the repair tissue maximally benefits when MSCs are injected in the initial phase of healing, therefore at least by four to five weeks following injury.
- The primary benefit of MSCs is thought to be a better-quality repair tissue that reduces the reinjury rate. Two studies in racehorses reported an 18 and 27% reinjury rate in treated horses compared to a 56% reinjury rate for horses receiving no intralesional therapy in one study.
- Use of allogenic MSCs have been reported in one study with adverse reactions reported in 10/230 injection sites – these were defined as pain, swelling, heat, and lameness.
- Tendon-derived progenitor cells harvested from a donor tendon site, such as the lateral digital extensor tendon, and then cultured have also been investigated in recent years as an alternative to bone marrow or stem cell therapies.

Blood-Derived Biologics: PRP, ACS, and Bone Marrow Aspirate

- The reasoning behind the use of PRP comes from the knowledge that growth factors are released from platelet α granules including PDGF, TGF-β, FGF, VEGF, IGF-I, and EGF.
- Many animal models have demonstrated positive effects on tissue healing of these growth factors, both alone and in combination.
- Current studies have reported beneficial effects of PRP on equine ligament and tendon, both in vitro and in vivo. A recent

in vivo study reported improved repair of the SDF tendon when core lesions were induced mechanical.

- In one clinical study, 80% of horses treated with PRP returned to performance after one-year compared to 50% of those treated with saline. However, another study found no benefit of PRP compared to more traditional treatments.
- ACS has also been reported to treat SDF tendinopathies. Recurrence of the tendon injury was not reported in any of the horses in the study up to 2–4 years post-diagnosis.
- Autologous bone marrow aspirate (ABMA) has been used in recent years as an inexpensive and fast intralesional treatment modality, by which stem cells and growth factors may be administered into a lesion without conditioning or culture.
- Two studies using ABMA to treat SDF tendon lesions in Thoroughbred and Standardbred racehorses reported that 59 and 62%, respectively, of treated horses had five or more starts.

Corticosteroids

- Perilesional CSs are occasionally used in acute cases to treat tendinitis/desmitis as an anti-inflammatory. A single perilesional dose of triamcinolone (6–9 mg) or methyl-prednisolone acetate (40 mg) is sometimes used in horses with peripheral tendon lesions or suspensory ligament desmitis.
- Use of CSs should probably be reserved for tendon or ligaments in which minimal or no structural damage is seen ultrasonographically.
- Numerous other uses have been described for local injection of CSs in areas of inflammation such as over splint bones, muscle/back soreness, and various soft-tissue inflammatory conditions. The choice and amount of steroid seem to be empirical and dependent on the clinician.

Sarapin

- Sarapin is an extract derived from the pitcher plant that is believed to have a numbing effect in chronic pain; however, one study could not detect analgesic effects of sarapin in a model of acute pain using heat.
- Sarapin is commonly utilized to treat various forms of desmitis and muscle soreness with a widely believed suspicion that a temporary analgesic effect is produced.
- Sarapin is often combined with other medications such as CSs and is used primarily to treat lameness conditions of the axial skeleton such as back and sacroiliac problems.

Oral/Nutritional

Nonsteroidal Anti-inflammatory Drugs (NSAIDs)

Overview

- NSAIDs are a large group of drugs with differing degrees of analgesic, anti-inflammatory, and antipyretic properties (Table 6.3).
- In a recent survey of horse owners and trainers, 96% of respondents stated that they use NSAIDs and 82% said they administer them without consulting a veterinarian.
- NSAIDs are also heavily prescribed by equine veterinarians.
- Oral formulations come in many varieties such as pills, paste, granules, and powder, allowing the consumer to choose the best formulation for each individual.
- NSAIDs act by inhibiting cyclooxygenase (COX) enzymes that convert arachidonic acid into prostaglandins and thromboxanes.
- There are two well-known isoenzymes of the COX enzymes: COX-1 and COX-2. COX-1 is considered the housekeeping isoenzyme responsible for producing prostaglandins involved in normal physiological functions such as gastric and renal function and hemostasis. The COX-2 isoenzyme is considered to be an important inducible mediator of inflammation in several organs and is also primarily responsible for the inflammatory pathway.

Table 6.3 Commonly used NSAIDs and their modes of action, formulations, and doses for equine musculoskeletal disorders.

Name of NSAID	Primary inhibitory action	Available formulations	Recommended dose
Phenylbutazone	Cox-1 and -2	Powder Tablets Paste Injectable solution	2.2–4.4 mg/kg SID or BID
Flunixin meglumine	Cox-1 and -2	Paste Granules Injectable solution	1.1 mg/kg SID
Acetylsalicylic acid	Cox-1 > Cox-2	Gel Powder Granules Paste Tablets	25–35 mg/kg SID or BID
Meclofenamic acid	Cox-1 and -2	Granules	2.2 mg/kg SID for 5–7 days
Naproxen	Cox-1 and -2	Granules Tablets Suspension	10 mg/kg SID or BID
Firocoxib	Cox-2	Paste Injectable solution Tablets	0.1 mg/kg SID and 0.09 mg/kg IV
Carprofen	Cox-2 > Cox-1	Tablets Injectable solution	0.7 mg/kg SID
Vedaprofen	Cox-2 > Cox-1	Gel Injectable solution	2 mg/kg loading dose followed by 1 mg/kg q 12 hours
Meloxicam	Cox-2 > Cox-1	Suspension Injectable solution Oral solution Tablets	0.6 mg/kg SID

- The variation in efficacy and toxicity of the different NSAIDs is closely related to inhibition of the different COX isoenzymes (Table 6.3).
- Some NSAIDS are more potent inhibitors of COX-1 than COX-2, some equally inhibit both, and others inhibit COX-2 more than COX-1.
- In general, the anti-inflammatory and analgesic properties of NSAIDs are believed to be mainly due to inhibition of the inducible COX-2, whereas the adverse effects seem to be caused by inhibition of the constitutive COX-1.
- Although used frequently, NSAIDs have a wide range of side effects, mainly involving the gastrointestinal, renal, and cardiovascular systems. These side effects can result from acute overdosing or extended duration of use and vary among the different drugs.
- In general, oral NSAIDs should be used at the lowest effective dose and frequency as possible, for the shortest period of time.

Phenylbutazone (PBZ; Butazolidin®, Butatron™, Bizolin®, Phenylbute™, Phenylzone®, Equiphen®, Butequine®, Superiorbute®, Equizone 100™)

- Oral PBZ is an inexpensive NSAID that has analgesic, antipyretic, and anti-inflammatory properties. It is available in several formulations (Table 6.3).
- It provides potent pain relief and reduction in inflammation in many common lameness problems in horses including chronic OA.
- PBZ is often used perioperatively to minimize pain and inflammation associated with orthopedic surgical procedures.
- The plasma half-life after oral administration has been reported to be between 6.2 and 6.7 hours. However, absorption can be influenced by the drug's formulation and its route of administration.
- Oral PBZ is considered relatively nontoxic at repeated doses of 2.2 mg/kg once or twice a day or less.
- The gastrointestinal tract is the most commonly affected site of toxicity following oral administration, contributing to ulcers (oral, esophageal, gastric, cecal, and right dorsal colon) and a protein-losing enteropathy.
- Some studies have shown a better clinical improvement in lameness when a combination of drugs is used compared to PBZ alone. However, caution should be used when combining NSAIDs to minimize the potential toxic effects.

Flunixin Meglumine (Banamine®)

- Flunixin meglumine is a derivative of nicotinic acid that exhibits analgesic, anti-inflammatory, and antipyretic activity.
- Oral flunixin meglumine can be used to treat musculoskeletal disorders in horses, but because of its cost compared to PBZ, oral formulations are used infrequently.
- After oral administration, the drug is rapidly absorbed with a peak in plasma levels within 30 minutes, and the plasma half-life is approximately 1.6 hours.

- The rapid absorption is thought to minimize its potential ulcerogenicity but similar to PBZ, recent feeding delays absorption.
- The onset of action after oral administration occurs after two hours, with the greatest effect obtained between 2 and 16 hours; some activity may persist for up to 30 hours.
- Oral administration of flunixin is relatively safe. However, high doses for long periods can cause gastrointestinal intolerance, hypoproteinemia, and hematological abnormalities.

Acetylsalicylic Acid (Aspirin)

- Acetylsalicylic acid is a weak acid that reduces platelet aggregation and has analgesic, anti-inflammatory, and antipyretic properties.
- It is only available in oral forms and has a limited clinical use in the horse.
- Aspirin has been reported to decrease platelet numbers and function and prolong bleeding time in horses with doses between 12 and 24 mg/kg. These effects can occur after a single dose and can last 48 hours.
- Due to its antiplatelet effects, aspirin has been used for the empirical treatment of navicular syndrome and laminitis. However, its therapeutic benefits for these diseases are not well defined.

Meclofenamic Acid (Arquel)

- Meclofenamic acid (MA) is another oral NSAID used to treat lameness and chronic musculoskeletal conditions such as navicular disease, OA, and laminitis in horses.
- Compared with other NSAIDs, MA has a slow onset of action of 36–96 hours for full effect.
- It is unclear whether feeding dramatically affects absorption – one study demonstrated that fasted and non-fasted ponies had similar oral absorption, whereas another study demonstrated that plasma levels could be delayed by feeding.
- MA may prove to be useful for horses with OA because high levels can be found in synovial fluid and articular cartilage.

- High doses produce clinical signs of toxicity similar to those of PBZ (at a dose 13–18 mg/kg).

Naproxen (Equiproxen®, Naprosyn)

- Naproxen is a nonselective NSAID with analgesic and antipyretic properties that has been used primarily to treat myositis and soft tissue problems.
- In a study using an equine myositis model, oral naproxen was reported to be superior to oral PBZ, with faster relief of inflammatory swelling and associated lameness.
- Successful use of naproxen in the human field for treating joint pain may suggest that it can also be used to treat inflammatory swelling and associated lameness in horses.
- Naproxen has a wide margin of safety. Oral administration of 4× the recommended dose for 42 days did not cause signs of toxicity.

Firocoxib (Equioxx®)

- Firocoxib is a COX-2 selective NSAID that has been approved by the FDA for controlling pain and inflammation associated with OA in horses.
- Oral firocoxib is thought to reduce inflammation, pain, and fever with lower risks of toxicities compared to other traditional NSAIDs.
- The bioavailability after oral administration in horses is 79%, with a time to peak concentration of 3.9 hours and elimination half-life of 30 hours. It is well distributed in the body, including synovial fluid, liver, fat, kidney, and muscle.
- In a study done in horses with chronic OA and navicular syndrome, no significant differences in clinical improvement were found between horses treated 14 days with firocoxib compared to PBZ.
- In a study of a large number and cross section of horses with musculoskeletal pain or lameness associated with OA, firocoxib paste significantly improved lameness scores, comfort, and mobility in horses with the most change occurring within the first 7 days of treatment.

- Compared with other NSAIDs, firocoxib is relatively safe, with no clinical and biochemical signs of toxicity reported using the recommended dose (0.1 mg/kg).
- The main downfall to firocoxib is that it is more expensive than PBZ, which may result in the off-label use of the canine tablets in horses.

Carprofen (Zenecarp, Rimadyl®)

- Carprofen is a propionic acid NSAID approved in Europe for oral use in horses.
- Its mechanism of action in horses is still unclear; however, it is described as being a more effective analgesic than anti-inflammatory agent.
- Carprofen in horses was well tolerated when given at twice the oral dose for 14 consecutive days.
- The benefit of using carprofen in horses compared to other available NSAIDs needs further investigation.

Vedaprofen (Quadrisol®)

- Vedaprofen is an arylpropionic acid NSAID with anti-inflammatory, antipyretic, and analgesic properties.
- Vedaprofen is approved in Europe for oral use and is recommended for musculoskeletal disorders and soft-tissue lesions.
- The main toxic effect is ulcer formation in the gastrointestinal tract, making it contraindicated for use in foals under 6 months of age. Other side effects are similar to other NSAIDs.

Meloxicam (Metacam®)

- Meloxicam is a relative COX-2-selective NSAID intended for the treatment of inflammatory orthopedic problems, including chronic musculoskeletal and soft-tissue disorders.
- Meloxicam is available for use in Europe and has been shown to be more effective than PBZ in decreasing pain in a synovitis model.
- Side effects are a similar to other NSAIDs, and oral doses of 0.6 mg/kg daily were well tolerated for up to 6 weeks.

- Increased doses (1.8–3 mg/kg) may result in decreased protein and albumin concentrations, GI and renal damage, or bone marrow dyscrasia.

Nutraceuticals

Overview

- A nutraceutical is basically any substance that is a food, or part of a food, that can be administered orally to provide or stimulate production of raw materials or biochemical pathways required for normal bodily functions.
- Although these substances are neither nutrients nor pharmaceuticals, they are generally used in an attempt to lower the dose of other drugs that are more problematic and provide medical benefits that prevent or treat disease.
- The FDA does not recognize nutraceuticals as foods or drugs and does not regulate these products unless they become unsafe or are associated with labels that claim a drug use.
- Nutraceuticals can be nutrients, dietary supplements, functional foods, and phytochemicals (including herbs), and there is no requirement to prove safety or efficacy of these products.
- Nutraceuticals/supplements are available in a variety of formulations and often used by many owners or trainers independent of their veterinarians.
- Quality control of these products is problematic as there can be considerable variability in purity, formulation, and consistency of ingredients between batches.
- Efficacy of these products in the horse is difficult to prove, and most of the information is anecdotal and based on the lack of any major adverse reactions after treatment.
- Safety of these products should not be assumed just because there is lack of published adverse reactions to a nutraceutical.

- Many nutraceutical products used in horses are directed toward preventing joint and musculoskeletal problems that may contribute to poor performance and/or lameness.

Glucosamine (GLN)

- Glucosamine is an aminosaccharide essential for normal growth and repair of articular cartilage.
- Glucosamine compounds have been used as nutraceuticals in horses due to their possible role in stimulating chondrocyte metabolism and reducing inflammation in the articular cartilage.
- Exogenous glucosamine can be produced synthetically or derived from marine exoskeletons or beef carcasses.
- There are three commercially available forms of exogenous GLN: hydrochloride (HCl), sulfate, and N-acetyl-D-glucosamine – GLN sulfate has been postulated to be more efficacious.
- Several studies have generally identified that GLN induces the production of new cartilage while protecting cartilage that is already present.
- GLN stimulates synthesis of proteoglycans (PG) and collagen while inhibiting PG degradation and may protect against some of the negative effects of steroids on cartilage.
- The levels of GLN used for in vitro experiments that were high enough to be effective and have never been achieved in experimental models in humans and animals.
- The most consistent information that can be extrapolated from human studies regarding GLN is that it appears to take four to eight weeks before it begins to work, and that GLN would likely give the best effects when used preventatively – when minor lesions are present prior to the advancement of the disease process.
- Variability in composition and dosing of GLN should be considered when evaluating product use.

Chondroitin Sulfate (CS)

- CS is a long-chain polysaccharide that constitutes about 80% of all GAG in articular cartilage.
- CS is often derived from shark and bovine cartilage, and it is rather expensive to synthesize and extract.
- The species or tissue of origin of CS can determine differences in the concentrations, pharmacokinetics profile, molecular composition and weight, metabolic fate, and therapeutic results. Because of these differences, it cannot be assumed that all CS products have the same clinical effect.
- CS is orally absorbed in horses; however, the molecular weight and source can have a direct influence on its permeability across the gastrointestinal tract and its bioavailability.
- Reports using radiolabeled CS have demonstrated that it achieves high concentrations in plasma, articular cartilage, and synovial fluid.
- Exogenous CS has been shown to reduce cartilage degradation and has profound anti-inflammatory effects on several tissues involved with joint metabolism.
- In a synovitis model in horses, CS was found to be less effective than PSGAG administered IM (Adequan®, Luitpold Pharmaceuticals, Inc.) for relief of lameness, stride length, and carpal flexion.
- Another study using the same model suggested that CS had therapeutic value irrespective of the route of administration (oral or IM). However, the time of onset of clinical improvement was slower with oral administration of CS.

Glucosamine and Chondroitin Sulfate (GLN-CS)

- Many equine nutraceuticals contain a combination of GLN and CS; this combination may be synergistic.
- It has been shown that the combination improves collagen synthesis in tenocytes and ligament cells, and it may be important for use in accessory joint structures.

- Studies suggest that GLN may work best for potentially inhibiting OA progression, whereas CS may be best for controlling symptomatic action of OA.
- GLN-CS has demonstrated equivocal success in research models, showing no clinical benefit in one study and an anti-inflammatory effect (reduced PGE2) in another.
- Results of studies of clinical cases treated with this GLN-CS are mixed, but with more demonstrating favorable responses – horses showed improved lameness, flexion, and stride length in one study and horses with navicular disease showed significant improvement in soundness compared to placebo controls.

Methylsulfonylmethane (MSM)

- Methylsulfonylmethane is a normal oxidative metabolite product of industrial-grade DMSO that is naturally found in small amounts in fruit, alfalfa, and corn. It is very soluble in water.
- MSM can be found as a product by itself or in combination with GLN and/or CS.
- MSM has been used as a nutraceutical because of its analgesic, anti-inflammatory, and antioxidant properties.
- Very little is known about the pharmacokinetics of oral MSM, or its safety, toxicity or clinical use to manage OA in horses.
- Horses receiving oral MSM, and vitamins demonstrated that MSM could exert some protective effect on oxidative and inflammatory exercise-induced injury related to jumping.
- In another uncontrolled non-peer-reviewed study, MSM administration was associated with improved performance in Standardbred racehorses in training.

Avocado and Soybean Unsaponifiable Extracts (ASU)

- The unsaponifiable portions of avocado and soybean oils are extracted via hydrolysis to make up fractions of one-third avocado oil and two-thirds soybean oil.

- It appears that this mixture has synergistic properties, but the active ingredient is still unknown.
- in vitro studies have suggested that ASU extracts may have a positive effect on both the inflammatory cascade and structural components of the cartilage matrix.
- One controlled study that used horses with induced OA in the middle carpal joint failed to demonstrate any significant clinical effects.
- ASU has been combined with GLN-CS in some products.

Fatty Acids

- Polyunsaturated fatty acids (PUFAs) are essential fatty acids that are found in fish and plants that potentially regulate inflammatory processes.
- The two principal essential fatty acids are linoleic acid and α-linolenic acid. In the body, they are desaturated and elongated to produce analogs of arachidonic acid (n-6 fatty acid) called eicosapentaenoic acid (EPA omega-3 fatty acids) and docosahexaenoic acid (DHA omega-3 fatty acids).
- When horses in one study received fish oil in their diet, there was an increase in the concentration EPA and DHA in their serum, compared to horses that received corn oil.
- Studies have demonstrated that n-3 fatty acid supplementation can reduce or inhibit the inflammatory and matrix degradative response elicited by chondrocytes during OA progression.
- Cetyl myristoleate (CM) is an ester, omega-5 fatty acid that may act by inhibition of the 5-lipo-oxygenase pathway, which is responsible for the metabolism of leukotrienes (potent inflammatory mediators from the arachidonic acid cascade).
- One equine product containing CM contributed to lower lameness scores compared to placebo horses in a double-blinded OA clinical trial.
- The clinical usefulness of essential fatty acids in the treatment of joint disease remains to be determined.

Collagen Hydrolysate (CH)

- Collagen hydrolysate is a food ingredient that has been used in humans to improve joint comfort and function.
- CH is derived from bovine or porcine skin and bones.
- Orally administered CH has been shown to be absorbed intestinally and accumulate in cartilage.
- In contrast with other nutraceuticals, no direct analgesic and anti-inflammatory effects have been found after using CH.
- The theory behind CH is that it provides amino acids specific to the collagen network, playing an important role in the structure and function of cartilage by directly stimulating chondrocytes to synthesize collagenous matrix.
- There are no published reports on the safety, absorption, metabolism, or clinical use of CH in the horse.
- Glycosylated undenatured type-II collagen is another collagen product that has been used as a nutraceutical and has primarily been used in horses with OA.

Resveratrol

- Resveratrol is a non-flavonoid, polyphenolic compound found in some fruits (such as grapes) and plants.
- Resveratrol has been shown to decrease IL-1 synthesis via inhibition of nuclear factor-κB, downregulating COX-2 pathways, and scavenging of reactive oxygen species.
- Resveratrol has been shown in experimental models of OA to protect cartilage due to balancing the oxidation–reduction (redox) reactions and preventing GAG release and cell death.
- In one placebo-controlled clinical trial, resveratrol supplementation for four months resulted in a significantly greater percentage of riders reporting that their horse's performance was improved at 2 (95 vs 70%) and 4 (86 vs 50%) months compared to the placebo group.

Manual Therapy

Overview

- Manual therapy is the application of the hands to the body with the goal to influence reparative or healing processes within the neuromusculoskeletal system.
- Chiropractic, osteopathy, physical therapy, massage therapy, and touch therapies are all considered forms of manual therapy techniques that have been developed for treatment of musculoskeletal disorders in humans and transferred for use in horses (Table 6.4).
- Manual therapy is believed to produce physiological effects within local tissues on sensory and motor components of the nervous system and at a psychological or behavioral level.

- Anecdotally, manual therapies have reported effectiveness in humans and horses but are often not supported by higher levels of evidence such as controlled clinical trials.

Massage Therapy

- Massage therapy is the manipulation of the skin and underlying soft tissues either manually (e.g. by rubbing, kneading, or tapping) or with an instrument or machine (e.g. mechanical vibration).
- Massage techniques include many named methods such as Swedish massage, sports massage, trigger point therapy, cross-fiber friction massage, lymphatic drainage, and acupressure.
- Clinically, massage and soft tissue mobilization are thought to increase blood flow,

Table 6.4 Types of manual therapy, proposed mechanisms of action, and possible clinical applications.

Manual therapies	Mechanisms of action	Clinical applications
Touch therapies	Psychological: Calming Behavioral deconditioning Novel cutaneous stimulation Mechanoreceptive stimulation	Behavioral issues Anxiety or nervousness Poor proprioception or body awareness Pain
Therapeutic massage	Psychological: Relaxation Mechanical: Soft tissues Neurophysiological: Pain	Anxiety or nervousness Soft-tissue restriction Muscle hypertonicity Pain
Passive stretching exercises	Mechanical: Articular and soft tissues Neuromotor learning	Soft tissue restriction Muscle hypertonicity Joint stiffness Pain
Mobilization		
Soft tissue	Mechanical: Soft tissues	Soft tissue restriction Muscle hypertonicity Pain
Articular	Mechanical: Articular and soft tissues	Restricted joint motion Joint effusion Pain
Manipulation	Mechanical: Articular and soft tissues Neurophysiological: Pain Mechanoreceptive stimulation	Restricted joint motion Joint motion asymmetry Muscle hypertonicity Pain

promote relaxation, relax muscles, increase tissue extensibility, reduce pain, and speed return to normal function.

- In horses, massage therapy has been shown to be effective at reducing stress-related behavior and pain thresholds within the thoracolumbar spine.

Passive Stretching

- Passive stretching consists of applying forces to a limb or body segment to lengthen muscles or connective tissues beyond their normal resting lengths, with the intent of increasing joint range of motion and flexibility.
- Stretching exercises are thought to increase joint range of motion, enhance flexibility, improve coordination and motor control, increase blood flow to muscles, and help to prevent injuries.
- Both positive and potential negative benefits of passive stretching have been reported in horses.

Mobilization

- Mobilization is manually induced movement of articulations or soft tissues for therapeutic purposes commonly used in physical therapy.
- Soft-tissue mobilization focuses on restoring movement to the skin, connective tissue, ligaments, tendons, and muscles with the goal of modulating pain, reducing inflammation, increasing extensibility, and improving function.
- Joint mobilization is characterized as non-impulsive, repetitive joint movements using passive range of joint motion with the goals of restoring symmetric joint range of motion, stretching connective tissues, and restoring normal joint end-feel.
- Few formal studies support the use of limb or spinal mobilization techniques in horses.

Manipulation/Mobilization

- In people, the chiropractic and osteopathic professions have many overlapping philosophies, techniques, and potential mechanisms of

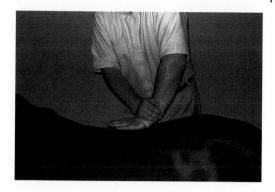

Figure 6.1 Thoracolumbar spinal extension mobilization. A gentle rhythmic force is applied over the dorsal spinous processes of the thoracolumbar junction in an effort to assess regional spinal flexibility and local pain or muscle hypertonicity. *Source:* Courtesy of Kevin Haussler.

action related to joint mobilization and manipulation.

- Chiropractic treatment is characterized primarily as the application of high-velocity, low-amplitude (HVLA) thrusts to induce therapeutic effects within articular structures, muscle function, and neurological reflexes (Figure 6.1).
- Chiropractic manipulation is most commonly focused on the axial skeleton in horses, and pilot work suggests that these techniques are able to produce substantial segmental spinal motion within the thoracolumbar region in horses.
- Manipulation on asymmetrical spinal movement patterns in horses with documented back pain suggests that chiropractic treatment elicits minor but significant changes in thoracolumbar and pelvic kinematics and that some of these changes are likely to be beneficial.

Rehabilitation/Physical Therapy

Overview

- Rehabilitation and physical therapy (PT) play an important role in performance enhancement, injury prevention, and restoration of full function during recovery from injury in any species.

- Veterinary medicine continues to follow the principles of human sports medicine and rehabilitation to encompass many professional fields, including PT.
- Rehabilitation encompasses broad-based concepts with a focus on tissue healing, biomechanics, and neuromotor control.
- Rehabilitation/PT techniques includes manual therapies, electrotherapy, functional retraining, proprioceptive exercises, application of various modalities, and therapeutic exercise-based treatments.
- Rehabilitation/PT is individually tailored to each patient rather than prescriptive for a given lesion or pathoanatomical diagnosis, and should consider the whole horse, short- and long-term goals, discipline, and overall prognoses.
- There is still a great need for further research on the effects of rehabilitation/PT in horses

to complement the considerable research in pathology and the high prevalence of injuries in athletic horses.

Soft Tissue and Joint Mobilization

- These techniques encompass the application of very specific passive and/or active assisted movements by the therapist to the horse to manage and/or alter pain and dysfunction of the articular, neural, and muscle systems.
- Passive range of motion exercises for joints are proposed to work at a cellular level by decreasing the random alignment of the collagen fibers through stimulation of physiologic motion enhancing parallel fiber orientation.
- Two very effective mobilization techniques often used to restore joint motion and reduce pain in the horse are (i) passive physiological mobilizations and (ii) passive accessory movements (Figure 6.2).

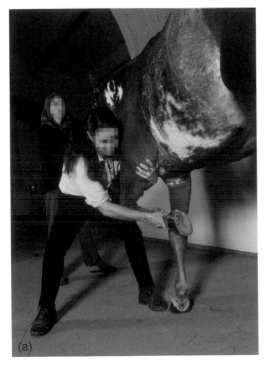 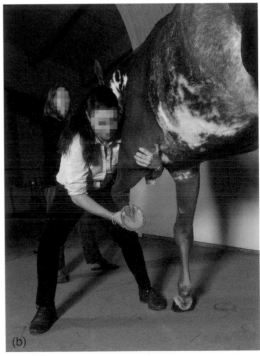

(a) (b)

Figure 6.2 Manual therapy mobilization technique. A combination of passive physiological and passive accessory mobilization techniques is applied to the carpus to increase the available range of motion into flexion. The carpus is flexed, the radius is stabilized, and medial (a) and lateral motion (b) are applied to the end of range via the third metacarpus. *Source:* Courtesy of Narelle Stubbs.

- Soft-tissue mobilization techniques are intended to normalize tissue irritability, muscle tone, extensibility, length, contractility, strength, and coordination, and ultimately improve motor control.

Mobilization with Movement Techniques/ Exercises

- Indirect mobilization with movement techniques/exercises in conjunction with direct manual therapy techniques are very effective clinically, especially in relation to functional motor control.
- Many of these mobilization techniques/exercises use neuromuscular reflexive responses along with muscular facilitation and inhibition and are useful in the majority of rehabilitation cases to maintain and improve mobility, strength, and dynamic stability (Figure 6.3).

- There are many combinations of these types of exercises that often use a food incentive or bait to encourage the horse to move in the desired posture (Figure 6.4).
- The aim of these exercises is not only to mobilize both the axial and distal skeletons but also to facilitate core muscle activity (thoracic sling, hypaxial/epaxial, and pelvic musculature), improve neuromuscular control, and strengthen over time.
- Physical therapy aides such as balance pads (Figure 6.5), ground poles, tactile stimulators, and incorporation of surface changes offer clinicians passive means of engaging neuromotor control during activities of daily rehabilitation or training.
- Many of these exercises can be used in horses with spinal pathology and back pain to strengthen the epaxial and core musculature.

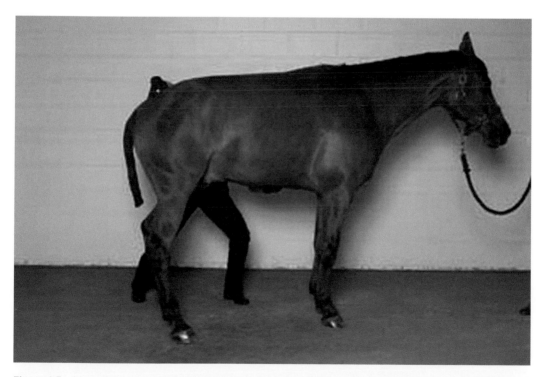

Figure 6.3 Manual therapy mobilization with movement technique. A combined rounding response into end-of-dorsoventral flexion range of motion of the thoracolumbar spine and pelvis. This is performed by manual finger pressure to the ventral midline with one hand and dorsally directly over the midline of the sacrum with the other hand. Depending on the size of the horse, this may need to be performed by two people. *Source:* Courtesy of Narelle Stubbs.

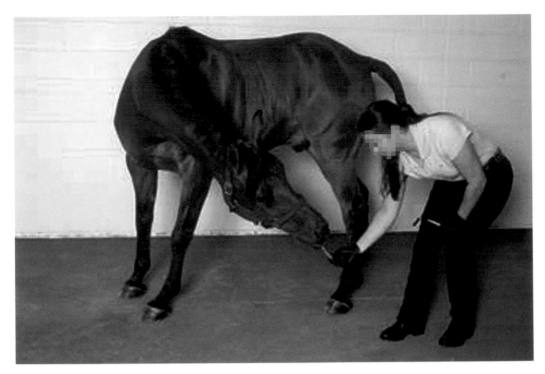

Figure 6.4 Baited mobilization with movement exercises; lateral bending coupled with flexion and rotation. The horse's functional end-of-range posture is attained by the horse's chin following the carrot toward its hock/fetlock. The position is held for 3–5 seconds to increase the activity of the core muscles of the thoracic sling, trunk, and pelvic sling, as seen in the photograph. *Source:* Courtesy of Narelle Stubbs.

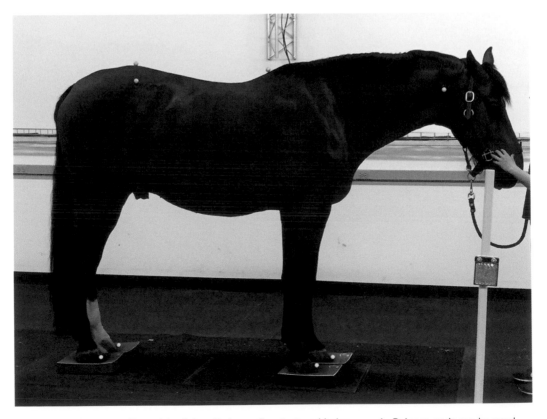

Figure 6.5 Horse standing with all four limbs on firm textured balance pads. Balance pads can be used during various stages of rehabilitation to engage the core and improve core strength and postural stability. *Source:* Courtesy of Melissa King.

Proprioceptive Facilitation/Neuromotor Control Techniques

- The application of various proprioceptive techniques can be utilized to increase joint range of motion, reestablish appropriate neuromuscular firing patterns, and improve the strength of targeted muscles that function to move and stabilize the joints.
- Because the horse has the ability to feel the smallest tactile stimulus such as a fly, tactile stimulants or cues can be applied to the skin over targeted regions, including the limbs or specific muscles, to alter mechanoreceptive/proprioception feedback and thus potentially alter motor control (Figure 6.6)
- A multitude of proprioceptive techniques are utilized from resistive bands and kinesiotape to ground poles and changes in ground surfaces (Figure 6.7).
- TheraBand, a two-piece equine elastic band system, is thought to stimulate core abdominal muscles with the abdominal band and engage hindlimb musculature with the hindquarter band.
- Many of these techniques may be combined with many forms of in-hand and ridden exercises and should be tailored to the individual horse.
- Any exercise program should be gradually increased with consideration given to exercise time, gaits, transitions, direction, surfaces, and gradients/slopes.

Physical Modalities

- There are a variety of ancillary therapies that can be used as part of any rehabilitation/PT program. Many of these modalities are thought to alter and/or accelerate tissue healing and minimize the effects of disuse atrophy, immobilization, and denervation. Several of them are listed below in no order of efficacy. The reader is referred to the main text of Adams and Stashak's Lameness in Horses for further details on these treatments.
  1) Cryotherapy
  2) Heat
  3) Contrast therapy (combination of heat and cold)
  4) Therapeutic ultrasound
  5) Radiofrequency diathermy
  6) Laser therapy
  7) Transcutaneous electrical nerve stimulation (TENS)
  8) Neuromuscular electrical stimulation (NMES)
  9) Pulsed electromagnetic field therapy (PEMF)
  10) Underwater treadmill
  11) Whole body vibration (WBV)

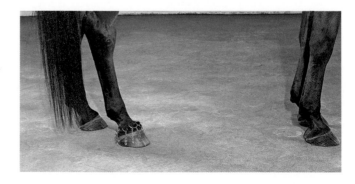

Figure 6.6 Sensory integration technique. A lightweight (55-g) tactile stimulation device is placed around the coronary band of a horse and worn during exercise to increase the peak height of the swing phase of gait. *Source:* Courtesy of Narelle Stubbs.

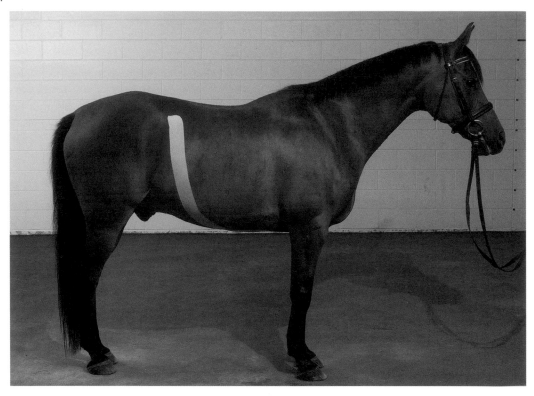

Figure 6.7 Sensory integration. In this example of a taping technique of the abdominal complex, Kinesio Tape™ is applied to stretch from the transverse processes of the lumbar vertebrae, following the line of the transverse abdominus, internal oblique, and rectus abdominus muscles. The tape finishes on the ventral aspect of the sternum and pectoral muscle complex. *Source:* Courtesy of Narelle Stubbs.

Bibliography

1 Aggarwal A, Sempowski IP: 2004. Hyaluronic acid injections for knee osteoarthritis. Systematic review of the literature. *Can Fam Physician* 50:249–256.

2 Aghighi SA, Tipold A, Piechotta M, et al.: 2012. Assessment of the effects of adjunctive gabapentin on postoperative pain after intervertebral disc surgery in dogs. *Vet Anaesth Analg* 39:636–646. doi: 10.1111/j.1467-2995.2012.00769.x.

3 Aktar MW, Karimi H, Gilani SA: 2017. Effectiveness of core stabilization exercises and routine exercise therapy in management of pain in chronic nonspecific low back pain: A randomized controlled clinical trial. *Pak J Med Sci* 33:1002–1006.

4 Anderson D, Kollias-Baker C, Colahan P, et al.: 2005. Urinary and serum concentrations of diclofenac after topical application to horses. *Vet Ther* 6:57–66.

5 Back W, Clayton HM: 2010. *Equine Locomotion, Second Edition*. Philadelphia, WB Saunders.

6 Baggot JD: 1992. Bioavailability and bioequivalence of veterinary drug dosage forms, with particular reference to horses: An overview. *J Vet Pharmacol Ther* 15:160–173.

7 Bell CD, Howard RD, Taylor DS, et al.: 2009. Outcomes of podotrochlear (navicular) bursa injections for signs of foot pain in horses evaluated via magnetic resonance imaging:

23 cases (2005–2007). *J Am Vet Med Assoc* 234:920–923.

8 Bolt DM, Burba DJ, Hubert JD, et al.: 2004. Determination of functional and morphologic changes in palmar digital nerves after nonfocused extracorporeal shock wave treatment in horses. *Am J Vet Res* 65:1714–1718.

9 Bowman S, Awad ME, Hamrick MW, et al.: 2018. Recent advances in hyaluronic acid-based therapy for osteoarthritis. *Clin Transl Med*;7:6. doi: 10.1186/s40169-017-0180-3.

10 Burns G, Dart A, Jeffcott L: 2018. Clinical progress in the diagnosis of thoracolumbar problems in horses. *Equine Vet Educ* 30:477–485.

11 Caldwell FJ, Mueller PO, Lynn RC, et al.: 2004. Effect of topical application of diclofenac liposomal suspension on experimentally induced subcutaneous inflammation in horses. *Am J Vet Res* 65:271–276.

12 Canada NC, Beard WL, Guyan ME, et al.: 2018. Effect of bandaging techniques on sub-bandage pressures in the equine distal limb, carpus, and tarsus. *Vet Surg* 47:640–647. doi: 10.1111/vsu.12914.

13 Caron JP, Peters TL, Hauptman JG, et al.: 2002. Serum concentrations of keratan sulfate, osteocalcin, and pyridinoline crosslinks after oral administration of glucosamine to Standardbred horses during race training. *Am J Vet Res* 63:1106–1110.

14 Caron JP: 2005. Intra-articular injections for joint disease in horses. *Vet Clin North Am Equine Pract* 21:559–573.

15 Carstanjen B, Balali M, Gajewski Z, et al.: 2013. Short-term whole body vibration exercise in adult healthy horses. *Pol J Vet Sci* 16:403–405.

16 Celeste C, Ionescu M, Robin PA, et al.: 2005. Repeated intraarticular injections of triamcinolone acetonide alter cartilage matrix metabolism measured by biomarkers in synovial fluid. *J Orthop Res* 23:602–610.

17 Chunekamrai S, Krook LP, Lust G, et al.: 1989. Changes in articular cartilage after intra-articular injections of methylprednisolone acetate in horses. *Am J Vet Res* 50:1733–1741.

18 Clayton HM, White AD, Kaiser LJ, et al.: 2010. Hind limb response to tactile stimulation of the pastern and coronet. *Equine Vet J* 42:227–233.

19 Clayton HM: 2004. *The Dynamic Horse. Sport Horse Publications*, Mason, MI, Sport Horse Publications.

20 Cohen SB: 2004. An update on bisphosphonates. *Curr Rheumatol Rep* 6:59–65.

21 Colles CM, Nevin A, Brooks J: 2014. The osteopathic treatment of somatic dysfunction causing gait abnormality in 51 horses. *Equine Vet Educ* 26:148–155.

22 Coudry V, Thibaud D, Riccio B, et al.: 2007. Efficacy of tiludronate in the treatment of horses with signs of pain associated with osteoarthritic lesions of the thoracolumbar vertebral column. *Am J Vet Res* 68: 329 337.

23 Curtis CL, Harwood JL, Dent CM, et al.: 2004. Biological basis for the benefit of nutraceutical supplementation in arthritis. *Drug Discov Today* 9: 165–172.

24 Da Costa Gomez TM, Radtke CL, Kalscheur VL, et al.: 2004. Effect of focused and radial extracorporeal shock wave therapy on equine bone microdamage. *Vet Surg* 33:49–55.

25 Dabareiner RM, Carter GK, Honnas CM: 2003. Injection of corticosteroids, hyaluronate, and amikacin into the navicular bursa in horses with signs of navicular area pain unresponsive to other treatments: 25 cases (1999–2002). *J Am Vet Med Assoc* 223: 1469–1474.

26 de Grauw JC, Visser-Meijer MC, Lashley F, et al.: 2016. Intra-articular treatment with triamcinolone compared with triamcinolone with hyaluronate: A randomized open-label multicenter clinical trial in 80 lame horses. *Equine Vet J* 48:152–158.

27 Del Bue M, Ricco S, Ramoni R, et al.: 2008. Equine adipose-tissue-derived mesenchymal stem cells and platelet concentrates: Their association in vitro and in vivo. *Vet Res Commun* 32 (Suppl):S51–S55.

28 Delguste C, Amory H, Doucet M, et al.: 2007. Pharmacological effects of tiludronate in horses after long-term immobilization. *Bone* 41:414–421.

29 Denoix JM, Thibaud D, Riccio B: 2003. Tiludronate as a new therapeutic agent in the treatment of navicular disease: A double-blind placebo-controlled clinical trial. *Equine Vet J* 35:407–413.

30 Dorna V, Guerrero RC: 1998. Effects of oral and intramuscular use of chondroitin sulfate in induced equine aseptic arthritis. *J Equine Vet Sci* 18:548–555.

31 Doucet MY, Bertone AL, Hendrickson D, et al.: 2008. Comparison of efficacy and safety of paste formulations of firocoxib and phenylbutazone in horses with naturally occurring osteoarthritis. *J Am Vet Med Assoc* 232:91–97.

32 Du J, White N, Eddington ND: 2004. The bioavailability and pharmacokinetics of glucosamine hydrochloride and chondroitin sulfate after oral and intravenous single dose administration in the horse. *Biopharm Drug Dispos* 25:109–116.

33 Duesterdieck-Zellmer KF, Larson MK, Plant TK, et al.: 2016. Ex vivo penetration of low-level laser light through equine skin and flexor tendons. *Am J Vet Res* 77:991–999.

34 Dunkel B, Pfau T, Fiske-Jackson A, et al.: 2017. A pilot study of the effects of acupuncture treatment on objective and subjective gait parameters in horses. *Vet Anaesth Analg* 44:154–162.

35 Dutton DW, Lashnits KJ, Wegner K: 2009. Managing severe hoof pain in a horse using multimodal analgesia and a modified composite pain score. *Equine Vet Educ* 21:37–43. doi: 10.2746/095777308 X382669.

36 Dyson SJ: 2010. Medical management of superficial digital flexor tendonitis: A comparative study in 219 horses (1992–2000). *Equine Vet J* 36:415–419. doi: 10.2746/0425164044868422.

37 Edmonds RE, Garvican ER, Smith RKW, et al.: 2017. Influence of commonly used pharmaceutical agents on equine bone marrow-derived mesenchymal stem cell viability. *Equine Vet J* 49:352–357.

38 Elmali N, Baysal O, Harma A, et al.: 2007. Effects of resveratrol in inflammatory arthritis. *Inflamm* 30:1–6.

39 Ewers BJ, Haut RC: 2000. Polysulphated glycosaminoglycan treatments can mitigate decreases in stiffness of articular cartilage in a traumatized animal joint. *J Orthop Res* 18:756–761.

40 Faber MJ, van Weeren PR, Schepers M, et al.: 2003. Long-term follow-up of manipulative treatment in a horse with back problems. *J Vet Med A Physiol Pathol Clin Med* 50:241–245.

41 Ferris DJ, Frisbie DD, Kisiday JD, et al.: 2014. Clinical outcome after intra-articular administration of bone marrow derived mesenchymal stem cells in 33 horses with stifle injury. *Vet Surg* 43: 255–265.

42 Ferris DJ, Frisbie DD, McIlwraith CW, et al.: 2011. Current joint therapies in equine practice: A survey of veterinarians, 2009. *Equine Vet J* 43:530–535.

43 Foland JW, McIlwraith CW, Trotter GW, et al.: 1994. Effect of betamethasone and exercise on equine carpal joints with osteochondral fragments. *Vet Surg* 23:369–376.

44 Foreman JH, Ruemmler R: 2011. Phenylbutazone and flunixin meglumine used singly or in combination in experimental lameness in horses. *Equine Vet J* 43(Suppl 40):12–17.

45 Fortier L, Barker J, Strauss E, et al.: 2011. The role of growth factors in cartilage repair. *Clin Orthop Relat Res* 469:2706–2715.

46 Fortier LA: 2005. Systemic therapies for joint disease in horses. *Vet Clin North Am Equine Pract* 21: 547–557.

47 Fradette ME, Celeste C, Richard H, et al.: 2007. Effects of continuous oral administration of phenylbutazone on biomarkers of cartilage and bone metabolism in horses. *Am J Vet Res* 68:128–133.

48 Frean SP, Cambridge H, Lees P: 2002. Effects of anti-arthritic drugs on proteoglycan synthesis by equine cartilage. *J Vet Pharmacol Ther* 25:289–298.

49 Frisbie DD, Kawcak CE, McIlwraith CW, et al.: 2009. Evaluation of polysulfated glycosaminoglycan or sodium hyaluronan administered intra-articularly for treatment of horses with experimentally induced osteoarthritis. *Am J Vet Res* 70:203–209.

50 Frisbie DD, Kawcak CE, McIlwraith CW: 2009. Evaluation of the effect of extracorporeal shock wave treatment on experimentally induced osteoarthritis in middle carpal joints of horses. *Am J Vet Res* 70: 449–454.

51 Frisbie DD, Kawcak CE, Werpy NM, et al.: 2007. Clinical, biochemical, and histologic effects of intra-articular administration of autologous conditioned serum in horses with experimentally induced osteoarthritis. *Am J Vet Res* 68:290–296.

52 Frisbie DD, McIlwraith CW, Kawcak CE, et al.: 2016. Efficacy of intravenous administration of hyaluronan, sodium chondroitin sulfate, and N-acetyl-d-glucosamine for prevention or treatment of osteoarthritis in horses. *Am J Vet Res* 77:1064–1070. doi: 10.2460/ajvr.77.10.1064.

53 Frisbie DD, McIlwraith CW, Kawcak CE, et al.: 2009. Evaluation of topically administered diclofenac liposomal cream for treatment of horses with experimentally induced osteoarthritis. *Am J Vet Res* 70:210–215.

54 Fuller CJ, Ghosh P, Barr AR: 2002. Plasma and synovial fluid concentrations of calcium pentosan polysulphate achieved in the horse following intramuscular injection. *Equine Vet J* 34:61–64.

55 Gaustad G, Larsen S: 1995. Comparison of polysulphated glycosaminoglycan and sodium hyaluronate with placebo in treatment of traumatic arthritis in horses. *Equine Vet J* 27:356–362.

56 Geburek F, Gaus M, van Schie HTM, et al.: 2016. Effect of intralesional platelet-rich plasma (PRP) treatment on clinical and ultrasonographic parameters in equine naturally occurring superficial digital flexor tendinopathies – a randomized prospective controlled clinical trial. *BMC Vet Res* 12:191. doi: 10.1186/s12917-016-0826-1.

57 Gillespie CC, Adams SB, Moore GE: 2016. Methods and variables associated with the risk of septic arthritis following intra-articular injections in horses: A survey of veterinarians. *Vet Surg* 45:1071–1076.

58 Godwin EE, Young NJ, Dudhia J, et al.: 2012. Implantation of bone marrow-derived mesenchymal stem cells demonstrates improved outcome in horses with overstrain injury of the superficial digital flexor tendon. *Equine Vet J* 44:25–32. doi: 10.1111/j. 2042-3306.2011.00363.x.

59 Goff L, Stubbs N: 2007. Equine Treatment and Rehabilitation. *In*: McGowan C, Goff L, Stubbs N (eds) *Animal Physiotherapy: Assessment, Treatment and Rehabilitation of Animals*, Ames, IA, Blackwell Publishing, 238–251.

60 Goff LM: 2009. Manual therapy for the horse—A contemporary perspective. *J Equine Vet Sci* 29:799–808.

61 Goggs R, Vaughan-Thomas A, Clegg PD, et al.: 2005. Nutraceutical therapies for degenerative joint diseases: A critical review. *Crit Rev Food Sci Nutr* 45:145–164.

62 Gomez Alvarez CB, L'Ami JJ, Moffat D, et al.: 2008. Effect of chiropractic manipulations on the kinematics of back and limbs in horses with clinically diagnosed back problems. *Equine Vet J* 40:153–159.

63 Goodrich LR, Nixon AJ: 2006. Medical treatment of osteoarthritis in the horse—A review. *Vet J* 171:51–69.

64 Halsberghe BT, Gordon-Ross P, Peterson R: 2017. Whole body vibration affects the cross-sectional area and symmetry of the m. Multifidus of the thoracolumbar spine in the horse. *Equine Vet Educ* 29:493–499.

65 Hamm D, Jones EW: 1988. Intra-articular (IA) and intramuscular (IM) treatment of noninfectious equine arthritis (DJD) with polysulphated glycosaminoglycan (PSGAG). *J Equine Vet Sci* 8:456–459.

66 Harvey A, Kilcoyne I, Byrne BA, et al.: 2016. Effect of dose on intra-articular amikacin sulfate concentrations following intravenous regional limb perfusion in horses. *Vet Surg* 45:1077–1082. doi: 10.1111/vsu.12564.

67 Haussler KK, Hill AE, Puttlitz CM, et al.: 2007. Effects of vertebral mobilization and manipulation on kinematics of the thoracolumbar region. *Am J Vet Res* 68:508–516.

68 Haussler KK: 2009. Review of manual therapy techniques in equine practice. *J Equine Vet Sci* 29:849–869.

69 Haussler KK: 2010. The role of manual therapies in equine pain management. *Vet Clin North Am Equine Pract* 26:579–601.

70 Higler MH, Brommer H, L'ami JJ, et al.: 2014. The effects of three-month oral supplementation with a nutraceutical and exercise on the locomotor pattern of aged horses. *Equine Vet J* 46: 611–617.

71 Hinchcliff KW, Kaneps AJ, Geor RJ: 2014. *Equine Sports Medicine and Surgery, Second Edition.* St. Louis, MO, Elsevier Saunders, 3061–3064.

72 Holland B, Fogle C, Blikslager AT, et al.: 2014. Pharmacokinetics and pharmacodynamics of three formulations of firocoxib in healthy horses. *J Vet Pharmacol Ther* 38:249–256.

73 Hovanessian N, Davis JL, McKenzie HC, et al.: 2013. Pharmacokinetics and safety of firocoxib after oral administration of repeated consecutive doses to neonatal foals. *J Vet Pharmacol Ther* 37:243–251.

74 Hyde RM, Lynch TM, Clark CK, et al.: 2013. The influence of perfusate volume on antimicrobial concentration in synovial fluid following intravenous regional limb perfusion in the standing horse. *Can Vet J* 54:363–367.

75 Jones EW, Hamm D: 1978. Comparative efficacy of phenylbutazone and naproxen in induced equine myositis. *J Equine Med Surg* 2:341–347.

76 Kawcak CE, Frisbie DD, McIlwraith CW, et al.: 2007. Evaluation of avocado and soybean unsaponifiable extracts for treatment of horses with experimentally induced osteoarthritis. *Am J Vet Res* 68:598–604.

77 Kawcak CE, Frisbie DD, Trotter GW, et al.: 1997. Effects of intravenous administration of sodium hyaluronate on carpal joint in exercising horses after arthroscopic surgery and osteochondral fragmentation. *Am J Vet Res* 58:1132–1140.

78 Kay AT, Bolt DM, Ishihara A, et al.: 2008. Anti-inflammatory and analgesic effects of intra-articular injection of triamcinolone acetonide, mepivacaine hydrochloride, or both on lipopolysaccharide-induced lameness in horses. *Am J Vet Res* 69:1646–1654.

79 Keegan K, Hughes F, Lane T, et al.: 2007. Effects of an oral nutraceutical on clinical aspects of joint disease in a blinded, controlled clinical trial: 39 horses. *Proc Am Assoc Equine Pract* 53:252–255.

80 Keegan KG, Messer NT, Reed SK, et al.: 2008. Effectiveness of administration of phenylbutazone alone or concurrent administration of phenylbutazone and flunixin meglumine to alleviate lameness in horses. *Am J Vet Res* 69:167–173.

81 Kilcoyne I, Dechant JE, Nieto JE: 2016. Evaluation of 10-minute versus 30-minute tourniquet time for intravenous regional limb perfusion with amikacin sulfate in standing sedated horses. *Vet Rec* 178:585. doi: 10.1136/vr.103609.

82 King MR, Haussler KK, Kawcak CE, et al.: 2013. Effect of underwater treadmill exercise on postural sway in horses with experimentally induced carpal joint osteoarthritis. *Am J Vet Res* 74:971–982.

83 King MR. Principles and application of hydrotherapy for equine athletes. *Vet Clin North Am Equine Pract* 2016;32:115–126.

84 Kivett L, Taintor J, Wright J: 2013. Evaluation of the safety of a combination of oral administration of phenylbutazone and firocoxib in horses. *J Vet Pharmacol Ther* 37:413–416.

85 Knych HK, Stanley SD, Arthur RM, et al.: 2014. Detection and pharmacokinetics of three formulations of firocoxib following

multiple administrations to horses. *Equine Vet J* 46:734–738.

86 Knych HK, Stanley SD, Seminoff KN, et al.: 2016. Pharmacokinetics of methocarbamol and phenylbutazone in exercised Thoroughbred horses. *J Vet Pharmacol Ther* 39:469–477. doi: 10.1111/jvp.12298.

87 Knych HK, Vidal MA, Chouicha N, et al.: 2017. Cytokine, catabolic enzyme and structural matrix gene expression in synovial fluid following intra-articular administration of triamcinolone acetonide in exercised horses. *Equine Vet J* 49:107–115.

88 Kollias-Baker C: 1999. Therapeutics of musculoskeletal disease in the horse. *Vet Clin North Am Equine Pract* 15:589–602.

89 Kraus KH, Kirker-Head C: 2006. Mesenchymal stem cells and bone regeneration. *Vet Surg* 35:232–242.

90 Kristiansen KK, Kold SE: 2007. Multivariable analysis of factors influencing outcome of 2 treatment protocols in 128 cases of horses responding positively to intra-articular analgesia of the distal interphalangeal joint. *Equine Vet J* 39:150–156.

91 Kvaternick V, Pollmeier M, Fischer J, et al.: 2007. Pharmacokinetics and metabolism of orally administered firocoxib, a novel second generation coxib, in horses. *J Vet Pharmacol Ther* 30:208–217.

92 Labens R, Mellor DJ, Voute LC: 2007. Retrospective study of the effect of intra-articular treatment of osteoarthritis of the distal tarsal joints in 51 horses. *Vet Rec* 161:611–616.

93 Laverty S, Sandy JD, Celeste C, et al.: 2005. Synovial fluid levels and serum pharmacokinetics in a large animal model following treatment with oral glucosamine at clinically relevant doses. *Arthritis Rheum* 52:181–191.

94 Lippiello L, Woodward J, Karpman R, et al.: 2000. In vivo chondroprotection and metabolic synergy of glucosamine and chondroitin sulfate. *Clin Orthop Relat Res* 381:229–240.

95 Macedo LG, Maher CG, Latimer J, et al.: 2009. Motor control exercise for persistent, nonspecific low back pain: A systematic review. *Phys Ther* 89:9–25.

96 Martin BB Jr., Klide AM: 2001. Acupuncture for Treatment of Chronic Back Pain in Horses. *In*: Schoen AM (ed) *Veterinary Acupuncture: Ancient Art to Modern Medicine*, St. Louis, MO, Mosby, Inc., 467–473.

97 McClure SR, Sonea IM, Evans RB, et al.: 2005. Evaluation of analgesia resulting from extracorporeal shock wave therapy and radial pressure wave therapy in the limbs of horses and sheep. *Am J Vet Res* 66:1702–1708.

98 Mcclure SR, Wang C: 2017. A preliminary field trial evaluating the efficacy of 4% polyacrylamide hydrogel in horses with osteoarthritis. *J Equine Vet Sci* 54:98–102.

99 McCluskey MJ, Kavenagh PB: 2004. Clinical use of triamcinolone acetonide in the horse (205 cases) and the incidence of glucocorticoid-induced laminitis associated with its use. *Equine Vet Educ* 16:86–89.

100 McIlwraith CW, Frisbie DD, Kawcak CE: 2012. Evaluation of intramuscularly administered sodium pentosan polysulfate for treatment of experimentally induced osteoarthritis in horses. *Am J Vet Res* 73:628–633. doi: 10.2460/ajvr.73.5.628.

101 McKellar QA, Bogan JA, von Fellenberg RL, et al.: 1991. Pharmacokinetic, biochemical and tolerance studies on carprofen in the horse. *Equine Vet J* 23:280–284.

102 Mendez-Angulo JL, Firschman AM, Groschen DM, et al.: 2013. Effect of water depth on amount of flexion and extension of joints of the distal aspects of the limbs in healthy horses walking on an underwater treadmill. *Am J Vet Res* 74:557–566.

103 Merial: 2009. Horse Owner Survey Shows NSAID Use Trends. https://thehorse.com/

104 Moraes APL, Moreira JJ, Brossi PM, et al.: 2015. Short- and long-term effects of

platelet-rich plasma upon healthy equine joints: clinical and laboratory aspects. *Can Vet J* 56:831–838.

105 Neil KM, Caron JP, Orth MW: 2005. The role of glucosamine and chondroitin sulfate in treatment for and prevention of osteoarthritis in animals. *J Am Vet Med Assoc* 226:1079–1088.

106 Nixon AJ, Dahlgren LA, Haupt JL, et al.: 2008. Effect of adipose-derived nucleated cell fractions on tendon repair in horses with collagenase-induced tendonitis. *Am J Vet Res* 69:928–937.

107 Noble G, Edwards S, Lievaart J, et al.: 2012. Pharmacokinetics and safety of single and multiple oral doses of meloxicam in adult horses. *J Vet Intern Med* 26:1192–1201.

108 Orsini JA, Ryan WG, Carithers DS, et al.: 2012. Evaluation of oral administration of firocoxib for the management of musculoskeletal pain and lameness associated with osteoarthritis in horses. *Am J Vet Res* 73:664–671.

109 Pacini S, Spinabella S, Trombi L, et al.: 2007. Suspension of bone marrow–derived undifferentiated mesenchymal stromal cells for repair of superficial digital flexor tendon in racehorses. *Tissue Eng* doi: 10.1089/ten.2007.0108.

110 Paulekas R, Haussler KK: 2009. Principles and practice of therapeutic exercise for horses. *J Equine Vet Sci* 29:870–893.

111 Pauwels FE, Schumacher J, Castro FA, et al.: 2008. Evaluation of the diffusion of corticosteroids between the distal interphalangeal joint and navicular bursa in horses. *Am J Vet Res* 69:611–616.

112 Pichereau F, Décory M, Cuevas Ramos G: 2014. Autologous platelet concentrate as a treatment for horses with refractory fetlock osteoarthritis. *J Equine Vet Sci* 34:489–493.

113 Pluim M, Martens A, Vanderperren K, et al.: 2018. Short- and long-term follow-up of 150 sports horses diagnosed with tendinopathy or desmopathy by ultrasonographic examination and treated with high-power laser therapy. *Res Vet Sci* 119:232–238.

114 Popot MA, Bonnaire Y, Guechot J, et al.: 2004. Hyaluronan in horses: Physiological production rate, plasma and synovial fluid concentrations in control conditions and following sodium hyaluronate administration. *Equine Vet J* 36:482–487.

115 Ramey DW, Eddington N, Thonar E: 2002. An analysis of glucosamine and chondroitin sulfate content in oral joint supplement products. *J Equine Vet Sci* 22:125–127.

116 Ramon T, Prades M, Armengou L, et al.: 2017. Effects of athletic taping of the fetlock on distal limb mechanics. *Equine Vet J* 236:764–768.

117 Richardson LM, Whitfield-Cargile CM, Cohen ND, et al.: 2018 Effect of selective versus nonselective cyclooxygenase inhibitors on gastric ulceration scores and intestinal inflammation in horses. *Vet Surg* 47:784–791.

118 Rungsri PK, Trinarong C, Rojanasthien S, et al.: 2009. The effectiveness of electro-acupuncture on pain threshold in sport horses with back pain. *Am J Traditional Chin Vet Med* 4:22–26.

119 Russell JW, Russell TM, Vasey JR, et al.: 2016. Autologous bone marrow aspirate for treatment of superficial digital flexor tendonitis in 105 racehorses. *Vet Rec* 179:69. doi: 10.1136/vr.103620.

120 Schnabel LV, Lynch ME, van der Meulen MC, et al.: 2009. Mesenchymal stem cells and insulin-like growth factor-I gene-enhanced mesenchymal stem cells improve structural aspects of healing in equine flexor digitorum superficialis tendons. *J Orthop Res* 27:1392–1398.

121 Schnabel LV, Papich MG, Watts AE, et al.: 2010. Orally administered doxycycline accumulates in synovial fluid compared to plasma. *Equine Vet J* 42:208–212. doi: 10.2746/042516409X478514.

122 Serena A, Schumacher J, Schramme MC, et al.: 2005. Concentration of

methylprednisolone in the centrodistal joint after administration of methylprednisolone acetate in the tarsometatarsal joint. *Equine Vet J* 37: 172–174.

123 Smith LCR, Wylie CE, Palmer L, et al.: 2018. A longitudinal study of fractures in 1488 Thoroughbred racehorses receiving intrasynovial medication: 2006–2011. *Equine Vet J* 50:774–780. doi: 10.1111/evj.12833.

124 Smith RK: 2008. Mesenchymal stem cell therapy for equine tendinopathy. *Disabil Rehabil* 30:1752–1758.

125 Soma LR, Robinson MA, You Y, et al.: 2018. Pharmacokinetics, disposition, and plasma concentrations of dimethyl sulfoxide (DMSO) in the horse following topical, oral, and intravenous administration. *J Vet Pharmacol Ther* 41:384–392. doi: 10.1111/jvp.12476.

126 Spriet M, Buerchler S, Trela JM, et al.: 2015. Scintigraphic tracking of mesenchymal stem cells after intravenous regional limb perfusion and subcutaneous administration in the standing horse. *Vet Surg* 44:273–280. doi: 10.1111/j.1532-950X.2014.12289.x.

127 Steel C, Pannirselvam R, Anderson G: 2013. Risk of septic arthritis after intra-articular medication: A study of 16,624 injections in Thoroughbred racehorses. *Aust Vet J* 91:268–273.

128 Stubbs NC, Clayton HM: 2008. *Activate Your Horse's Core: Unmounted Exercises for Dynamic Mobility, Strength, and Balance*, Mason, MI, Sport Horse Publications.

129 Stubbs NC, Kaiser LJ, Hauptman J, et al.: 2011. Dynamic mobilization exercises increase cross sectional area of musculus multifidus. *Equine Vet J* 43:522–529.

130 Sullivan KA, Hill AE, Haussler KK: 2008. The effects of chiropractic, massage and phenylbutazone on spinal mechanical nociceptive thresholds in horses without clinical signs. *Equine Vet J* 40: 14–20.

131 Textor JA, Tablin F: 2013. Intra-articular use of a platelet-rich product in normal horses: clinical signs and cytologic response. *Vet Surg* 42:499–510.

132 Tnibar A, Schougaard H, Camitz L, et al.: 2015. An international multicentre prospective study on the efficacy of an intraarticular polyacrylamide hydrogel in horses with osteoarthritis: A 24-month follow-up. *Acta Vet Scand* 57:20–22.

133 Tnibar A, Schougaard H, Koene M, et al.: 2014. A controlled clinical trial on the efficacy of an intra-articular polyacrylamide hydrogel in horses with osteoarthritis [abstract]. *Vet Surg* 43:s138.

134 Trumble TN: 2005. The use of nutraceuticals for osteoarthritis in horses. *Vet Clin North Am Equine Pract* 21:575–597.

135 Ursini TL, Amelse LL, Elkhenany HA, et al.: 2018. Retrospective analysis of local injection site adverse reactions associated with 230 allogenic administrations of bone marrow-derived mesenchymal stem cells in 164 horses. *Equine Vet J* doi: 10.1111/evj.12992.

136 Usha PR, Naidu MU: 2004. Randomized, double-blind, parallel, placebo-controlled study of oral glucosamine, Methylsulfonylmethane and their combination in osteoarthritis. *Clin Drug Investig* 24:353–363.

137 Van de Water E, Oosterlinck M, Dumoulin M, et al.: 2017. The preventative effects of two nutraceuticals on experimentally induced acute synovitis. *Equine Vet J* 49:532–538.

138 van Eps AW, Orsini JA: 2016. A comparison of seven methods of continuous therapeutic cooling of the equine digit. *Equine Vet J* 48:120–124.

139 Vandeweerd J-M, Coisnon C, Clegg P, et al.: 2012. Systemic review of efficacy of nutraceuticals to alleviate clinical signs of osteoarthritis. *J Vet Intern Med* 26:448–456.

140 Wakeling JM, Barnett K, Price S, et al.: 2006. Effects of manipulative therapy on the longissimus dorsi in the equine back. *Equine Comp Exerc Physiol* 3:153–160.

141 Wehling P, Moser C, Frisbie D, et al.: 2007. Autologous conditioned serum in the treatment of orthopedic diseases: The orthokine therapy. *BioDrugs* 21:323–332.

142 Whitton RC, Jackson MA, Campbell AJD, et al.: 2014. Musculoskeletal injury rates in Thoroughbred racehorses following local corticosteroid injection. *Vet J* 200:71–76.

143 Witte S, Dedman C, Harriss F, et al.: 2016. Comparison of treatment outcomes for superficial digital flexor tendonitis in National Hunt racehorses. *Vet J* 216:157–163. doi: 10.1016/J. TVJL.2016.08.003.

144 Xie H, Colahan P, Ott EA: 2005. Evaluation of electroacupuncture treatment of horses with signs of chronic thoracolumbar pain. *J Am Vet Med Assoc* 227:281–286.

Revised from "Principles of Therapy for Lameness" in *Adams and Stashak's Lameness in Horses, 7ᵗʰ Edition,* by Laurie R. Goodrich, Drew W. Koch, Lauren E. Smanik, Sara K.T. Steward, Nicolas S. Ernst, Troy N. Trumble, Melissa King, Katherine Ellis, Narelle C. Stubbs and Kevin K. Haussler.

7

Musculoskeletal Emergencies

Severe Unilateral Lameness

Overview

- Non-weight-bearing lameness of a single limb is usually due to an infection somewhere in the limb or a fracture/luxation.
- Periarticular infections and soft-tissue injuries typically cause less severe swelling and lameness than fractures and improve more quickly over time.
- Horses with infections usually worsen over time vs. those with soft-tissue injuries will usually improve with time.
- Resolution of the severe lameness as quickly as possible is important to prevent supporting limb laminitis in the contralateral foot.

Etiology

- Severe lameness from infection is usually associated with a hoof abscess or synovial sepsis.
- Fractures or joint luxations anywhere in the limb may cause non-weight-bearing lameness. Fractures are more common than luxations.
- Penetrating injuries of the foot and synovial cavities usually lead to severe lameness.

Clinical Signs

- Acute onset of non-weight-bearing lameness is the typical clinical sign of severe unilateral lameness.

- Limb deviation, abnormal posture, crepitus with manipulation, and pain on palpation are often present in horses with fractures/ luxations (Figures 3.78, 3.92 and 7.1).
- Horses with foot abscesses may have no visible swelling but will be extremely painful to hoof testers at the site of the infection.
- Synovial infections often have synovial effusion, peri-synovial edema, heat, and pain on palpation.
- Purulent drainage from synovial cavities is usually present with chronic penetrating injuries (Figure 7.2).

Diagnosis

- Horses with suspected fractures should have the limb radiographed as soon as possible. Ultrasonography is often helpful to identify fractures in the proximal limb and pelvic region.
- Synoviocentesis with evaluation of the fluid for white blood cell count and total protein remains the most expedient method to document synovial infection.
- Radiography (including contrast radiography) and ultrasonography can be used to document osteomyelitis and other soft-tissue injuries within the synovial cavities.
- Physical examination of the foot together with hoof tester application are usually the primary methods used to document the location of a hoof abscess.
- Perineural anesthesia should not be used in horses with suspected fractures but can be

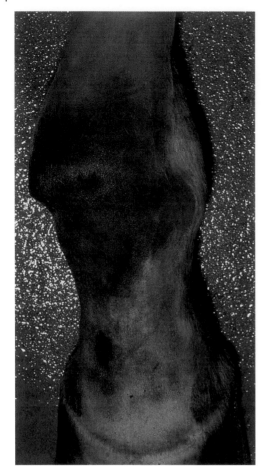

Figure 7.1 Horse with a closed luxation of the fetlock joint with deviation of the distal limb and extensive soft-tissue bruising.

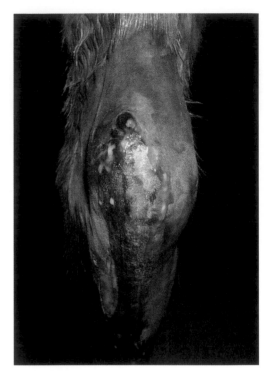

Figure 7.2 Horse with a puncture wound and established infection within the calcaneal bursa. Purulent drainage is exiting the wound and the horse was non-weight-bearing on the limb.

helpful to localize the lameness to the foot in cases of suspected sole abscesses.

Treatment

- Fractured limbs should be immobilized to reduce anxiety and pain and for transport if surgical treatment is warranted. Some fractures of the upper forelimb and hind limb cannot be adequately immobilized. Further details are discussed in a later section in this chapter.
- Hoof abscesses are usually treated by drainage, ± soaking, and foot protection until the hoof defect has cornified.
- Synovial infections are best treated with arthroscopic or endoscopic lavage; parenteral, regional, and intrasynovial antimicrobials; and systemic NSAIDs. Further details are discussed in a later section in this chapter.

Prognosis

- The prognosis is variable, depending on the type and location of the fracture and the severity and location of the infection.
- Most horses with foot abscesses have a very good prognosis. Other conditions within the foot such as keratomas, chronic laminitis, osteomyelitis, etc. should be suspected in horses with recurring abscesses.
- Most horses with synovial infections that are treated aggressively have a good prognosis.
- In general, synovial infections with secondary osteomyelitis have a much worse prognosis than those without bone involvement.

Severely Swollen Limb

Overview

- Numerous conditions can result in local or generalized limb swelling.
- The severity of lameness is very important in the initial assessment of the horse and in determining the potential cause of the swelling.
- Horses with fractures, luxations, and synovial infections usually have severe lameness together with localized swelling at the affected site.
- Less severe lameness with generalized limb swelling is often seen with cellulitis, lymphangitis, traumatic wounds, or hematomas.
- Horses with traumatic soft-tissue injuries usually have localized swelling, can bear weight on the limb, and usually respond quickly to first-aid treatment.

Etiology

- The cause is usually either traumatic or infectious.

Clinical Signs

- The clinical signs include localized or diffuse swelling of the limb with or without edema, pain, and heat.
- Diffuse, painful swellings are often associated with cellulitis, lymphangitis, or small puncture wounds.
- Effusion together with edema and local swelling around the synovial cavity are often present with synovial infections (Figure 7.3).
- Crepitus may be felt or heard during manipulation of complete long bone fractures.
- The severity of lameness can be variable, but most acute cases are often lame at the walk or non-weight-bearing.
- Diffuse swelling with serum oozing through the skin may be present in horses with lymphangitis and cellulitis.

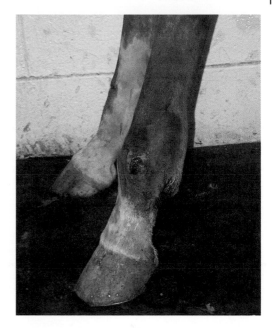

Figure 7.3 This wound, on the dorsal aspect of the fetlock healed by second intention and trapped infection within the fetlock joint. Joint effusion, soft-tissue swelling, and periarticular edema were present.

Diagnosis

- A tentative diagnosis can usually be made based on physical findings and the severity of the lameness.
- Radiography is used to document a fracture/luxation and the presence of secondary osteomyelitis in synovial infections.
- Ultrasonography is very helpful to evaluate soft-tissue swelling from any cause.
- Bacterial culturing should be performed whenever possible in horses with suspected diffuse or localized infection.

Treatment

- The definitive treatment depends on the cause, but initial first-aid treatment of soft-tissue swelling is often similar and usually consists of hydrotherapy/cryotherapy, topical and systemic NSAIDs, bandaging, and systemic antimicrobials if infection is suspected.
- Fractures should be immobilized if possible and the horses sent to a hospital for definitive treatment.

- Horses with synovial infections should be treated with synovial lavage (preferably with the arthroscope), and systemic, regional, and intrasynovial antimicrobials.

Prognosis

- The prognosis usually is very good for horses with cellulitis, except for horses with lymphangitis.
- Horses with soft-tissue injuries usually respond well to first-aid treatment, but the prognosis depends on the structure that is damaged (i.e. muscle vs. tendon).
- Horses with fractures/luxations and synovial infections have a worse prognosis than horses with cellulitis.

Long Bone Fractures/Luxations

Overview

- Complete long bone fractures usually result in a severe non-weight-bearing lameness and soft-tissue swelling in the region.
- Fractures of the phalanges and MC/MT occur most commonly.
- Fractures in any location can be complete or incomplete, displaced or non-displaced, and open or closed.

- Horses with incomplete and stress fractures can usually bear weight on the limb and the fractures are not always easily diagnosed.
- The most common sites for joint luxations include the fetlock, pastern, tarsus (PIT or TMT joints), carpus, and hip (Figures 3.17, 4.9, 4.55, 7.1 and 7.4).

Etiology

- Repetitive overloading of the bone associated with exercise is the most common cause of incomplete and stress fractures in performance horses.
- Repetitive overloading of the bone can also predispose to complete loss of the structural support of the bone with complete fractures.
- Single-event traumatic injury such as an awkward step, fall, kick, or strenuous event also is a cause of many complete fractures.
- Luxations/subluxations are often associated with the foot getting caught between two immovable objects, or an awkward step or fall.

Clinical Signs

- Acute onset of severe non-weight-bearing lameness is the characteristic sign of complete fractures.

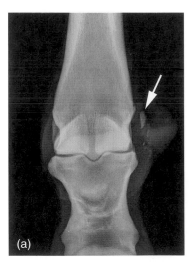 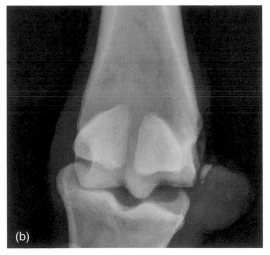

Figure 7.4 (a) Standing and (b) stressed radiographs of a horse with subluxation of the fetlock with fragmentation of the collateral ligament origin (arrow). *Source:* Courtesy of Matt Brokken.

- Limb deviation, abnormal limb posture, crepitus with manipulation, swelling, and pain on palpation are also often present with complete fractures.
- Horses with incomplete and stress fractures can usually bear weight on the limb, are lame at the walk, and may have minimal external signs suggestive of a fracture.
- Abnormal rotation or angulation of the joint often can be identified with complete joint luxations. Pain is obvious with manipulation. Joint subluxations are usually more difficult to document, and limb manipulation is often required.
- Both fractures and luxations can be open or closed.

Diagnosis

- The diagnosis of complete fractures is usually confirmed with radiography. The radiographic characteristics of the fracture are very important to determine whether repair is possible, the type of repair, and the prognosis if repair is attempted.
- Incomplete and stress fractures may not be evident with routine radiography and may require scintigraphy, CT, or PET/CT to document the fracture.
- Repeat radiographs taken 10–14 days or later after the injury may also be able to identify the fracture lines (Figure 7.5).
- Stress radiographs are helpful to identify joint luxations/subluxations and loss of collateral ligament support in many locations (Figures 4.9 and 7.4).
- Ultrasound can be used to identify fractures of the upper limb and pelvic region and to identify concurrent soft-tissue injuries associated with joint luxations.

First-Aid Fracture Management

- Horses are not readily ambulatory on three limbs and often become very anxious when they are unable to place weight on a fractured limb.

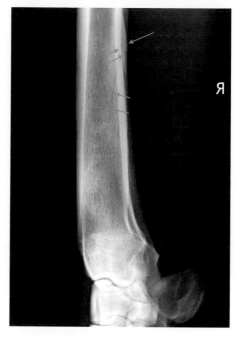

Figure 7.5 Incomplete, non-displaced fracture of the radius that was not identified until nearly four weeks after the initial injury (hoof strike from another horse; red and green arrows). *Source:* Courtesy of Kathryn Seabaugh.

- First-aid measures should be directed toward minimizing further damage to the fractured limb and maintaining it in a condition that will facilitate repair (Table 7.1).
- The goals of first-aid fracture management are to:
  1) Prevent damage to neural and vascular elements
  2) Keep the fractured bone from penetrating the skin and becoming an open fracture or protecting the limb from contamination through any existing skin opening
  3) Stabilize the limb to relieve anxiety that accompanies an uncontrolled limb in a horse
  4) Minimize any further damage to the fractured bone ends and surrounding soft tissues
- Fractures of the upper forelimb and hind limb in horses are inherently stabilized with the surrounding musculature and are difficult to stabilize with external splints.

Table 7.1 Recommended contents of fracture first-aid kit for horses.

Material	Purpose	Examples
Rigid material	To stabilize the fracture	PVC splints (varying lengths), aluminum rods, fiberglass cast material, wooden boards
Cotton	Padding for under the splint or cast Robert-Jones bandage	Roll cotton Sheet cotton Combine roll
Brown gauze vetrap	Compress the bandage/padding	
Sterile gauze	Cover any open wounds	Kerlix AMD
Razor and/or portable clippers	To remove the hair from around any open wounds	
Elastic tape	Secure the top and bottom of the bandage/padding	Elasticon
Nonelastic tape	Secure the splint to the bandage/padding	Athletic tape Duct tape
Pre-made splints	Stabilize lower limb fractures	Kimzey splint
Sedation	Ease anxiety Decrease activity	Xylazine, detomidine Butorphanol Acepromazine
Pain management	Reduce inflammation, pain, swelling	Phenylbutazone Flunixin meglumine
Antibiotics	To initiate if there is a wound or if the fracture has punctured the skin	Parenteral and oral options Dictated by case and veterinarian
Antibiotic ointment	Topical dressing for open wounds	Silver sulfadiazine Triple antibiotic ointment

PVC = polyvinyl chloride.

- Fractures of the distal and proximal aspects of the horse's limbs rarely become open, suggesting that fractures involving the MC/MT, radius, and tibia are the most critical to proper immobilization during transport.
- A good rule of thumb is that the joint above and below the fracture site should be immobilized, and the splint should never end at the same level as the fracture.
- For immobilization purposes, the limbs of the horse can be divided into four functional segments based on anatomy and biomechanical forces (Figure 7.6).

Methods of Immobilization Based on Location (Figure 7.6)

Phalanges and Distal Metacarpus
- The phalanges and distal MC are the most common locations for fractures to occur.
- The splinting techniques should attempt to counteract the bending force at the fetlock since biomechanically, the distal limb is dominated by the angle of the fetlock joint with minimal medial/lateral forces.
- A compression bandage combined with a dorsally placed splint (PVC) or a fiberglass cast applied with the limb maintained in a straight line from the carpus to the hoof provides the optimal dorsal cortical alignment (Figure 7.7).

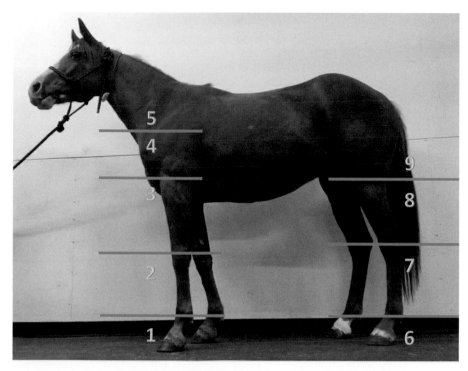

Figure 7.6 Functional divisions of the horse's limbs that can be used as a guide for appropriate application of external support to stabilize fractures for transport. They can be divided into five regions in the forelimb and four regions in the hind limb. Forelimb: (1) dorsal splint, (2) compression bandage with caudal and lateral splint, (3) compression bandage with extended lateral splint, (4) caudal splint to the level of the elbow to lock the carpus in extension, (5) no immobilization necessary, (6) plantar splint, (7) compression bandage with plantar and lateral splint, (8) compression bandage with extended lateral splint, (9) no immobilization necessary. *Source:* Courtesy of Kathryn Seabaugh.

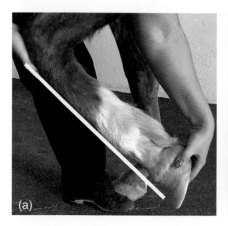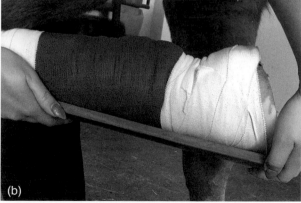

Figure 7.7 Dorsal cortical alignment is represented by the white line on the left image (a). This can be achieved with PCV placed on the dorsal aspect of the limb over a compression bandage (b). This stabilization is ideal for phalangeal fractures. The splint should be held in place with non-elastic tape. *Source:* Courtesy of Kathryn Seabaugh.

- Over-padding should be avoided because fracture fragments can move within a large bulky bandage.
- A bandage cast is another alternative—fiberglass casting material placed circumferentially over a lightly padded bandage striving to maintain dorsal cortical alignment.
- Commercially available splints such as the Kimzey Leg Saver (Kimzey Welding Works, Woodland, CA) are also available and can be utilized for distal limb fractures (Figure 7.8).

Mid-Forelimb (Mid-Metacarpus to Distal Radius)

- Fractures of this region include subluxation/luxation of the carpus, as well as fractures of the proximal metacarpus and distal radius.
- Fractures in this location are stabilized best with a compression-type bandage combined with full-limb PVC splints applied caudally and laterally (Figure 7.9).
- The bandage should contain only enough padding to help reduce swelling in the limb and protect the limb from the splint material.
- The bandage and splints should extend from the ground to the elbow with the splints placed at 90° angle to each other and tightly secured to the bandage using non-elastic white tape.

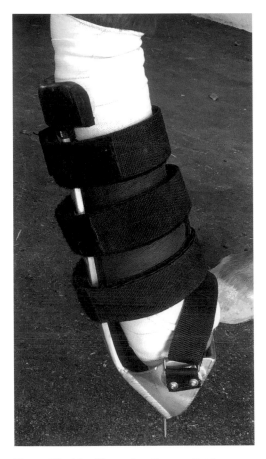

Figure 7.8 The Kimzey Leg Saver splint is a commercially available device used to stabilize phalangeal fractures or break-down injuries in the distal limb of racehorses. *Source:* Courtesy of Kathryn Seabaugh.

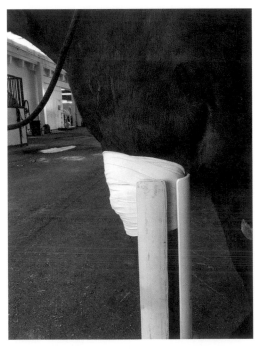

Figure 7.9 Placement for a caudal and lateral splint for a mid-forelimb fracture. Both splints should extend from the ground to the proximal radius/ulna. They can then be held in place by non-elastic tape or casting material. *Source:* Courtesy of Kathryn Seabaugh.

- If PVC material is not available, any light-weight, rigid material such as wood, aluminum, or flat steel may be used effectively for splinting.

Middle and Proximal Radius

- Preventing abduction of the distal limb is the goal when immobilizing fractures in this location. Limb abduction allows the proximal fracture fragment to penetrate the skin on the medial aspect of the radius.
- Fracture stabilization is best achieved by applying a compression-type bandage (including the caudal PVC splint) similar to

that used with mid-forelimb fractures, but the lateral splint is extended up the lateral aspect of the shoulder, scapula, and chest.

- A wide board (15–20 cm) or metal rod appears to work better than PVC for this lateral splint because it can lay flat against the muscles of the upper limb, but PVC can also be used (Figure 7.10).

Proximal to the Elbow

- The humerus, ulna, and scapula are well protected with muscles, which inherently stabilize and protect fractures in this location.

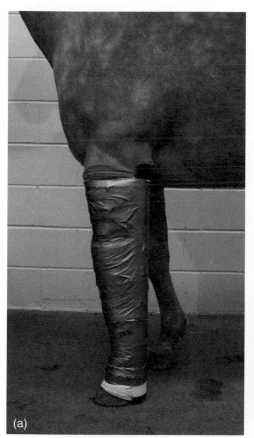 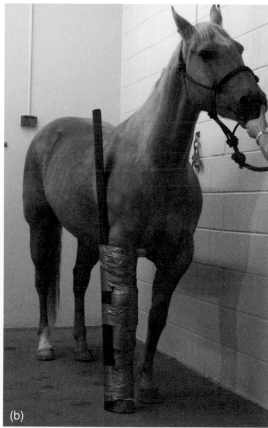

Figure 7.10 Stabilization for middle and proximal radius fractures. The tall lateral splint prevents abduction of the distal limb. A bandage and caudal splint are applied (a), and then a lateral splint extending proximal to the shoulder is applied (b). The tall lateral splint prevents abduction of the distal limb. A flat board or metal splint is best, but PVC can be used. *Source*: Courtesy of Jeremy Hubert.

- Complete fractures of these bones disable the triceps muscle apparatus, making it impossible for the horse to fix the elbow in extension for weight-bearing.
- A full-limb compression bandage with a full-limb caudally applied PVC splint will keep the carpus extended and help restore triceps muscle function (Figure 7.11).
- Not all fractures in these locations require stabilization as the risk of skin penetration is extremely low, and foals may not have the upper forelimb strength to move the limb with a splint in place.

Phalanges and Distal Metatarsus

- Fractures in this location can be managed similarly to those in the forelimb except that the PVC splint is best placed on the plantar surface of the limb and secured with either cast material or non-elastic tape (Figure 7.12).
- Splints applied to the dorsal surface of the hind limb over a bandage are less useful than in the forelimb and tend to break more readily.
- Due to the reciprocal apparatus, application of a bandage cast in the hind limb can be difficult because of the inability to keep the limb steady and in proper alignment while the cast material hardens.
- The Kimzey splint may be used to stabilize fractures in this location, similar to that in the forelimb (Figure 7.8).

Middle and Proximal Metatarsus

- A compression-type bandage with PVC splints applied laterally and caudally using the calcaneus as a caudal extension of the

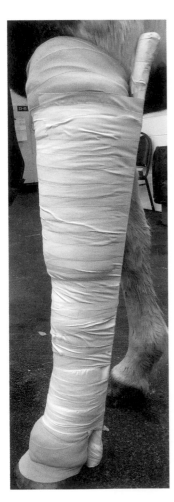

Figure 7.11 Caudal splint used to lock the carpus in extension and restore the triceps apparatus. *Source:* Courtesy of Valerie Moorman.

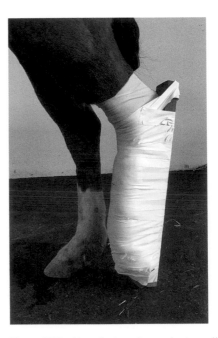

Figure 7.12 Use of a board as a plantar splint for stabilization of a distal limb fracture in the hind limb. Note that the splint extends proximally to include the calcaneus. *Source:* Courtesy of Kathryn Seabaugh.

metatarsus provides adequate support for fractures in this location.

- The bandage should be less extensive than in the forelimb because it will be difficult to secure the splints to the limb if the bandage is too bulky.

Tarsus and Tibia

- Fractures in this location are difficult to stabilize because of the reciprocal apparatus and its effect on joint motion in the tarsus and stifle.
- The main principal for stabilization is similar to that of the radius, which involves preventing abduction of the distal aspect of the limb.
- A single laterally placed splint that is bent to follow the angulation of the limb and extends proximally above the stifle joint works well to prevent abduction. The splint is applied over the full-limb compression bandage and is best made of lightweight metal such as aluminum that can be bent into the correct position (Figure 7.13).
- An alternative to the metal splint is a wide board (15–20 cm) that extends from the ground to the ilium and is applied to the lateral aspect of the bandage.

Transportation

- Ideally, horses should be loaded into a trailer with a ramp since ambulation can be difficult in the splinted limb.
- When possible, horses should travel facing forward for hind-limb fractures and facing backward for forelimb fractures.
- The use of dividers is recommended as the horse can brace against them during transport.

Definitive Treatment

- Treatment options for horses with fractures/ luxations range from stall confinement (with or without splinting) to euthanasia.
- Variable periods of rest and rehabilitation are recommended for most horses with incomplete or stress fractures depending on their location.

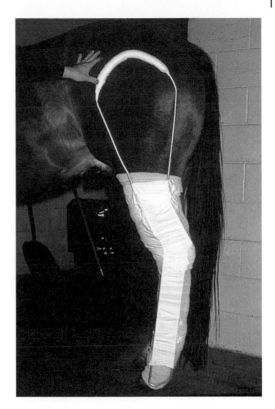

Figure 7.13 An aluminum rod has been shaped to extend from the ground up over the stifle and hip in this horse with a tibial fracture. Similar to radial fractures in the forelimb, the splint prevents abduction of the limb distal to the fracture, further stabilizing fractures of the tibia. A wide board could be used instead of the aluminum rod. *Source: Courtesy of Chris Ray.*

- Fractures of the phalanges, MC/MT, and ulna are the most amenable to some type of internal fixation.
- Casting alone can be used for some fractures of the phalanges, MC/MT, and distal radius, and for some luxations of the fetlock, carpus, and tarsus.
- In general, the smaller and younger the horse, the more likely that any type of treatment will be successful.

Prognosis

- The prognosis is extremely variable, depending on age, size, and temperament of the horse, and the type and location of the fracture/luxation.

- Horses with incomplete and/or stress fractures typically have a good prognosis with adequate rest and rehabilitation.
- In general, the prognosis for open fractures is much worse than for closed fractures and worse for adults than for foals.
- Comminuted long bone fractures in adults have a poor prognosis and are usually not amenable to treatment.

Synovial Infections

Overview

- Synovial infections are often associated with penetrating injuries to the coffin, pastern, fetlock, carpal, and TC joints, the digital flexor tendon and tarsal sheaths, and the navicular and calcaneal bursae.
- Synovial infections without external trauma are often associated with previous treatments (i.e. injections) or hematogenous spread (joint–ill in foals).
- Any wound affecting a synovial structure greater than 48 hours old should be considered to have an established synovial infection.

Etiology

- Trauma associated with a wound is a common cause of synovial infection.
- The cause may also be iatrogenic from previous intrasynovial injections or surgery.
- Hematogenous synovial infections occur most commonly in foals and are often associated with failure of passive transfer or other type of immunocompromise.

Clinical Signs

- Adult horses with infected synovial structures usually present because of severe lameness. With traumatic wounds, the increase in lameness may coincide with the healing of the wound.
- Synovial effusion is usually present together with concurrent soft-tissue edema, periarticular swelling, and heat (Figure 7.3).
- Those with concurrent open wounds often have a yellowish to clear, sticky fluid consistent with synovial fluid exiting the wound (Figure 7.2).
- The severity of lameness in foals is less consistent than in adults and multiple synovial cavities can be involved in the same foal.

Diagnosis

- Synoviocentesis combined with cytological evaluation of the fluid will provide useful information regarding synovial involvement.
- Synovial fluid white blood cell counts greater than 30×10^9/L and total protein concentrations greater than 4 g/L are highly consistent with infection (Table 7.2).
- Wound involvement of synovial cavities can also be documented by probing with a finger or cannula (Figure 7.14), injecting sterile fluid into the synovial structure at a site remote from the wound and observing for fluid exiting the wound, or using contrast radiography (Figure 2.40).

Table 7.2 Synovial fluid parameters used to aid diagnosis of synovial sepsis.

Fluid analysis parameter	Normal joint	Traumatic synovitis	Septic synovitis
Total protein (g/L)	18 ± 3 Less than 20	20–40	>40
Total nucleated cell count ($\times 10^9$/L)	<1.0 <3.5 (tendon sheath)	<10.0	>30.0
Neutrophils (%)	<10	<10	>80

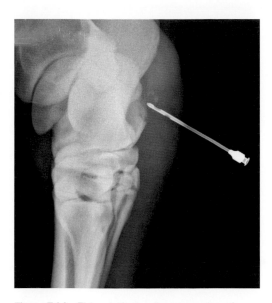

Figure 7.14 This relatively minor wound on the medial aspect of the tarsus was associated with fractures of the sustentaculum tali and a probe went directly to the bone and entered the tarsal sheath.

- Documentation of air within the synovial space using radiographs or ultrasound will also confirm synovial involvement provided this was done before synoviocentesis.
- The presence of abundant fibrin, severe synovial effusion, and thickening of the synovial lining on ultrasound also is suggestive of infection.
- Culturing the synovial fluid, fibrin, synovial membrane, or bone is the most definitive method to document infection, but not all cultures are positive.
- Foals with joint-ill with fibrinogen values of 900 mg/dL or greater should be suspected of having concurrent osteomyelitis.
- Radiographs should always be taken to rule out the presence of osteomyelitis since it is significantly associated with non-survival in cases with synovial sepsis.

Treatment
- Early recognition and treatment of synovial penetrating wounds are imperative to reduce the risk of developing synovial sepsis since

duration before treatment is thought to affect prognosis.
- Systemic and intrasynovial antimicrobials are the cornerstone of treatment of an established synovial infection (Table 7.3). IV or IM administration is recommended for a minimum of five days, with oral antimicrobials continued for two to three weeks based on culture results.
- A combination of penicillin (22 000 IU/kg every six hours IV, every 12 hours IM) and gentamicin (6.6 mg/kg every 24 hours IV) are often used initially.
- IV regional perfusion of antimicrobials is also recommended to increase the concentration of the antimicrobials to the site of the infection (Figure 7.15). Amikacin is commonly used for this purpose.
- Some type of synovial lavage/drainage is recommended. Methods include through-and-through lavage with needles/cannula or arthroscopic/endoscopic exploration.
- If osteomyelitis is suspected or diagnosed, arthroscopic/endoscopic debridement is recommended together with IV regional perfusion to aggressively treat the infection.

Prognosis
- In general, the quicker synovial involvement can be identified and treated, the better the prognosis.
- The absence of secondary bone or tendinous injuries usually improves the prognosis regardless of the location of the injury.
- In one study of horses treated with arthroscopy/endoscopy, 90% of the horses survived and 81% of the horses returned to performance.
- Another report found 84% of horses with infection of a synovial structure survived to discharge and 54% returned to athletic function.
- About 60% of foals with hematogenous synovial infections alone survive compared to only about 35–40% that have concurrent osteomyelitis.

Table 7.3 Systemic antimicrobials used to treat horses with synovial wounds and infections.

Antimicrobial	Dosage	Combinations and indications
Penicillin	22 000–44 000 IU/kg q 6–12 hours IV or IM	Combined with aminoglycoside, ceftiofur, or enrofloxacin (gram-positive infections)
Ampicillin	22 mg/kg IV q 8 hours	Combined with aminoglycoside
Cefazolin	10 mg/kg q 8 hours IV or IM	Can be used alone; usually combined with gentamicin or amikacin
Gentamicin	6.6 mg/kg q 24 hours IV or IM	Combined with penicillin, cephalosporin, or ampicillin (gram-negative infections)
Amikacin	7 mg/kg q 12 hours or 14 mg/kg q 24 hours IV or IM	Combined with penicillin, cephalosporin, or ampicillin (gram-negative infections)
Ceftiofur	2.2 mg/kg q 12 hours	Can be used alone or combined with penicillin or aminoglycoside (staphylococcus infections)
Enrofloxacin	7 mg/kg q 24 hours IV or PO	Not recommended for foals (resistant gram-negative infections; poor for anaerobes)
Doxycycline	10 mg/kg PO q 12 hours	Used as follow-up to parenteral antimicrobials
Trimethoprim-sulfonamides	30 mg/kg q 12 hours PO or 3–5 mg/kg q 12 hours PO (based on trimethoprim)	Used as follow-up to parenteral antimicrobials
Vancomycin	7.5 mg/kg IV q 8 hours	Methicillin-resistant staphylococcal and enterococcal infections

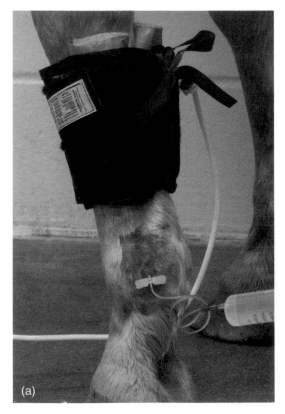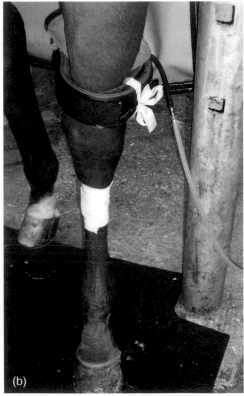

Figure 7.15 Intravenous regional limb perfusions using a pneumatic tourniquet. The tourniquet is placed above the site of the lesion and a vessel is selected to infuse the antimicrobials, the palmar vein in (a) and the saphenous in (b). Rolls of gauze can be applied over the vessels for extra pressure; these can be seen under the tourniquet in both (a and b). A pneumatic tourniquet is preferred while wide rubber tourniquets (i.e. Esmarch) are acceptable, but narrow rubber tubing is not. *Source:* Courtesy of Jeremy Hubert.

- Factors that have been associated with a negative prognosis include increased TP concentrations, a positive synovial fluid culture, and the presence of osteomyelitis.

Tendon and Ligament Lacerations

Overview

- The distal limb is prone to deep lacerations that may involve tendons and ligaments because of the horse's flight response, kicking defense, and high speeds.
- Tendon lacerations occur more commonly in the hind limbs than in the forelimbs.
- Most tendon lacerations/wounds occur in the mid-MC/MT region and involve the extensor tendons most frequently (common digital extensor tendon in the forelimb and long digital extensor tendon in the hind limb) or the flexor tendons (SDFT and/or DDFT).
- Extensor tendon injuries are often avulsion-type trauma with loss of skin over the dorsal aspect of the cannon bone (Figure 7.16).
- Laceration of both flexor tendons in the MC/MT region is a medical emergency similar to a fracture.
- Ligament lacerations may accompanied tendon lacerations, but this is less common.

Etiology

- These injuries usually result from external trauma from sharp objects.
- Extensor tendon injuries may result from the limb getting caught between objects that avulse the skin and soft tissues from the dorsal aspect of the MC/MT.
- Horses may jump sharp objects, fences, or often pull excessively if their lower limb is trapped, inciting significant tendon injury.
- Lacerations to CLs and branches of the SL do occur but are much less common than either extensor or flexor tendon lacerations.

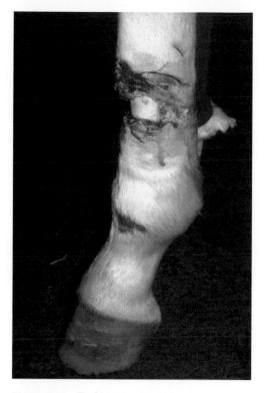

Figure 7.16 The dorsal metatarsus is a common location for extensor tendon lacerations, and many injuries also involve the metatarsus.

- Tendon and ligament rupture may occur from excessive exercise, but this is less common than external trauma.

Clinical Signs

- Characteristic gait deficits occur following complete tendon lacerations.
- If the extensor tendons are severed, the foot may move more freely than normal, and the horse may intermittently knuckle at the fetlock due to failure to extend the digit during limb placement (Figure 7.17).
- Horses are often not lame on weight-bearing with extensor tendon injuries but may have difficulty advancing the limb.
- Complete severance of both the DDFT and SDFT will result in hyperextension of the fetlock with the toe coming off the ground

422 | *Musculoskeletal Emergencies*

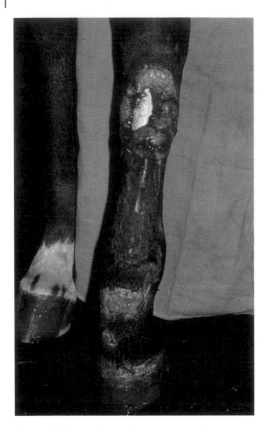

Figure 7.17 Avulsion injuries on the dorsal aspect of the metacarpus/metatarsus, resulting in dorsal knuckling of the fetlock. Note the wound on the dorsal fetlock and the sequestrum in the proximal MTIII.

during limb placement (Figures 7.18a and 7.19).

- Laceration of just the SDFT will cause the fetlock to drop with normal foot placement (Figure 7.18b).
- If the suspensory ligament is also severed, the fetlock will drop almost to the ground.
- Severe lameness accompanies flexor tendon lacerations, and the limb should be immobilized as quickly as possible.
- Palmar/plantar lacerations of the tendons around the fetlock region may involve the DFTS.
- Immobilization of limbs with lacerated DDFT and SDFT to support the fetlock and prevent further injury should be performed similar to those with fractures.

Diagnosis

- Often, a tentative diagnosis can be made based on the location of the wound and the characteristic limb posture and/or gait abnormality (Figures 7.17–7.19).
- Digital palpation of the wound can often reveal the extent of the laceration to the tendons and ligaments (Figure 7.20).
- Radiography should be performed to detect secondary bone abnormalities such as fractured splint bones or sequestration of the dorsal aspect of the MC/MT.
- Ultrasound examination may be used to define partial tears of the tendon or ligament and possibly locate foreign material in the wound.

Treatment

- Routine first-aid management of all wounds is recommended initially. Immobilization of limbs with lacerated DDFT and SDFT to support the fetlock and prevent further injury should be performed similar as with fractures of the distal limb.
- The optimal approach for acute extensor tendon injuries is to re-appose the tendon ends, close the wound, and provide support to the fetlock, such as a caudal splint to prevent knuckling, for at least the first four to six weeks.
- Unfortunately, many extensor tendon lacerations cannot be closed due to the severity of trauma and are treated with second intention healing.
- Weight-bearing can be permitted for extensor tendon lacerations, but external coaptation may be needed to prevent dorsal knuckling of the fetlock (Figure 7.17).
- Removal of sequestra from the dorsal MC/MT may be necessary in severe avulsion injuries (Figure 7.17).
- The optimal treatment of flexor tendon lacerations is wound debridement and closure, tendon apposition with suture, and cast application for four–six weeks (Figure 7.20).

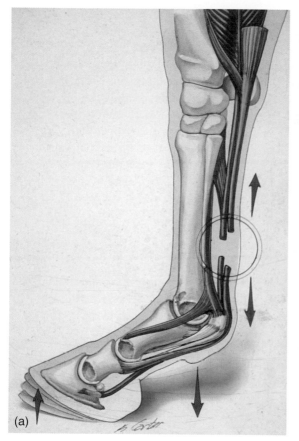 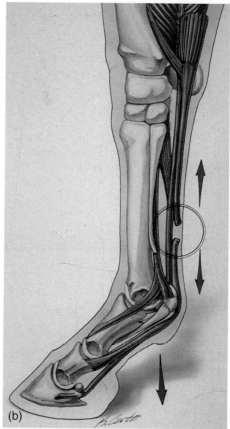

Figure 7.18 Illustration of the biomechanical effects of lacerations of both the SDFT and DDFT (a) and just the SDFT (b) in horses with flexor tendon lacerations. *Source:* Courtesy of K. Carter.

- The six-strand Savage or the three-loop pulley suture patterns are recommended for repair of the flexor tendons.
- If the tendon ends cannot be re-apposed, wound debridement and closure can still be performed because the tendons will heal with gap healing, provided they are adequately immobilized with a half-limb cast.
- If the digital sheath is concurrently involved with the laceration, tenoscopic exploratory of the sheath or lavage of the sheath should be performed. Closure of the tendon laceration and sheath are indicated in most cases unless gross contamination is present.

Prognosis

- Horses with extensor tendon lacerations have a good-to-excellent prognosis (more than 70%) for return to full function with conservative management.
- Horses with flexor tendon lacerations have a good prognosis for pasture or breeding soundness and a guarded to fair prognosis for athletic soundness.
- Two different studies reported that 55–59% of treated horses with tendon lacerations returned to some level of work.
- Complications include restrictive fibrosis, infection, fetlock hyperextension, delayed healing, and chronic lameness.

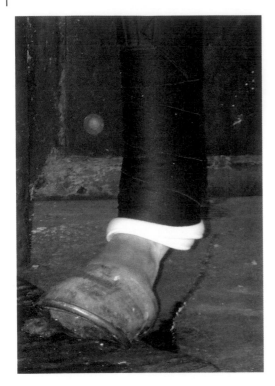

Figure 7.19 Characteristic elevation of the toe during weight-bearing following laceration or rupture of the DDFT. *Source:* Courtesy of Kathryn Seabaugh.

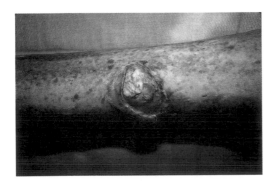

Figure 7.20 Typical location and appearance of a laceration of the flexor tendons in the mid-metatarsal region. The SDFT can be seen outside the wound and digital palpation revealed a lacerated DDFT as well.

Bibliography

1 Baxter GM: 2008. Management and Treatment of Wounds Involving Synovial Structures in Horses. *In:* Stashak TS, Theoret CL (eds) *Equine Wound Management, Second Edition.* Ames, Blackwell Publishing, 463–488.

2 Baxter GM: 2004 Management of wounds involving synovial structures in horses. *Clin Tech Equine Pract* 3:204–214.

3 Belknap JK, Baxter GM, Nickels FA: 1993. Extensor tendon lacerations in horses: 50 cases (1982–1988). *J Am Vet Med Assoc* 203:428–431.

4 Bramlage LR: 1983. Current concepts of emergency first aid treatment and transportation of equine fracture patients. *Comp Cont Educ Pract Vet* 5:S564–S574.

5 Bramlage LR: 1996. First Aid and Transportation of Fracture Patients. *In:* Nixon AJ (ed) *Equine Fracture Repair.* Philadelphia, WB Saunders Co, 36–42.

6 Cousty M, David Stack J, Tricaud C, et al.: 2017. Effect of arthroscopic lavage and repeated intra-articular administrations of antibiotic in adult horses and foals with septic arthritis. *Vet Surg* 46:1008–1016.

7 Cruz AM, Rubio-Martinez L, Dowling T: 2006. New antimicrobials, systemic distribution, and local methods of antimicrobial delivery in horses. *Vet Clin North Am Equine Pract* 22:297–322, vii–viii

8 Dyson S, Bertone AL: 2003. Tendon Lacerations and Repair. *In:* Dyson SJ, Ross MW (eds) *Diagnosis and Management of Lameness in Horses.* Philadelphia, WB Saunders, Part VIII:712–716.

9 Everett E, Barrett JG, Morelli J, et al.: 2012. Biomechanical testing of a novel suture pattern for repair of equine tendon lacerations. *Vet Surg* 41:278–285.

10 Foland JW, Trotter GW, Stashak TS, et al.: 1991. Traumatic injuries involving tendons of the distal limbs in horses: A retrospective study of 55 cases. *Equine Vet J* 23:422–425.

11 Fraser BS, Bladon BM: 2004. Tenoscopic surgery for treatment of lacerations of the digital flexor tendon sheath. *Equine Vet J* 36:528–531.

12 Fürst AE: 2012. Emergency Treatment and Transportation of Equine Fracture Patients. *In:* Auer JA (ed) *Equine Surgery, Fourth Edition.* Elsevier, 1015–1025.

13 Gibson KT, McIlwraith CW, Turner AS, et al.: 1989. Open joint injuries in horses: 58 cases (1980–1986). *J Am Vet Med Assoc* 194:398–404.

14 Goodrich LR, Nixon AJ: 2004. Treatment options for osteomyelitis. *Equine Vet Educ* 16:267–280.

15 Jordana M, Wilderjans H, Boswell J, et al.: 2011. Outcome after lacerations of the superficial and deep digital flexor tendons, suspensory ligament and/or distal sesamoidean ligaments in 106 horses. *Vet Surg* 40:277–283.

16 Kilcoyne I, Nieto JE, Knych HK, et al.: 2018. Time required to achieve maximum concentration of amikacin in synovial fluid of the distal interphalangeal joint after intravenous regional limb perfusion in horses. *Am J Vet Res* 79:282–286.

17 Loftin PG, Beard WL, Guyan ME, et al.: 2016. Comparison of arthroscopic lavage and needle lavage techniques, and lavage volume on the recovery of colored microspheres from the tarsocrural joints of cadaver horses. *Vet Surg* 45:240–245.

18 Mespoulhes-Riviere C, Martens A, Bogaert L, et al.: 2008. Factors affecting outcome of extensor tendon lacerations in the distal limb of horses. A retrospective study of 156 cases (1994–2003). *Vet Comp Orthop Traumatol* 21:358–364.

19 Milner PI, Bardell DA, Warner L, et al.: 2014. Factors associated with survival to hospital discharge following endoscopic treatment for synovial sepsis in 214 horses. *Equine Vet J* 46:701–705.

20 Mudge MC, Bramlage LR: 2007. Field fracture management. *Vet Clin North Am Equine Pract* 23:117–133.

21 Newquist J, Baxter GM: 2009. Plasma fibrinogen as an indicator of physeal/epiphyseal osteomyelitis in foals: A Retrospective Study (2000–2007). *J Am Vet Med Assoc* 235:415–419.

22 Orsini, JA, Divers T: 2008. *Equine Emergencies: Treatment and Procedures, Third Edition*. Philadelphia, Elsevier, 231–233, 280–283.

23 Schoonover MJ, Moser DK, Young JM, et al.: 2017. Effects of tourniquet number and exsanguination on amikacin concentrations in the radiocarpal and distal interphalangeal joints after low volume intravenous regional limb perfusion in horses. *Vet Surg* 46:675–682.

24 Schneider RK: 1999. Orthopedic Infections. *In:* Auer JA, Stick JA (eds) *Equine Surgery, Second Edition*. Philadelphia, Saunders, 727–736.

25 Smith JJ: 2006. Emergency fracture stabilization. *Clin Tech Equine Pract* 5:154–160.

26 Stashak TS: 2002. Lateral and Medial Luxation of the Metacarpophalangeal and Metatarsophalangeal Joints. *In*: Stashak TS (ed) *Adams' Lameness in Horses*. Philadelphia, Lippincott Williams & Williams, 790–792.

27 Taylor AH, Mair TS, Smith LJ, et al.: 2010. Bacterial culture of septic synovial structures of horses: Does a positive bacterial culture influence prognosis? *Equine Vet J* 42:213–218.

28 Walmsley EA, Anderson GA, Muurlink MA, et al.: 2011. Retrospective investigation of prognostic indicators for adult horses with infection of a synovial structure. *Aust Vet J* 89:226–231.

29 Wereszka MM, White NA, Furr MO: 2007. Factors associated with outcome following treatment of horses with septic tenosynovitis: 51 cases (1986–2003). *J Am Vet Med Assoc* 230:1195–1200.

30 Wright IM, Smith MR, Humphrey DJ, et al.: 2003. Endoscopic surgery in the treatment of contaminated and infected synovial cavities. *Equine Vet J* 35:613–619.

31 Wright IM, Phillips TJ, Walmsley JP: 1999. Endoscopy of the navicular bursa: A new technique for the treatment of contaminated and septic bursae. *Equine Vet J* 31:5–11.

32 Yovich JV, Turner AS, Stashak TS, et al.: 1987. Luxation of the metacarpophalangeal and metatarsophalangeal joints in horses. *Equine Vet J* 19:295–298.

Revised from "Musculoskeletal Emergencies" in *Adams and Stashak's Lameness in Horses, 7th Edition*, by Kathryn A. Seabaugh.

Index

Manual of Equine Lameness, Second Edition. Gary M. Baxter.
© 2022 John Wiley & Sons, Inc. Published 2022 by John Wiley & Sons, Inc.
Companion website: www.wiley.com/go/baxter/manual